UICC International Union Against Cancer
Union Internationale Contre le Cancer

TNM Atlas

Illustrated Guide to the TNM/pTNM Classification of Malignant Tumours

Edited by
B. Spiessl O. H. Beahrs P. Hermanek R. V. P. Hutter
O. Scheibe L. H. Sobin G. Wagner

Third Edition · Corrected Reprint

With 452 Figures and an insert with summaries of the T and N definitions by site

Springer-Verlag 1990
Berlin Heidelberg New York
London Paris Tokyo
Hong Kong Barcelona

Illustrations:

Ulrike Kerl-Jentzsch, Militschstraße 67, D-3300 Brunswick, FRG
Jörg Kühn, Handschuhsheimer Landstraße 71, D-6900 Heidelberg, FRG

1st Edition 1982
2nd Edition 1985

ISBN 3-540-17721-3
3. Auflage Springer-Verlag Berlin Heidelberg New York
ISBN 0-387-17721-3
3rd edition Springer-Verlag New York Berlin Heidelberg

ISBN 3-540-13443-3 2. Auflage Springer-Verlag Berlin Heidelberg New York
ISBN 0-387-13443-3 2nd edition Springer-Verlag New York Heidelberg Berlin

Library of Congress Cataloging-in-Publication Data
TNM-atlas : illustrated quide to the TNM/pTNM-classification of malignant tumors / edited by B. Spiessl ... [et al.]. - 3rd ed. corr. reprint. p cm.
At head of title: UICC, International Union Against Cancer.
ISBN 0-387-17721-3 (U.S.)
1. Tumors-Classification. 2. Cancer-Atlases. I. Spiessl, Bernd. II. International Union against Cancer.
[DNLM: 1. Neoplasms-classification-atlases. QZ 17 T626]
RC258.T58 1990 616.99'4'0012 DNLM/DLC
for Library of Congress 88-31846

Typesetting printing and binding: Appl, Wemding
2121/3145-543210 - Printed on acid-free paper

Preface to the Corrected Reprint 1990

This corrected reprint of the *TNM Atlas* was necessitated because of changes made by the Fédération Internationale de Gynécologie et d'Obstétrique (FIGO) in their classifications for corpus uteri and vulva carcinomas[1, 2] since the publication of the fourth edition of the *TNM Classification* in 1987. We have issued this corrected reprint so that there will continue to be complete agreement between the TNM and FIGO classifications. The changes appearing in this reprint compared to the previous issue are marked by a wavy line at the left-hand side of the page.

---

[1] FIGO (1989) Annual report on the results of treatment of gynecological cancer. Int J Gynecol Obstet 28: 189–193

[2] FIGO (1990) Changes in gynecologic staging by the International Federation of Gynecology and Obstetrics. Am J Obstet Gynecol 162: 610–611

Preface to the Third Edition

In 1938 the League of Nations Health Organization published an *Atlas Illustrating the Division of Cancer of the Uterine Cervix into Four Stages* (edited by J. Heymann, Stockholm). Since this work appeared, the idea of visual representation of the anatomical extent of malignant tumours at the different stages of their development has been repeatedly discussed.

At its meeting in Copenhagen in July 1954, the UICC adopted as part of its programme "the realization of a clinical atlas". However, the time to publish the planned book of illustrations was not ripe until the national committees and international organizations had officially recognized the 28 classifications of malignant tumours at various sites as presented in the third edition of the *TNM* Booklet edited by M. Harmer *(TNM Classification of Malignant Tumours, 1978)*. This was all the more important since publication of the Booklet was followed in 1980 by publication of *A Brochure of Checklists,* edited by A. H. Sellers, a further aid in the practical application of the TNM system.

The *TNM Atlas* (first edition 1982, second edition 1985) was the third of the aids intended to fulfil the one ultimate purpose of making the classification of the anatomical extent of malignant tumours as much a routine procedure as histological typing and grading.

A strong interest in the *TNM Atlas* manifested itself in the unexpectedly large demand for copies. Its strength in publicizing the use of the TNM system is encouraging and demonstrates the urgency of making the abbreviations of tumour findings easily understandable. The busy doctor is then in a position to comprehend at a glance not only the principle of the system, but also to put together easily the correct finding formulations in individual cases.

The public aimed at by the *Atlas* is, in the first instance, those doctors working in the field of oncology who should be interested in the general acceptance and use of the TNM rules. These

rules are considered to be an internationally accepted, uniform, generally binding and understood system which describes tumour stages exactly and thus facilitates the collection and the exchange of comparable data.
The third edition of the *TNM Classification of Malignant Tumours* appeared in 1978. Since then, the diagnosis of tumours has made great progress thanks to the wide application of computer tomography and through the introduction of endoscopic sonography and nuclear magnetic resonance imaging. Different studies have resulted in new knowledge about the relationship between the extent of the tumour at the time of diagnosis and the later course of disease.
As can be ascertained, some users of the TNM system changed the official definitions according to their own conceptions. In order to counteract this development and in order to take into account the scientific progress of the last 10 years, the national TNM committees agreed in 1982 to revise the 1978 *TNM Classification* and also to introduce new classifications for organs which had not yet been considered in the TNM system. The desired objective is to once again create generally accepted and internationally unified rules.
This objective was attained in 1986 after numerous national and international meetings. The result of these meetings - the fourth edition of the international *TNM Classification*, which was accepted by the TNM Committee of the UICC - was published in English in the spring of 1987.[1]
Malignant tumours of the following organs were newly classified:

- Head and neck: Salivary glands and maxillary sinus
- Gastrointestinal tract: Liver, gallbladder, extrahepatic biliary ducts, ampulla of Vater, pancreas
- Urological tumours: Renal pelvis and ureter, urethra
- Bones
- Brain

In the fourth edition, the TNM classification of gynaecological tumours coincides with the classification of the Fédération In-

[1] UICC: TNM Classification of Malignant Tumours, 4th edn. P. Hermanek, L. H. Sobin (eds) (1987) Springer, Berlin Heidelberg New York London Paris Tokyo

ternationale de Gynécologie et d'Obstétrique (FIGO). The classification of paediatric tumours is identical to that of the Sociéte Internationale d'Oncologie Pédiatrique (SIOP). The definitions which appear in the fourth edition were accepted by all national TNM committees including the American Joint Committee on Cancer (AJCC), so that now an internationally unified, up-to-date classification of tumours by anatomical extent is at our disposal.

The publication of the fourth edition of the *TNM Classification* necessitated the revision of the *TNM Atlas*. The present, third edition of the *TNM Atlas* takes into consideration all the additions and changes made in the fourth edition of the *TNM Classification* and, therefore, represents the current state of TNM classification as accepted world-wide by all the national committees and as it appears in the third edition of the *AJCC Manual for Staging of Cancer* (1988).

The editorial board was expanded by the inclusion of the Chairman of the TNM Project Committee of the UICC, L. H. Sobin, as well as two representatives of the AJCC.

The third edition of the *TNM Atlas* follows the sound principles on which previous editions were based. The structure of the *TNM Atlas* is similar to that of the *TNM Classification*. The Atlas' text is limited to the essentials, so that the original *Booklet* should be consulted for detailed information, principles and general rules of the TNM system.

For practical reasons, the format chosen is as similar as possible to that of the *TNM Booklet*. The one is not supposed to replace but rather to supplement the other. A major aim of the *TNM Atlas* is, therefore, to promote understanding of and interest in the application of the TNM system and to show how simply, uniformly and precisely the system is structured.

January 1989

B. Spiessl, Basel
O. H. Beahrs, Rochester, Minn
P. Hermanek, Erlangen
R. V. P. Hutter, Livingstone, NJ
O. Scheibe, Stuttgart
L. H. Sobin, Washington, DC
G. Wagner, Heidelberg

Foreword to the First Edition

Confronted with a myriad of T's, N's and M's in the UICC TNM booklet, classifying a malignancy may seem to many cancer clinicians a tedious, dull and pedantic task. But with a look at the *TNM Atlas* all of a sudden lifeless categories become vivid images, challenging the clinicians's know-how and investigational skills.

Birgit van der Werf-Messing, M.D.
Professor of Radiology
Chairman of the International
TNM-Committee of the UICC

Rotterdam, July 1982

Acknowledgements

The editors wish to express their thanks to Mrs. J. Wagner, Erlangen, for her help with the preparation of the manuscript. They are equally grateful to Mrs. U. Kerl, Braunschweig, who took great care in drawing the anatomical illustrations.
Financial support for the publication of the *TNM Atlas* was provided by the Federal German Ministry of Science and Technology, Bonn. The editors are indebted to this authority. Support of the TNM Project by the National Cancer Institute (USA) through grants CA 05096 and CA 38193 is gratefully acknowledged.
Finally, the editors wish to thank Springer-Verlag and its staff for their speedy handling of the matter as well as for the excellent presentation of this *Atlas*.

Contents

Editors

Professor Dr. Dr. B. Spiessl
Department für Chirurgie, Kantonspital, Universitätskliniken,
Spitalstraße 21, CH-4031 Basel, Switzerland

Professor Dr. O. H. Beahrs
Section on Surgery, Mayo Clinic and Mayo Foundation,
Mayo Medical School, Rochester, Minn, USA

Professor Dr. P. Hermanek
Abteilung für Klinische Pathologie,
Chirurgische Universitätsklinik Erlangen,
Maximiliansplatz, D-8520 Erlangen,
FRG

Dr. R. V. P. Hutter
Clinical Professor of Pathology, University of Medicine
and Dentistry of New Jersey, New Jersey Medical School,
Department of Pathology, Saint Barnabas Medical Center,
Old Short Hills Road, Livingston, NJ 07039, USA

Professor Dr. O. Scheibe
Chirurgische Klinik des Bürgerhospitals, Krankenhaus Feuerbach,
Stuttgarter Straße 151, D-7000 Stuttgart 3, FRG

Dr. L. H. Sobin
Department of Gastrointestinal Pathology,
Armed Forces Institute of Pathology,
Washington, DC 20306, USA

Professor Dr. G. Wagner
Deutsches Krebsforschungszentrum, Institut für Epidemiologie
und Biometrie, Im Neuenheimer Feld 280, D-6900 Heidelberg,
FRG

Contributors to the Third Edition

Baker, H. W., Portland, Ore, USA	Head and neck surgery
Beahrs, O. H., Rochester, Minn, USA	General surgery
Drepper, H., Münster-Handorf, FRG	Maxillofacial surgery
Gemsenjäger, E., Basel, Switzerland	General surgery
Genz, T., Berlin	Gynaecology
Glanz, H., Marburg, FRG	Otorhinolaryngology
Hasse, J., Freiburg, FRG	Thoracic surgery
Hermanek, P., Erlangen, FRG	Pathology
Hutter, R. V. P., Livingston, NJ, USA	Pathology
Kindermann, G., München, FRG	Gynaecology
Kleinsasser, O., Marburg, FRG	Otorhinolaryngology
Lang, G., Erlangen, FRG	Ophthalmology
Naumann, G. O. H., Erlangen, FRG	Ophthalmology
Remagen, W., Basel, Switzerland	Pathology
Scheibe, O., Stuttgart, FRG	General surgery
Schmitt, H. P., Heidelberg, FRG	Neuropathology
Sobin, L. H., Washington, DC, USA	Pathology
Spiessl, B., Basel, Switzerland	Maxillofacial surgery
Wagner, G., Heidelberg, FRG	Documentation and epidemiology

Contributors to the Second Edition

Adolphs, H. D., Höxter, FRG	Urology
Amberger, H., Heidelberg, FRG	General surgery
Baumann, R. P., Neuchâtel, Switzerland	Pathology
Berger, H., Göttingen, FRG	Dermatology
Bokelmann, D., Essen, FRG	General surgery
Brandeis, W. F., Heidelberg, FRG	Paediatric oncology
Dold, U., Gauting, FRG	Internal medicine
Drepper, H., Münster-Handorf, FRG	Maxillofacial surgery
Drings, P., Heidelberg, FRG	Internal medicine
Gemsenjäger, E., Basel, Switzerland	General surgery
Hasse, J., Basel, Switzerland	Thoracic surgery
Heitz, Ph., Basel, Switzerland	Pathology
Hermanek, P., Erlangen, FRG	Pathology
Karrer, K., Wien, Austria	Oncological epidemiology
Kuehnl-Petzold, C., Freiburg i. B., FRG	Dermatology
Liebenstein, J., Mannheim, FRG	Gynaecology
Molitor, D., Bonn, FRG	Urology
Nidecker, A., Basel, Switzerland	Radiology
Rohde, H., Köln FRG	General surgery
Scheibe, O., Stuttgart, FRG	General surgery
Schmitt, A., Mannheim, FRG	Gynaecology
Spiessl, B., Basel, Switzerland	Maxillofacial surgery
Thomas, C., Marburg, FRG	Pathology
Vogt-Moykopf, J., Heidelberg, FRG	Thoracic surgery
Wagner, G., Heidelberg, FRG	Documentation and epidemiology

Preliminary Note

The TNM system for describing the anatomical extent of disease is based on the assessment of three components:

T – The extent of the *primary tumour*

N – The absence or presence and extent of *regional lymph node metastasis*

M – The absence or presence of *distant metastasis*

The addition of numbers to these three components indicates the extent of the malignant disease, thus:

T0, T1, T2, T3, T4   N0, N1, N2, N3   M0, M1

In effect, the system is a "shorthand notation" for describing the extent of a particular malignant tumour.

Each site is described under the following headings:

1. *Anatomy.* Drawings of the anatomical sites and subsites are presented with the appropriate ICD-O topography numbers.[1]
2. *Regional Lymph Nodes.* The regional lymph nodes are listed and shown in drawings.
3. *T/pT Clinical and Pathological Classification of the Primary Tumour.* Above all, the definitions for T and pT categories are presented. Because in the fourth edition of the *TNM Classification* the clinical and pathological classification (T and pT) generally coincide, the same illustrations are valid for the T and pT classification. Exceptions to this are the carcinoma of the vulva, some tumours of the eye and the paediatric tumours.
4. *N/pN Clinical and Pathological Classification of Regional Lymph Nodes.* The N and pN categories are presented in a fashion similar to the T and pT categories. Differences between N and pN definitions in the fourth edition arise only in the case of cancer of the breast and with paediatric tumours.
5. *M/pM Clinical and Pathological Classification of Distant Metastasis.* The presentation of the many possible variables of the M localization is given only in some selected cases.

---

[1] ICD-O International Classification of Diseases for Oncology (1976). WHO, Geneva.

C-Factor

The C-factor, or certainty factor, reflects the validity of classification according to the diagnostic methods employed. Its use is *optional.* The C-factor definitions are:

C1 Evidence from standard diagnostic means (e.g. inspection, palpation and standard radiography, intraluminal endoscopy for tumours of certain organs)

C2 Evidence obtained by special diagnostic means (e.g. radiographic imaging in special projections, tomography, computerized tomography [CT], ultrasonography, lymphography, angiography; scintigraphy; magnetic resonance imaging [MRI]; endoscopy, biopsy, and cytology)

C3 Evidence from surgical exploration, including biopsy and cytology

C4 Evidence of the extent of disease following definitive surgery and pathological examination of the resected specimen

C5 Evidence from autopsy

Example: Degrees of C may be applied to the T, N and M categories. A case might be described as T3C2, N2C1, M0C2.

The TNM clinical classification is, therefore, equivalent to C1, C2 and C3 in varying degrees of certainty, while the pTNM pathological classification is equivalent to C4.

HEAD AND NECK TUMOURS

Introductory Notes

The following sites are included:

- Lip, oral cavity
- Pharynx
- Larynx
- Maxillary sinus
- Salivary glands
- Thyroid gland

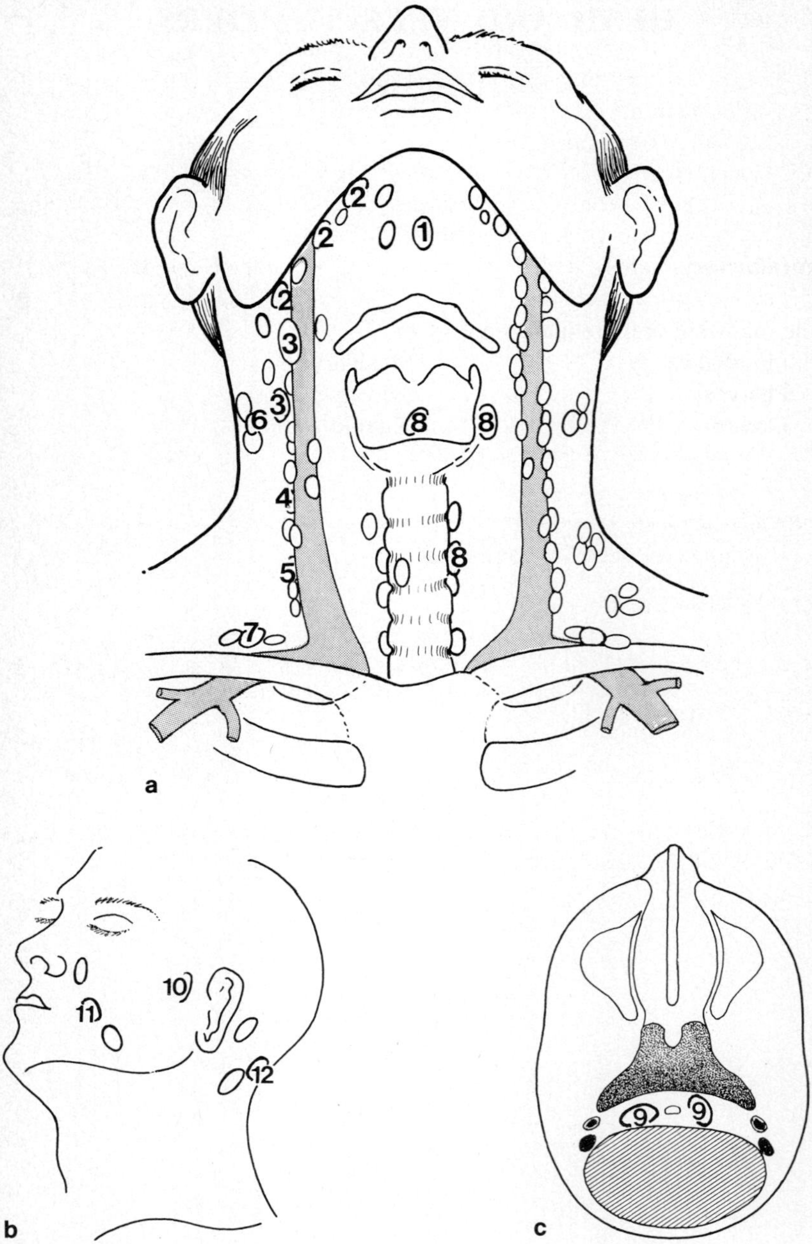

Fig. 1 a–c

Regional Lymph Nodes (Fig. 1)

The regional lymph nodes are the cervical nodes. These include
(1) submental nodes
(2) submandibular nodes
(3) cranial jugular (deep cervical) nodes
(4) medial jugular (deep cervical) nodes
(5) caudal jugular (deep cervical) nodes
(6) dorsal cervical (superficial cervical) nodes along the accessory nerve
(7) supraclavicular nodes
(8) prelaryngeal and paratracheal nodes
(9) retropharyngeal nodes
(10) parotid nodes
(11) buccal nodes
(12) retroauricular and occipital nodes

N/pN Classification

The definitions of the N categories for all head and neck sites *except thyroid gland* are:

N/pN - Regional Lymph Nodes

N/pNX Regional lymph nodes cannot be assessed
N/pN0 No regional lymph node metastasis

N/pN1 Metastasis in a single ipsilateral lymph node, 3 cm or less in greatest dimension (Fig. 2)

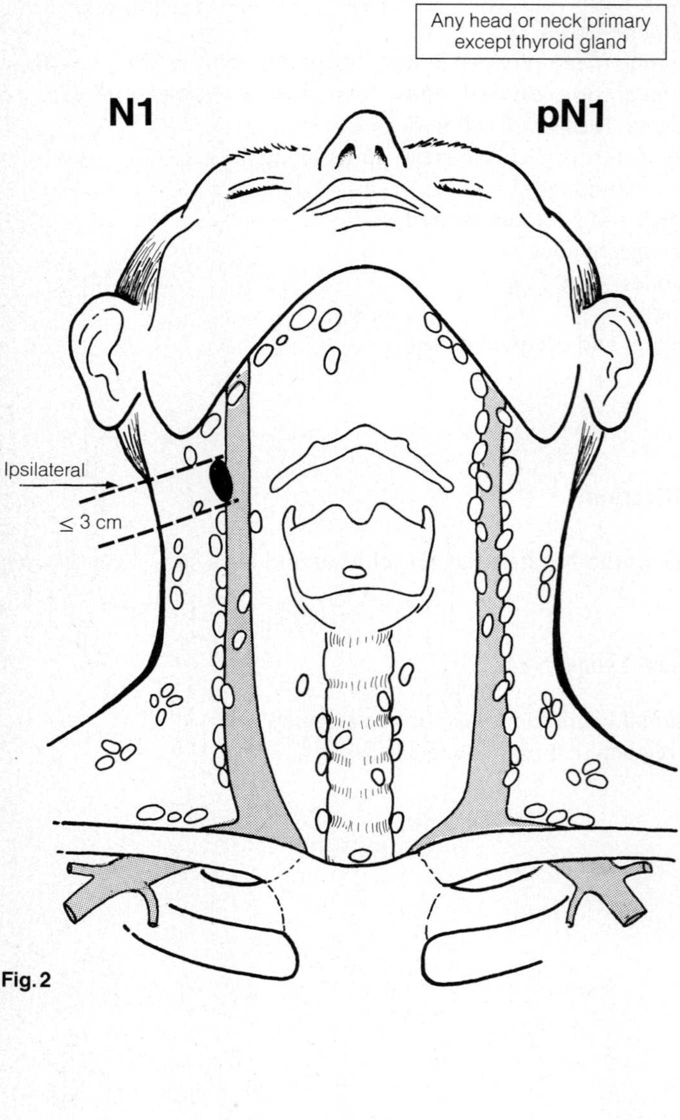

Fig. 2

N/pN2 Metastasis in a single ipsilateral lymph node, more than 3 cm but not more than 6 cm in greatest dimension; *or* in multiple ipsilateral lymph nodes, none more than 6 cm in greatest dimension; *or* in bilateral or contralateral lymph nodes, none more than 6 cm in greatest dimension

N/pN2a Metastasis in a single ipsilateral lymph node, more than 3 cm but not more than 6 cm in greatest dimension (Fig. 3)

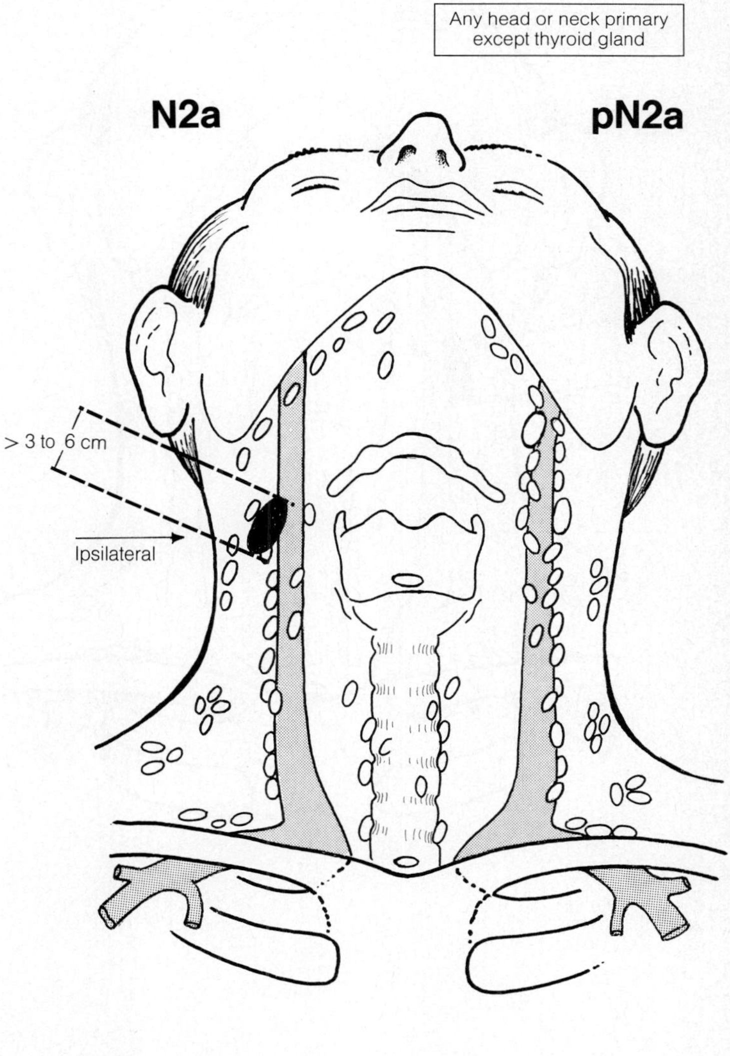

Fig. 3

N/pN2b Metastasis in multiple ipsilateral lymph nodes, none more than 6 cm in greatest dimension (Fig. 4)

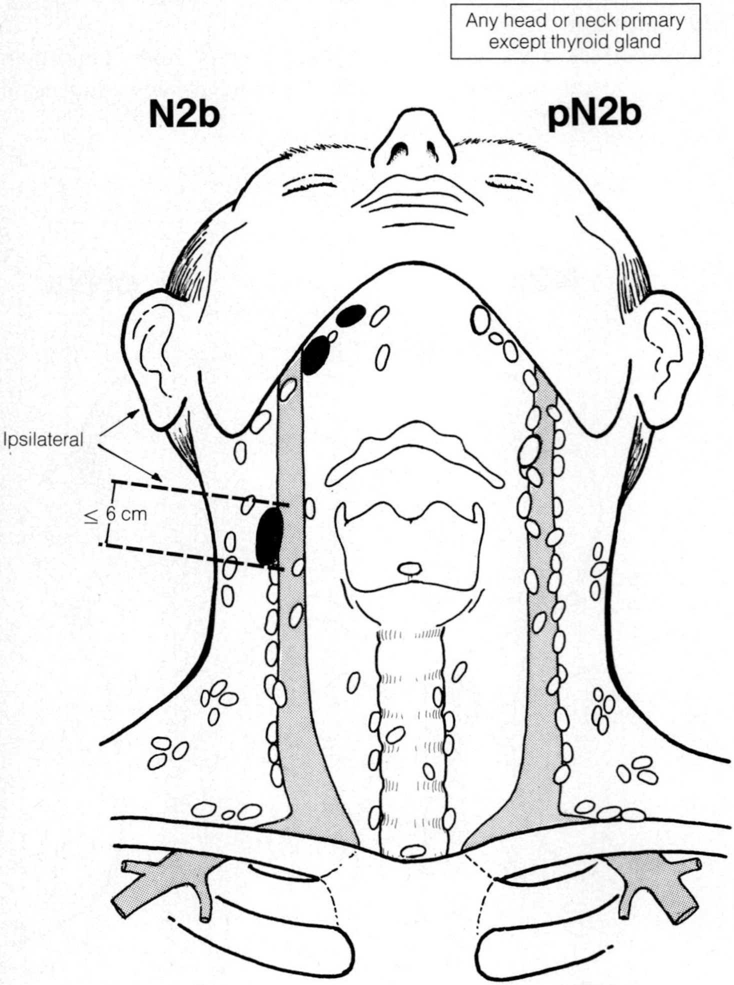

Fig. 4

N/pN2c Metastasis in bilateral or contralateral lymph nodes, none more than 6 cm in greatest dimension (Fig. 5)

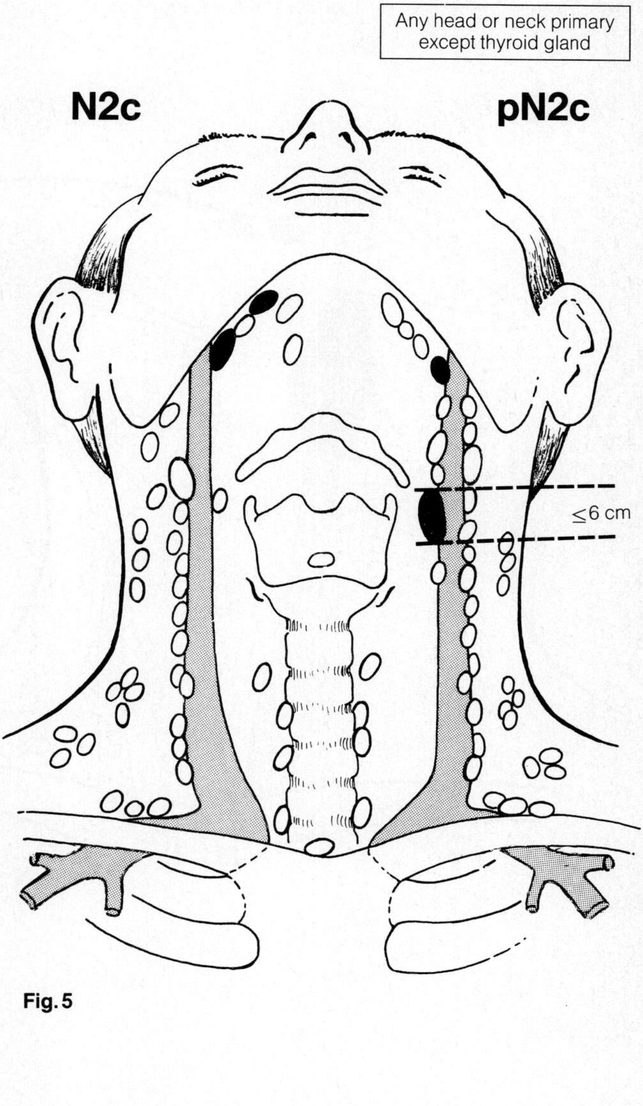

Fig. 5

N/pN3 Metastasis in a lymph node, more than 6 cm in greatest dimension (Fig. 6)

Note: Midline nodes are considered ipsilateral nodes.

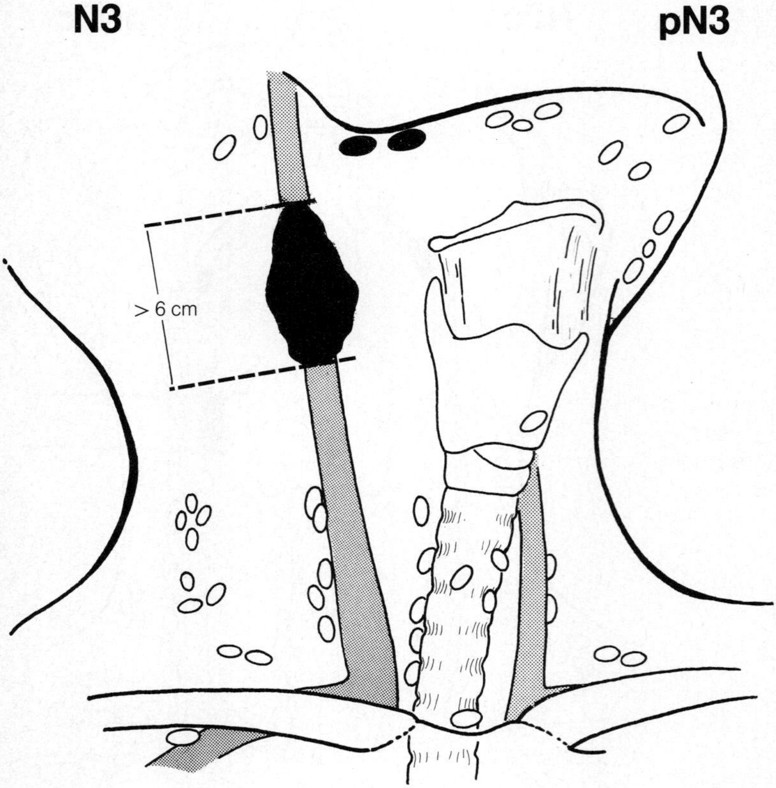

Fig. 6

Lip and Oral Cavity (ICD-O 140, 141, 143–145)

Rules for Classification

The classification applies only to squamous cell carcinoma of the vermilion surfaces of the lips and to carcinoma of the oral cavity.
There should be histological confirmation of the disease.

Anatomical Sites and Subsites

Lip (Fig. 7)

1. Upper lip, vermilion surface (140.0)
2. Lower lip, vermilion surface (140.1)
3. Commissures (140.6)

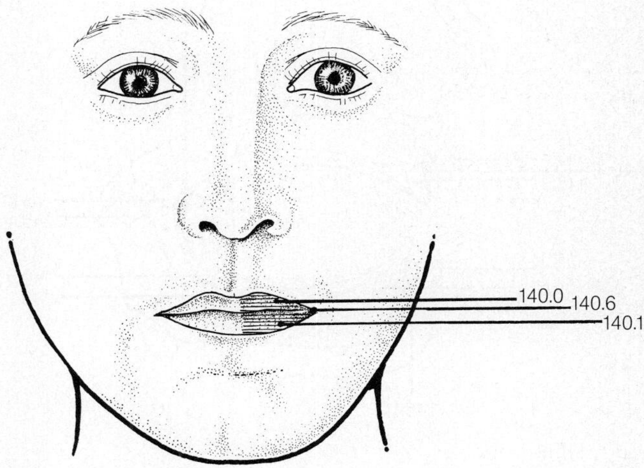

Fig. 7

Oral Cavity (Figs. 8–10)

1. Buccal mucosa
   i) Mucosal surfaces of upper and lower lips (140.3, 4)
   ii) Mucosal surface of cheeks (145.0)
   iii) Retromolar areas (145.6)
   iv) Bucco-alveolar sulci, upper and lower (145.1)
2. Upper alveolus and gingiva (143.0)
3. Lower alveolus and gingiva (143.1)
4. Hard palate (145.2)
5. Tongue
   i) Dorsal surface and lateral borders anterior to vallate papillae (anterior two-thirds) (141.1, 2)
   ii) Inferior surface (141.3)
6. Floor of mouth (144)

Regional Lymph Nodes

See p. 5

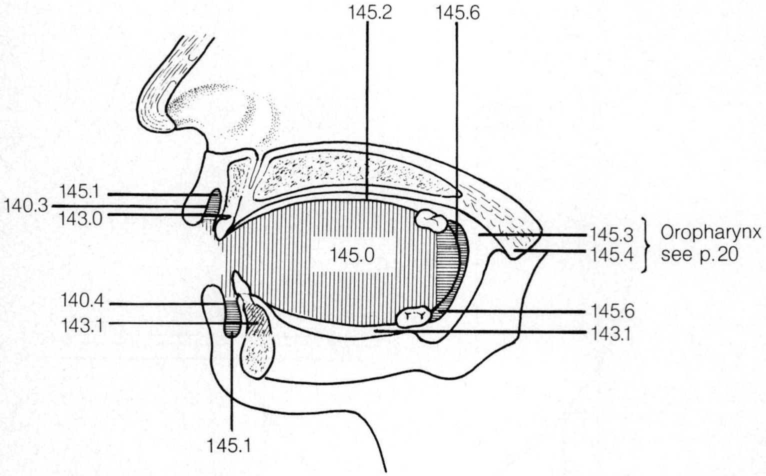

Fig. 8

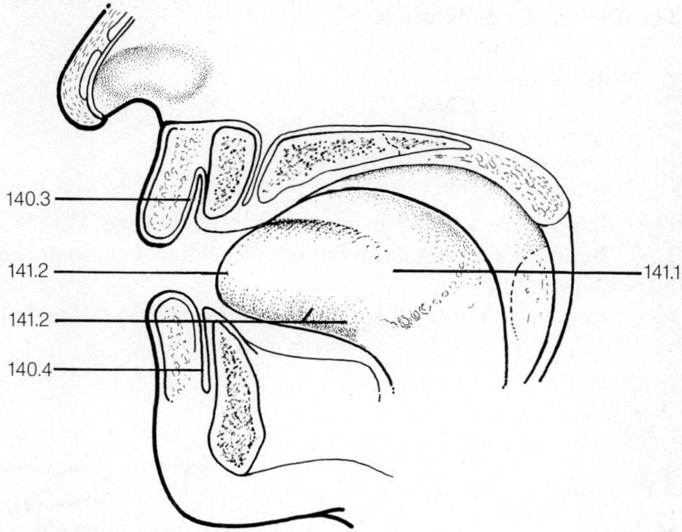

Fig. 9

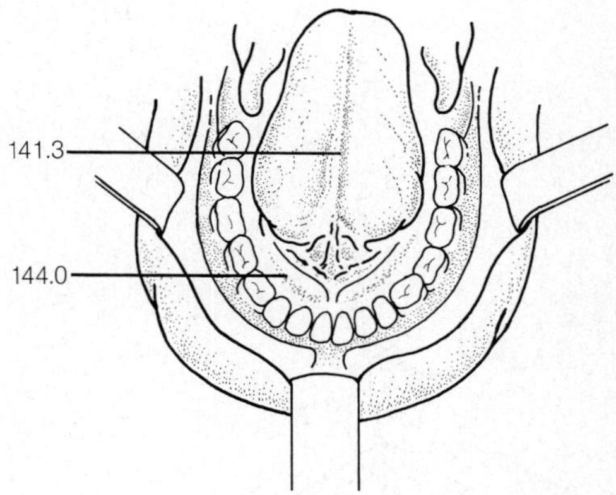

Fig. 10

TN Clinical Classification

T - Primary Tumour

TX Primary tumour cannot be assessed
T0 No evidence of primary tumour
Tis Carcinoma in situ

T1 Tumour 2 cm or less in greatest dimension (Figs. 11, 12)
T2 Tumour more than 2 cm but not more than 4 cm in greatest dimension (Figs. 13, 14)
T3 Tumour more than 4 cm in greatest dimension (Figs. 15, 16)

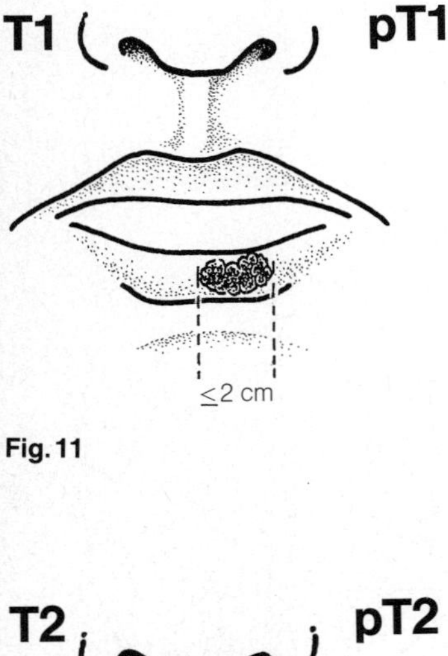

Fig. 11

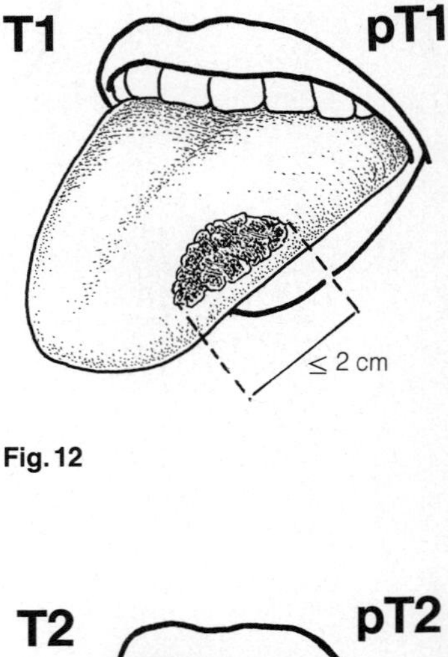

Fig. 12

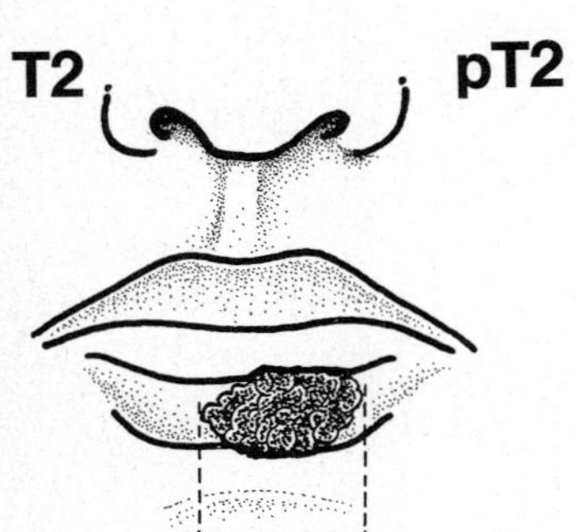

Fig. 13

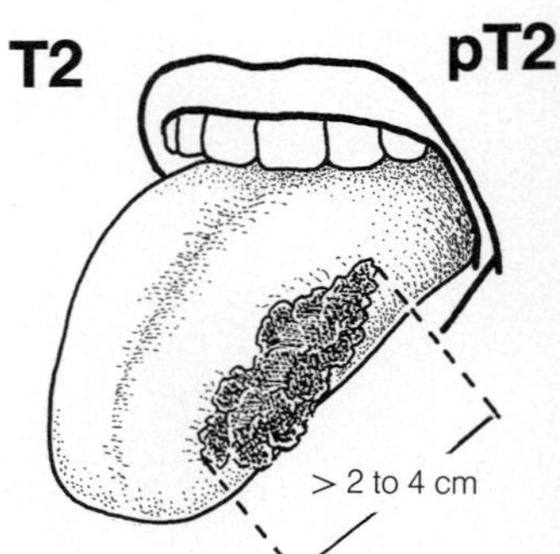

Fig. 14

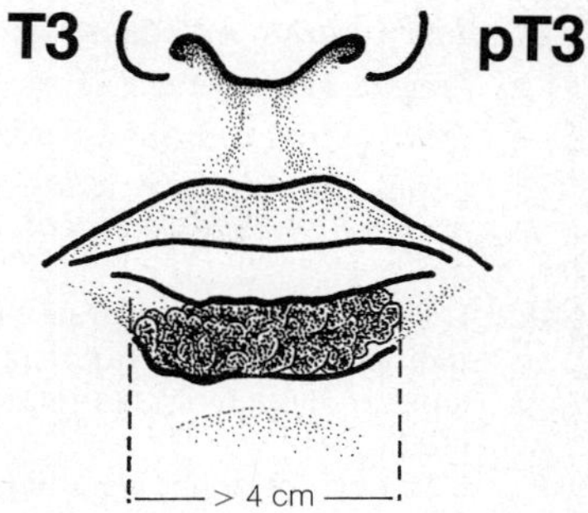

Fig. 15

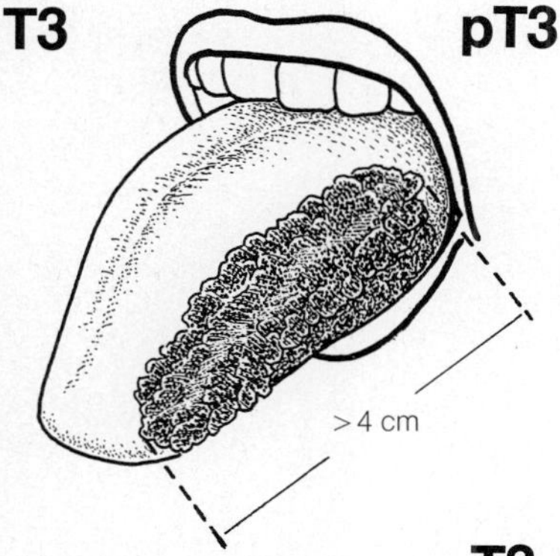

a

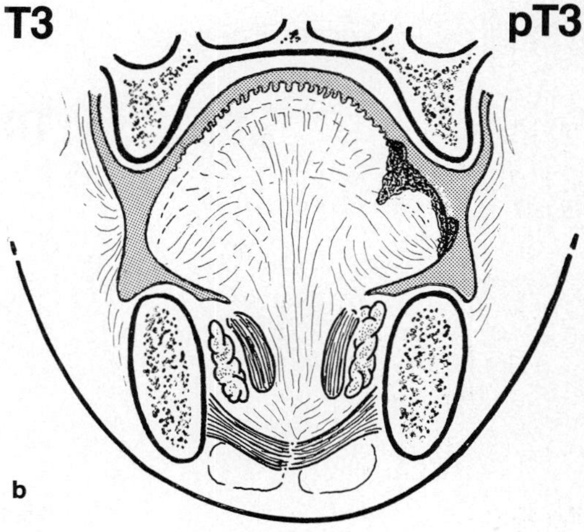

b

Fig. 16 a, b

T4 *Lip:* tumour invades adjacent structures, e.g. through cortical bone, tongue, skin of neck (Figs. 17, 18)

Oral cavity: tumour invades adjacent structures, e.g. through cortical bone, into deep *(extrinsic)* muscle of tongue, maxillary sinus, skin (Figs. 19–21)

Notes: 1. The *extrinsic* musculature of the tongue includes musculi hyo-, stylo-, genio- and palatoglossus. Invasion of the *intrinsic muscle alone* (musculi longitudinalis superior and inferior, transversus linguae and verticalis linguae) is not classified T4 (Fig. 16b).

2. In cases of doubt regarding the invasion through cortical bone, such as that of Fig. 20a, paragraph 4 of the General Rules of the TNM System (TNM Booklet, p. 6) should be applied: "If there is doubt concerning the correct T, N or M category to which a particular case should be allotted, the lower (i.e. less advanced) category should be chosen. This will also be reflected in the stage grouping". If scintigraphy is feasible and the resultant finding is conclusive as shown in Fig. 20b, the tumor must be classified as T4.

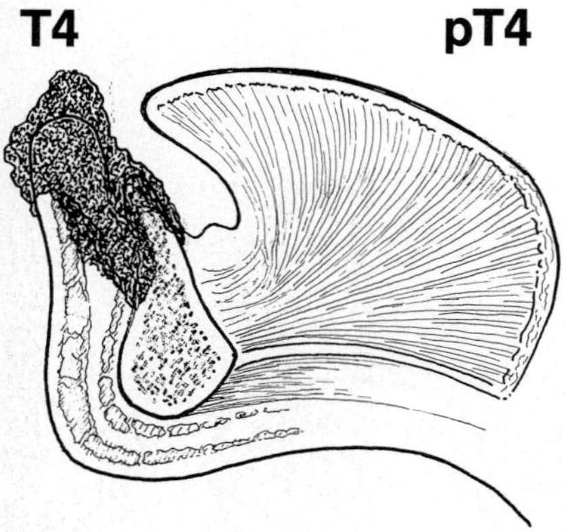

Fig. 17

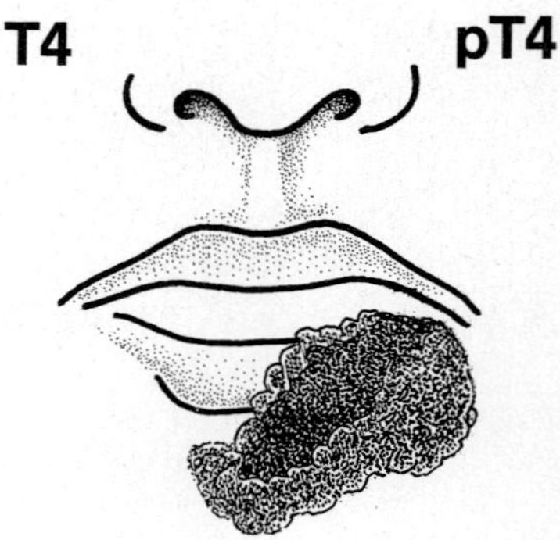

Fig. 18

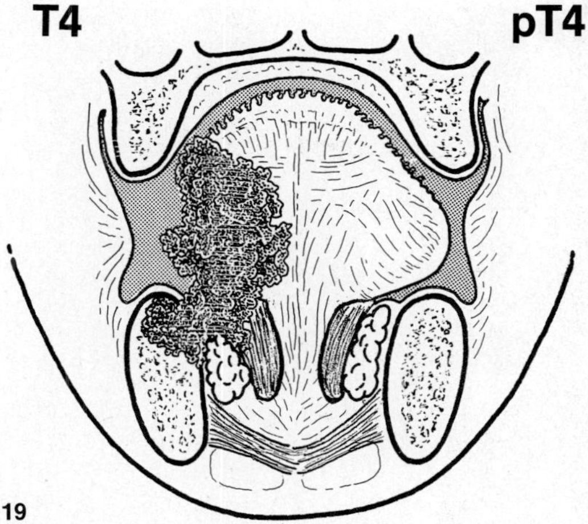

Fig. 19

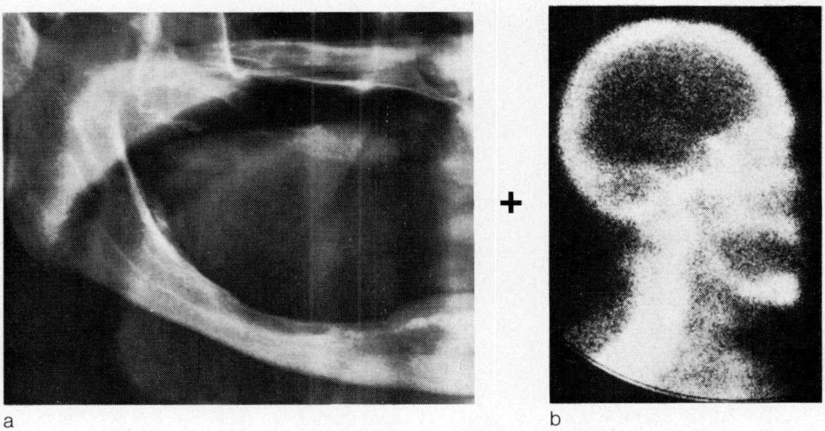

Fig. 20. **a** Radiographical suspicion but no evidence of invasion through the cortical bone; the tumour must be classified as non-T4 in correspondence with the definitions T1, T2 and T3. **b** Evidence of invasion through cortical bone by uptake, which corresponds with the suspected area in the premolar region of the radiograph shown in **a**. On the basis of the scintigraphic finding the tumour must be classified as T4

T4

a

T4

b

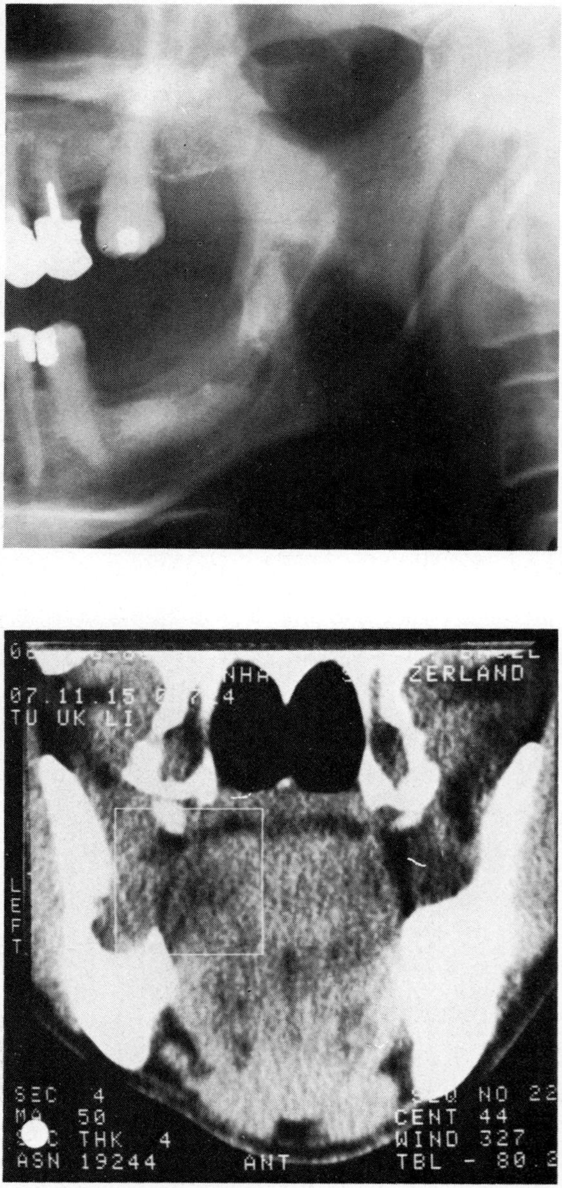

Fig. 21. **a** Evidence of invasion through cortical bone of the mandibula. **b** CT of case shown in **a**. The carcinoma of the floor of the mouth invades through the cortical bone and into the *extrinsic* muscle of the tongue (m. hyoglossus)

N – Regional Lymph Nodes

See p. 5

pTN Pathological Classification

The pT and pN categories correspond to the T and N categories.

Pharynx (ICD-O 141.0, 145.3, 4, 146–148)

Rules for Classification

The classification applies only to carcinoma. There should be histological confirmation of the disease.

Anatomical Sites and Subsites

Oropharynx (141.0, 145.3, 4, 146) (Figs. 22, 23)

1. Anterior wall (glosso-epiglottic area)
   i) Tongue posterior to the vallate papillae (base of tongue or posterior third) (141.0)
   ii) Vallecula (146.3)
2. Lateral wall (146.6)
   i) Tonsil (146.0)
   ii) Tonsillar fossa (146.1) and faucial pillars (146.2)
   iii) Glossotonsillar sulci (146.2)
3. Posterior wall (146.7)
4. Superior wall
   i) Inferior surface of soft palate (145.3)
   ii) Uvula (145.4)

Note: The anterior (lingual) surface of the epiglottis (146.4) is included with the larynx, suprahyoid epiglottis.

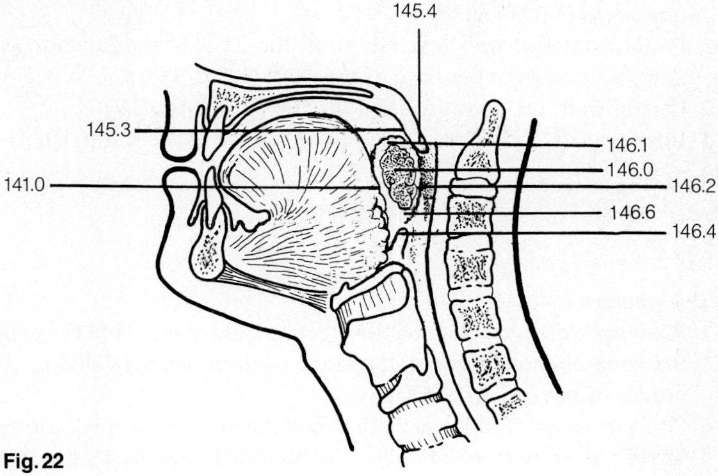
145.4
145.3
146.1
146.0
141.0
146.2
146.6
146.4

Fig. 22

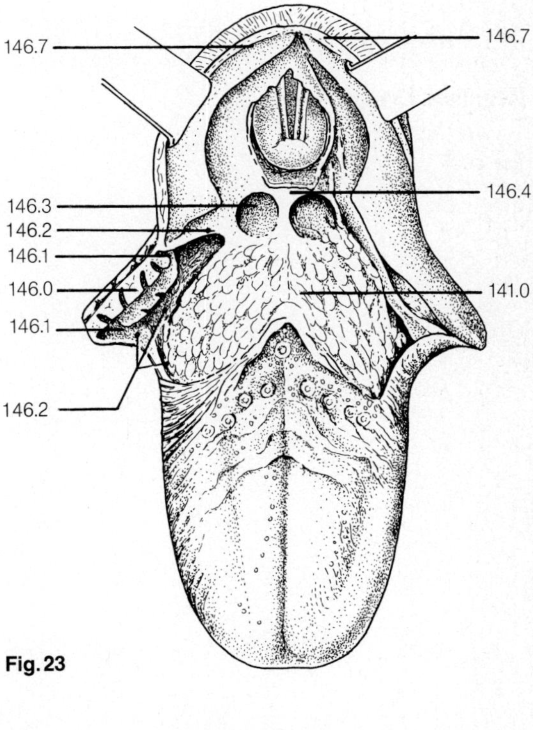
146.7
146.7
146.4
146.3
146.2
146.1
146.0
141.0
146.1
146.2

Fig. 23

Nasopharynx (147) (Fig. 24)

1. Postero-superior wall: extends from the level of the junction of the hard and soft palates to the base of the skull (147.0, 1)
2. Lateral wall: includes the fossa of Rosenmüller (147.2)
3. Inferior wall: consists of the superior surface of the soft palate (147.3)

Note: The margin of the choanal orifices, including the posterior margin of the nasal septum, is included with the nasal fossa.

Hypopharynx (148) (Fig. 24)

1. Pharyngo-oesophageal junction (postcricoid area) (148.0): extends from the level of the arytenoid cartilages and connecting folds to the inferior border of the cricoid cartilage
2. Piriform sinus (148.1): extends from the pharyngo-epiglottic fold to the upper end of the oesophagus. It is bounded laterally by the thyroid cartilage and medially by the surface of the aryepiglottic fold (148.2) and the arytenoid and cricoid cartilages
3. Posterior pharyngeal wall (148.3): extends from the level of the floor of the vallecula to the level of the crico-arytenoid joints

Regional Lymph Nodes

See p. 5

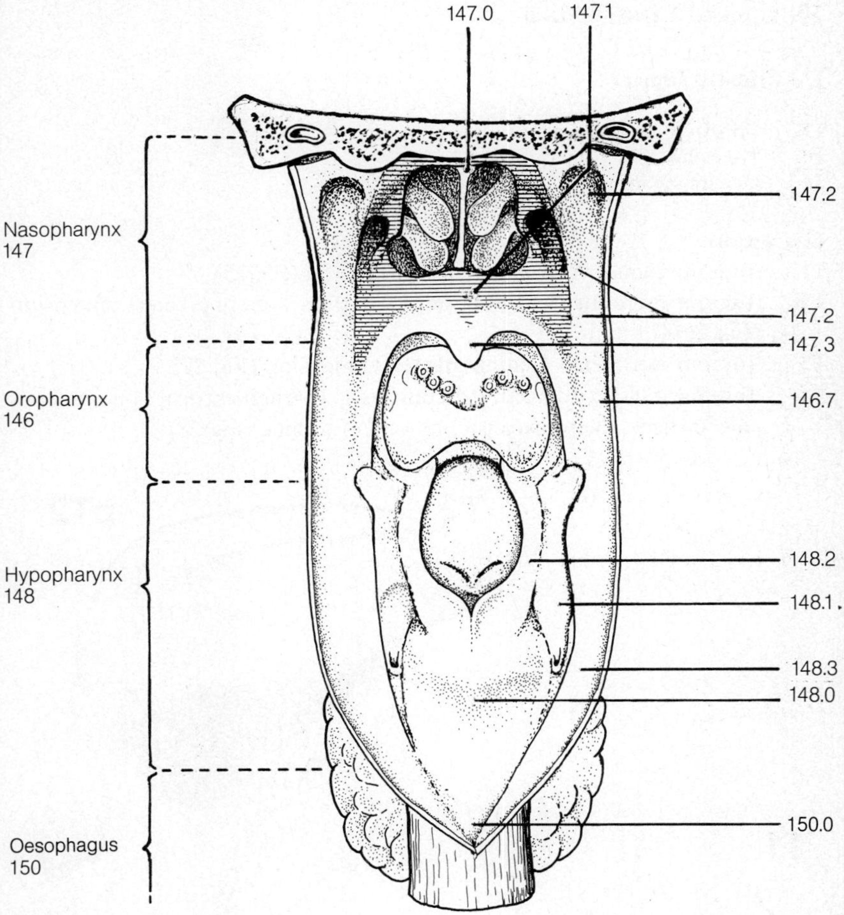
147.0
147.1
147.2
147.2
147.3
146.7
148.2
148.1
148.3
148.0
150.0
Nasopharynx
147
Oropharynx
146
Hypopharynx
148
Oesophagus
150

Fig. 24

TN Clinical Classification

T – Primary Tumour

TX Primary tumour cannot be assessed
T0 No evidence of primary tumour
Tis Carcinoma in situ

Oropharynx

T1 Tumour 2 cm or less in greatest dimension (Fig. 25)
T2 Tumour more than 2 cm but not more than 4 cm in greatest dimension (Fig. 26)
T3 Tumour more than 4 cm in greatest dimension (Fig. 27)
T4 Tumour invades adjacent structures, e.g. through cortical bone, soft tissues of neck, deep (extrinsic) muscle of tongue (Fig. 28)

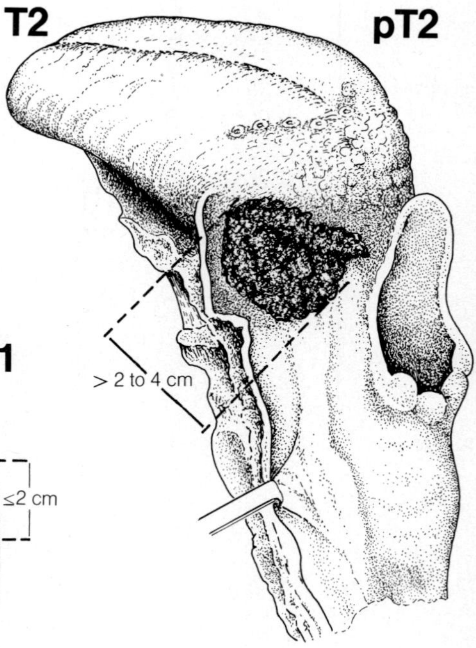

Fig. 26

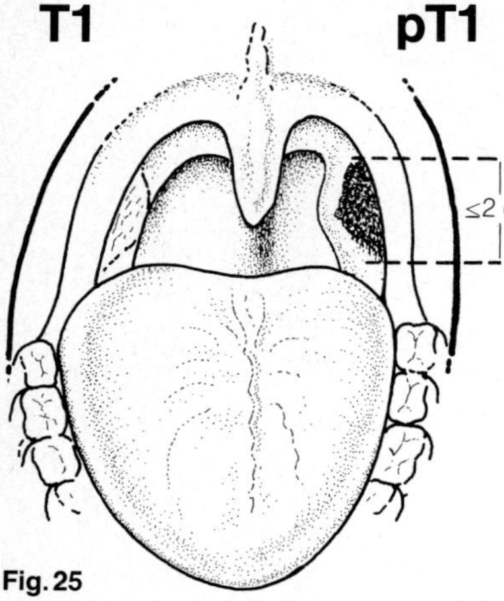

Fig. 25

T3 pT3

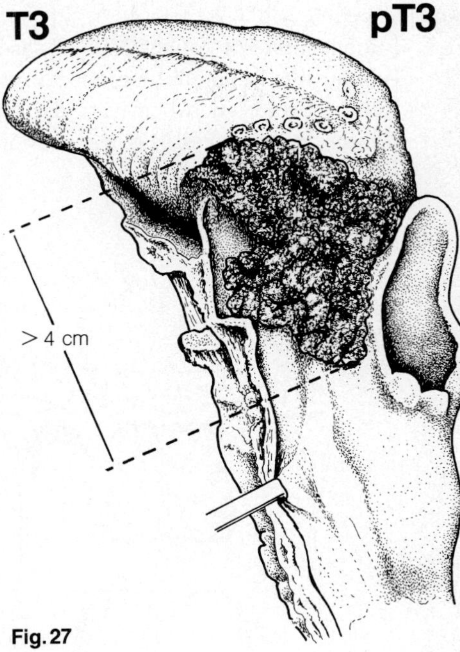

Fig. 27

T4 pT4

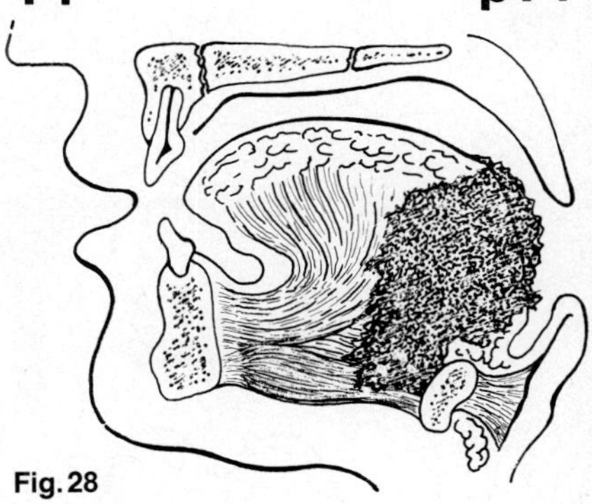

Fig. 28

Nasopharynx

T1 Tumour limited to one subsite of nasopharynx (Fig. 29)
T2 Tumour invades more than one subsite of nasopharynx (Fig. 30)
T3 Tumour invades nasal cavity and/or oropharynx (Fig. 31)
T4 Tumour invades skull (Fig. 32) and/or cranial nerve(s) (Fig. 33)

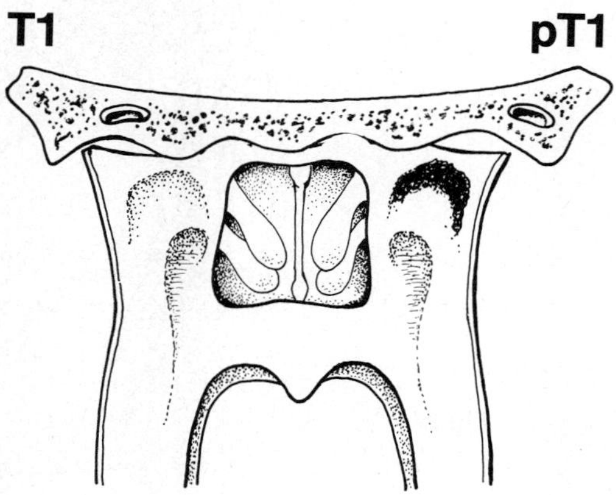

Fig. 29

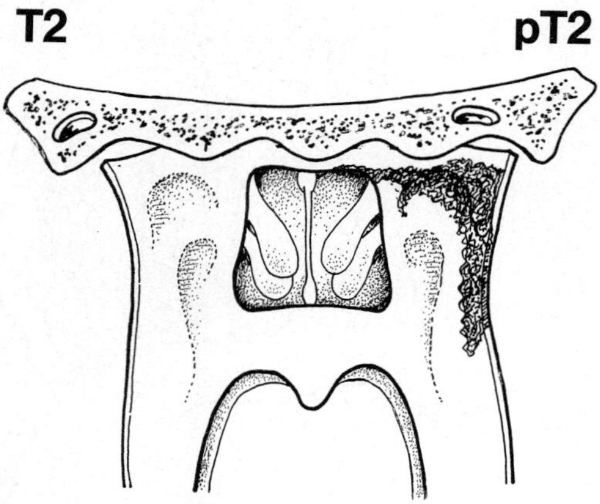

Fig. 30

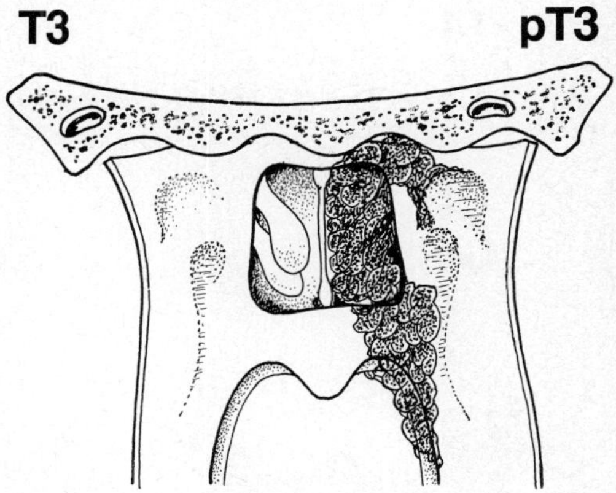

Fig. 31

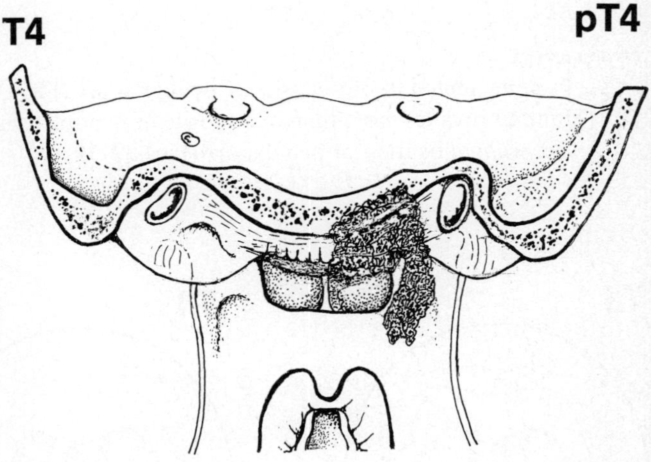

Fig. 32

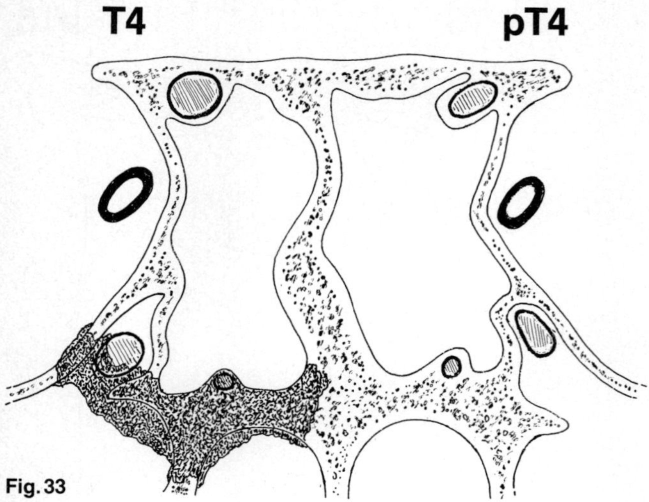

Fig. 33

Hypopharynx

T1 Tumour limited to one subsite of hypopharynx (Figs. 34–36)

T2 Tumour invades more than one subsite of hypopharynx or an adjacent site, *without* fixation of hemilarynx (Figs. 37–39)

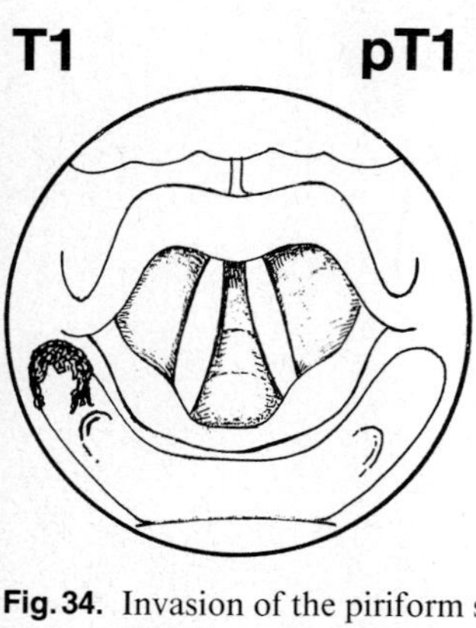

Fig. 34. Invasion of the piriform sinus (148.1)

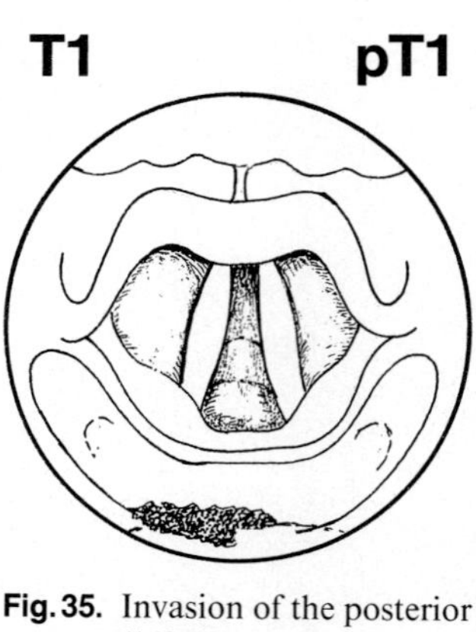

Fig. 35. Invasion of the posterior wall (148.3)

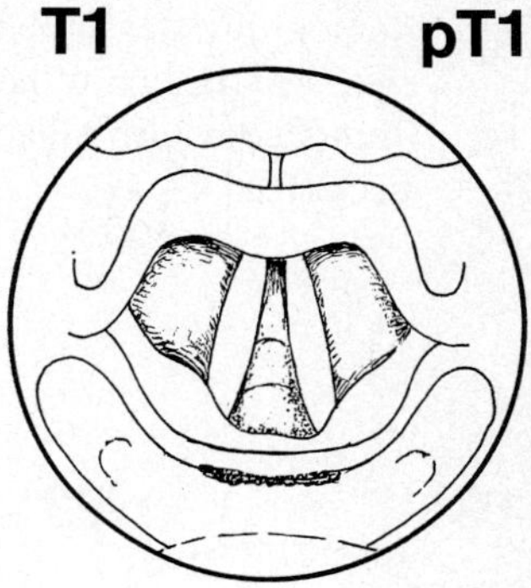

Fig. 36. Invasion of the post-cricoid area (148.0)

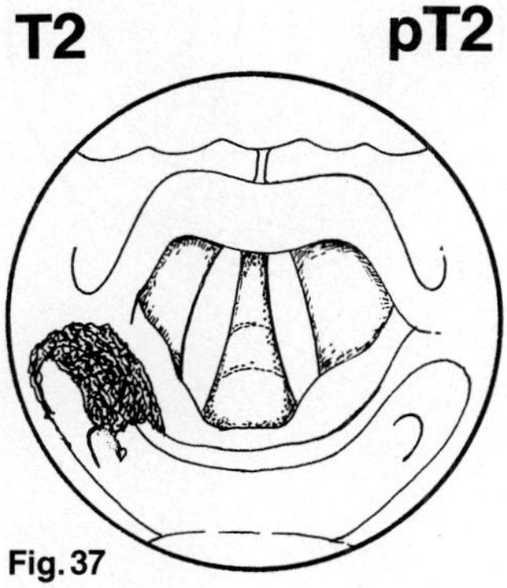

Fig. 37

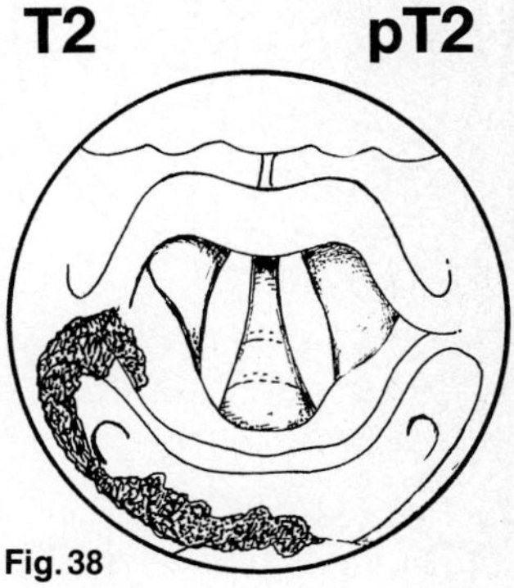

Fig. 38

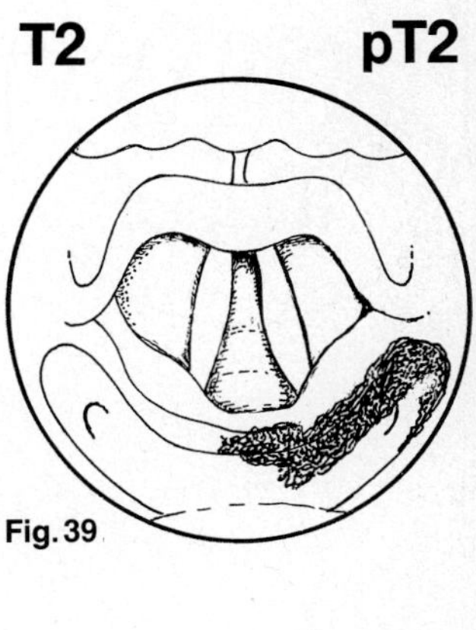

Fig. 39

Fig. 37. Invasion of the piriform sinus (148.1) and the aryepiglottic fold (148.2)

Fig. 38. Invasion of the piriform sinus (148.1) and the posterior wall (148.3)

Fig. 39. Invasion of the piriform sinus (148.1) and the postcricoid area (148.0)

T3 Tumour invades more than one subsite of hypopharynx or an adjacent site, *with* fixation of hemilarynx (Figs. 40–42)

T4 Tumour invades adjacent structures, e.g. cartilage or soft tissues of neck (Figs. 43, 44)

T3 **pT3**

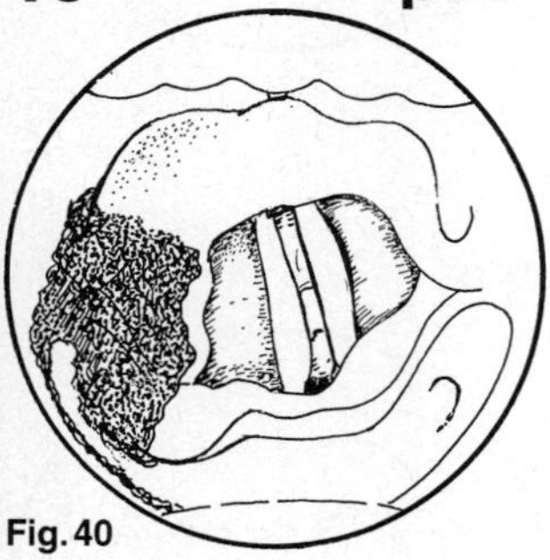

Fig. 40

T3 **pT3**

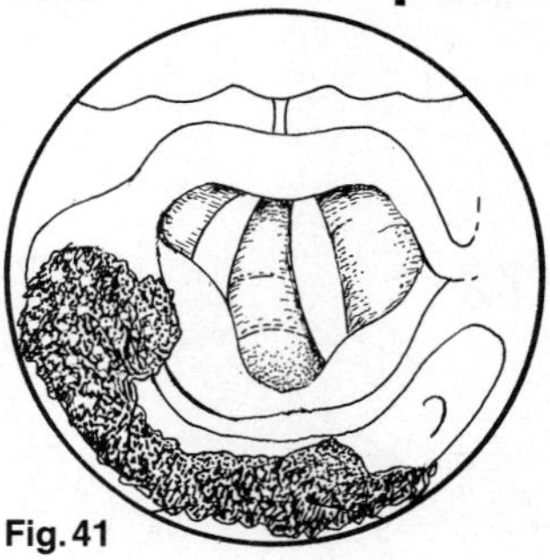

Fig. 41

T3 **pT3**

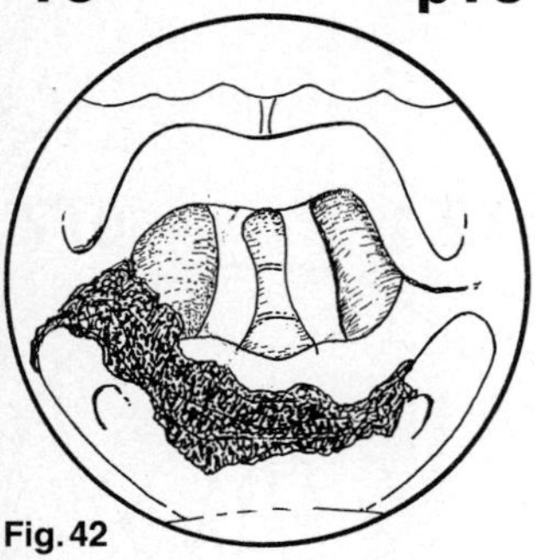

Fig. 42

Fig. 40. Invasion of the piriform sinus (148.1) and the aryepiglottic fold (148.2) with fixation of the hemilarynx

Fig. 41. Invasion of the piriform sinus (148.1), the aryepiglottic fold (148.2) and the posterior wall (148.3) with fixation of the hemilarynx

Fig. 42. Invasion of the piriform sinus (148.1) and postcricoid area (148.0) with fixation of the hemilarynx

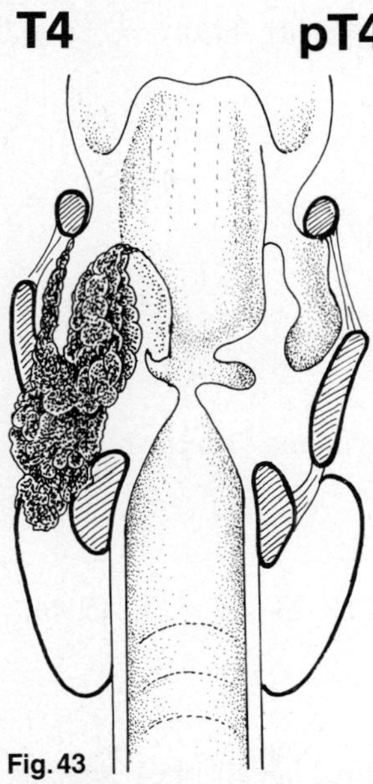

Fig. 43

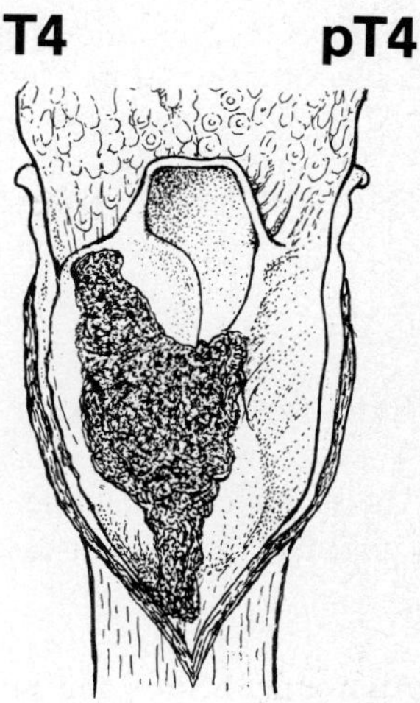

Fig. 44

Fig. 43. Invasion of the piriform sinus involving the cartilage of the epiglottis

Fig. 44. Invasion of the postcricoid area involving the cervical oesophagus and the arytenoid area

N – Regional Lymph Nodes

See p. 5

pTN Pathological Classification

The pT and pN categories correspond to the T and N categories.

Larynx (ICD-O 161, 146.4)

Rules for Classification

The classification applies only to carcinoma. There should be histological confirmation of the disease.

Anatomical Sites and Subsites (Figs. 22, 23 [see p. 21], 45, 46)

1. Supraglottis (161.1)
   Epilarynx (including marginal zone)
   i) Suprahyoid epiglottis [including tip, lingual (146.4) and laryngeal surfaces]
   ii) Aryepiglottic fold
   iii) Arytenoid
   Supraglottis excluding epilarynx
   iv) Infrahyoid epiglottis
   v) Ventricular bands (false cords)
   vi) Ventricular cavities

2. Glottis (161.0)
   i) Vocal cords
   ii) Anterior commissure
   iii) Posterior commissure

3. Subglottis (161.2)

Regional Lymph Nodes

See p. 5

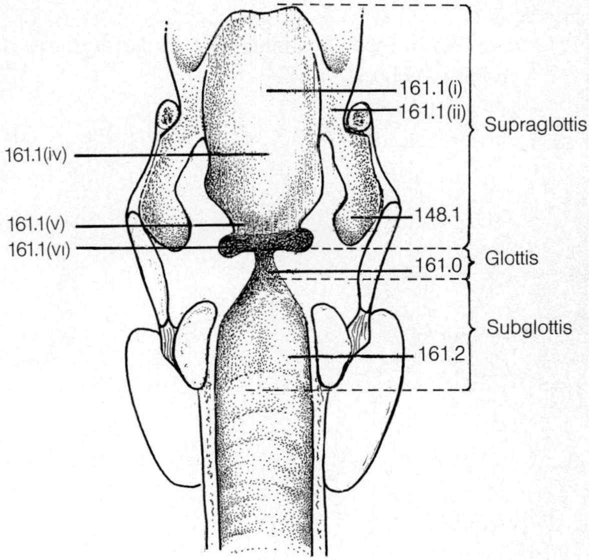

Fig. 45

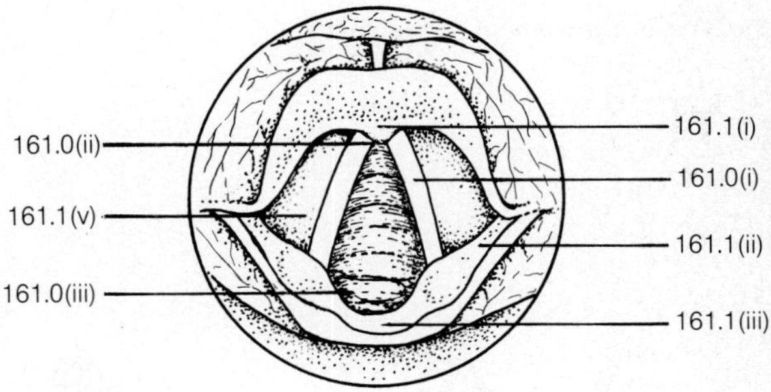

Fig. 46

TN Clinical Classification

T - Primary Tumour

TX Primary tumour cannot be assessed
T0 No evidence of primary tumour
Tis Carcinoma in situ

Supraglottis

T1 Tumour limited to one subsite of supraglottis with normal vocal cord mobility (Figs. 47, 48)

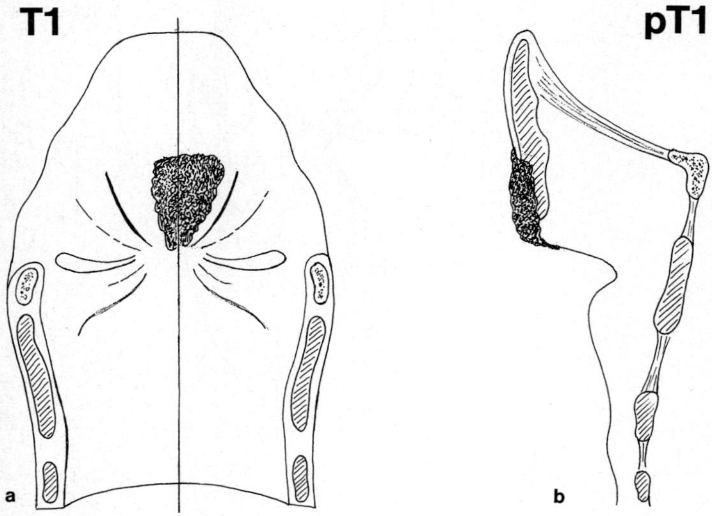

Fig. 47 a, b. Invasion of the epiglottis

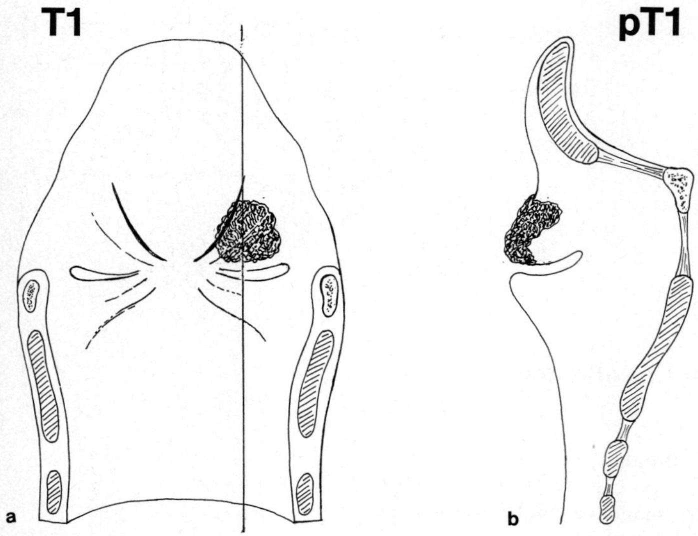

Fig. 48 a, b. Invasion of the false cord

T2 Tumour invades more than one subsite of supraglottis or glottis, with normal vocal cord mobility (Figs. 49, 50)

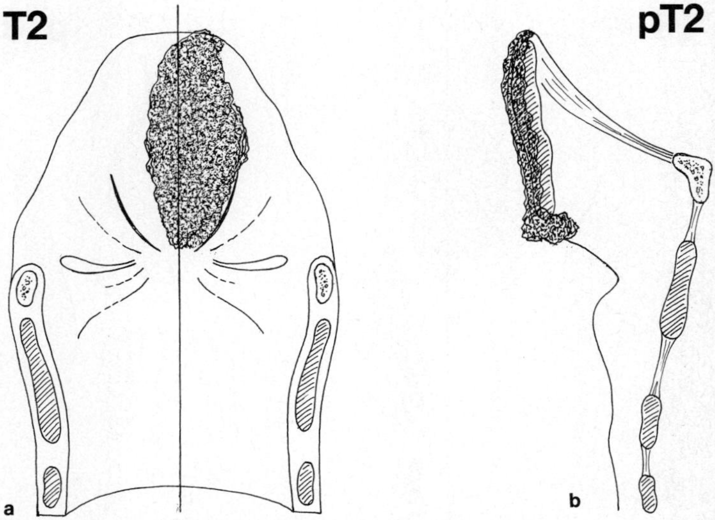

Fig. 49 a, b. Invasion of the suprahyoid and the infrahyoid epiglottis

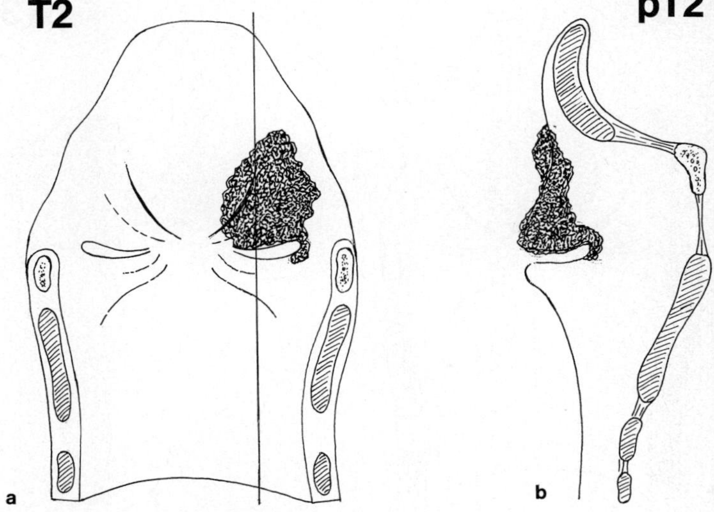

Fig. 50 a, b. Invasion of the false cord and the epiglottis

T3 Tumour limited to larynx with vocal cord fixation and/or invades postcricoid area, medial wall of piriform sinus or pre-epiglottic tissues (Figs. 51, 52)

T3 **pT3**

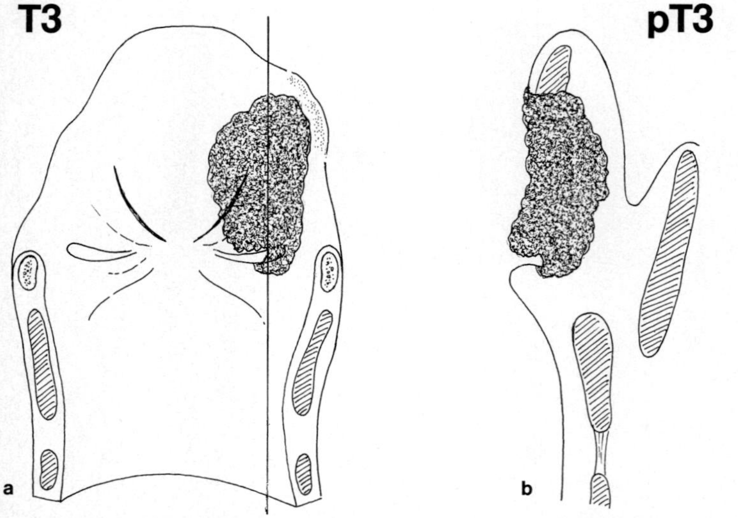

Fig. 51 a, b. Invasion of the vocal cord, the aryepiglottic fold and the medial wall of the piriform sinus

T3 **pT3**

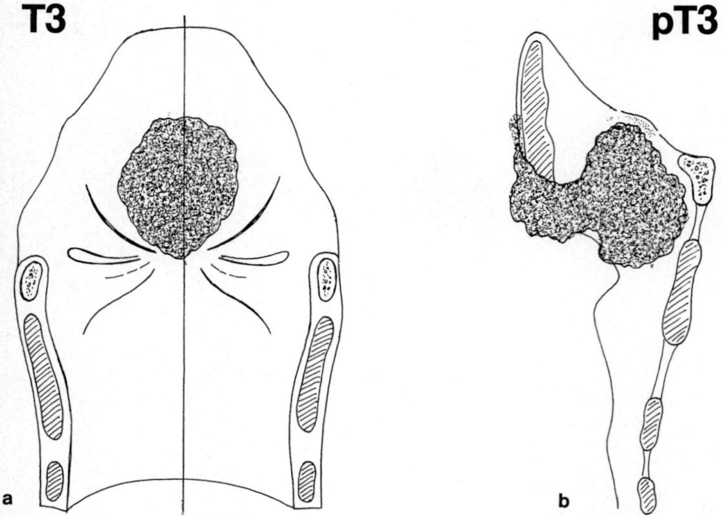

Fig. 52 a, b. Invasion of the pre-epiglottic tissues with vocal cord fixation

T4 Tumour invades through thyroid cartilage and/or extends to other tissues beyond the larynx, e.g. to oropharynx, soft tissues of neck (Fig. 53)

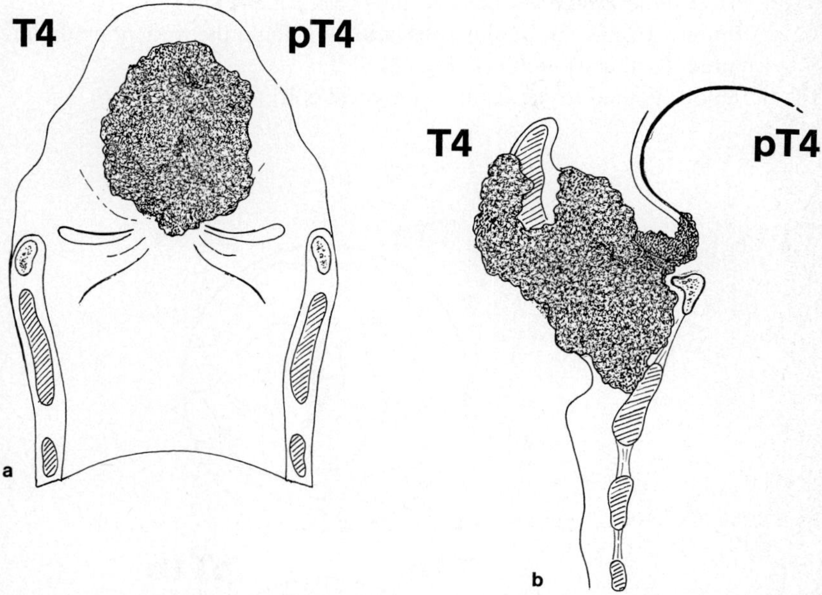

Fig. 53 a, b. Invasion beyond the larynx: oropharynx (vallecula and base of the tongue) and soft tissues of the neck (prelarynx)

Glottis

T1 Tumour limited to vocal cord(s) (may involve anterior or posterior commissures) with normal mobility (Fig. 54a)

 T1a Tumour limited to one vocal cord (Fig. 54b)

 T1b Tumour involves both vocal cords (Fig. 54c)

T2 Tumour extends to supraglottis and/or subglottis, and/or with impaired vocal cord mobility (Fig. 55)

T3 Tumour limited to the larynx with vocal cord fixation (Fig. 56)

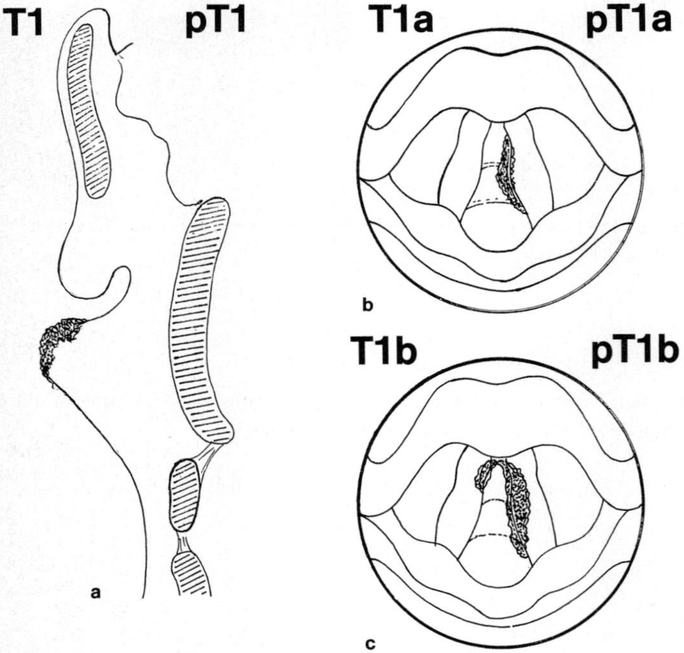

Fig. 54a, b. Tumour limited to vocal cord. **c** Tumour limited to vocal cords with invasion of the anterior commissure

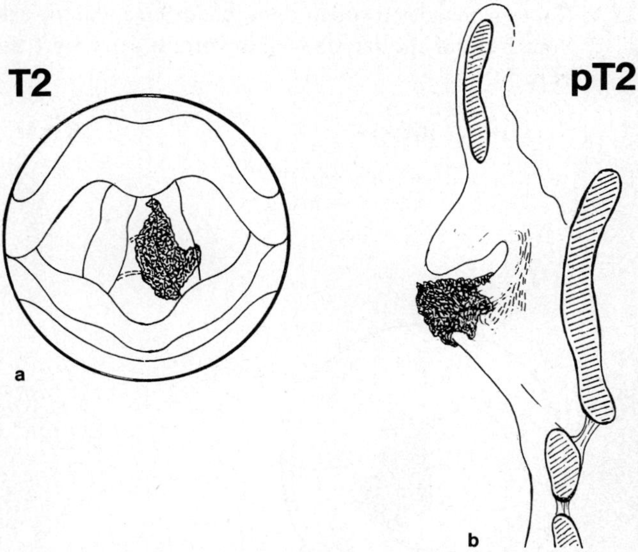

Fig. 55 a, b. Tumour extends to supraglottis with impaired vocal cord mobility by invasion of the superficial m. vocalis

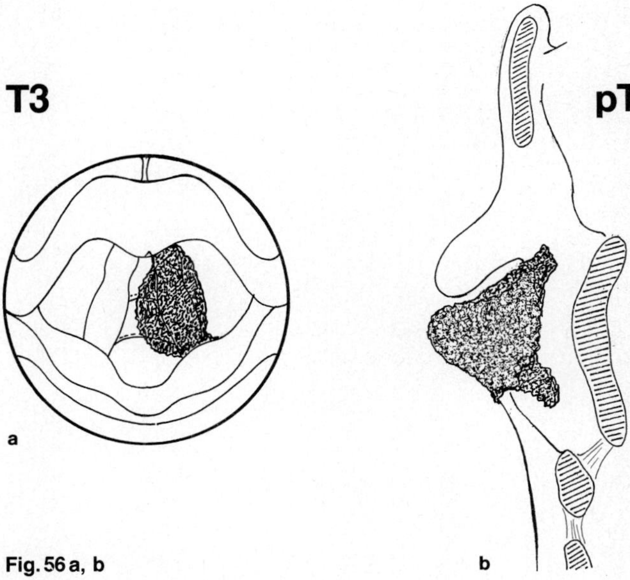

Fig. 56 a, b

T4 Tumour invades through thyroid cartilage and/or extends to other tissues beyond the larynx, e.g. to oropharynx, soft tissues of the neck (Fig. 57)

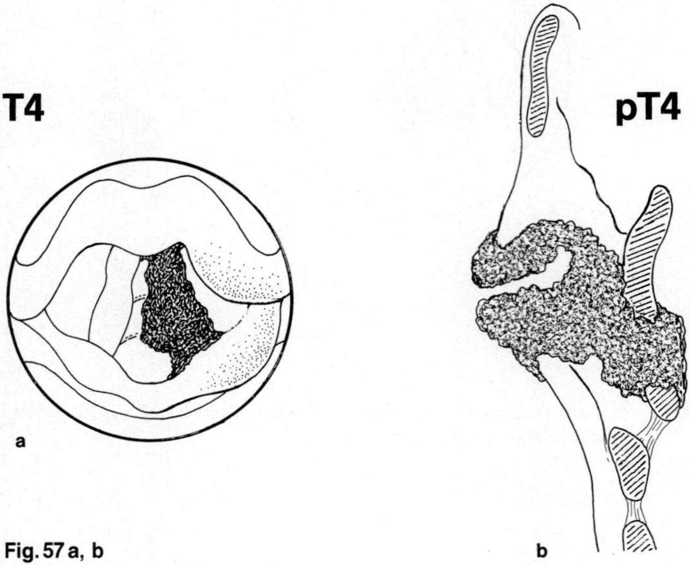

Fig. 57 a, b

Subglottis

T1 Tumour limited to the subglottis (Fig. 58)

T2 Tumour extends to vocal cord(s) with normal or impaired mobility (Fig. 59)

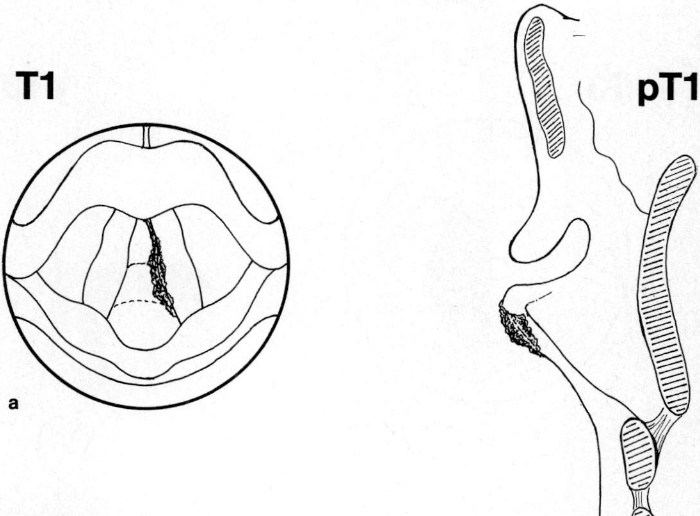

Fig. 58 a, b

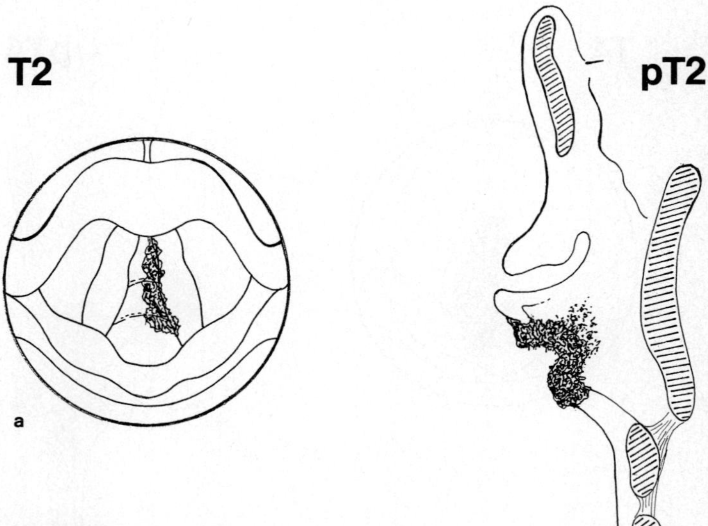

Fig. 59 a, b

T3 Tumour limited to the larynx with vocal cord fixation (Fig. 60)

T4 Tumour invades through cricoid or thyroid cartilage and/or extends to other tissues beyond the larynx, e.g. to oropharynx, soft tissues of the neck (Fig. 61)

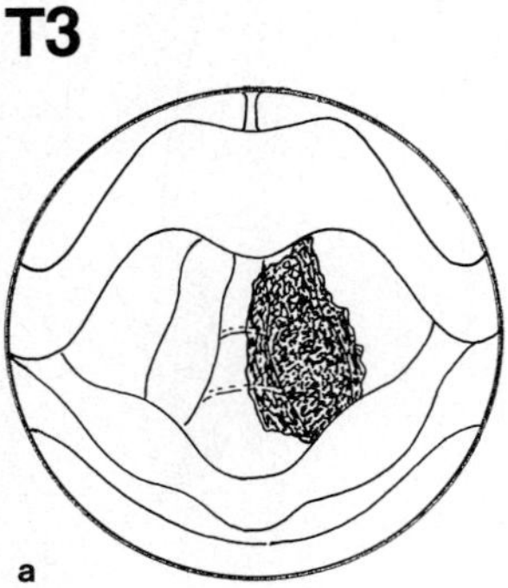

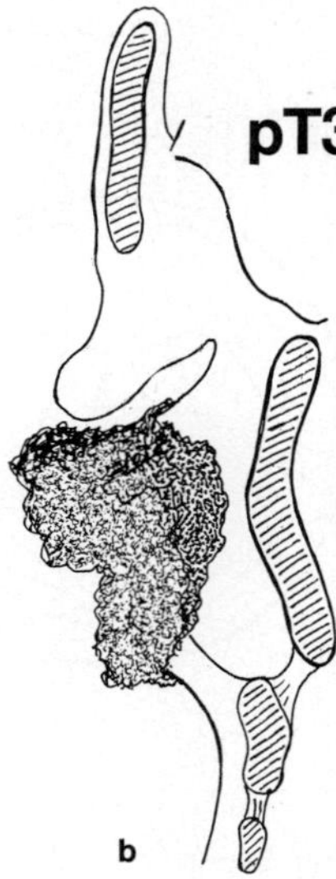

Fig. 60 a, b

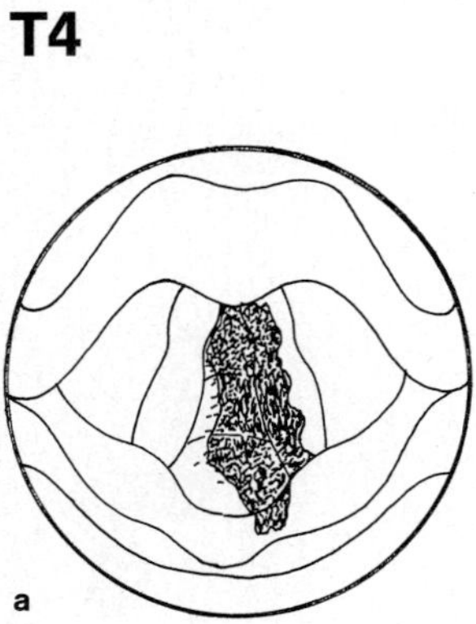

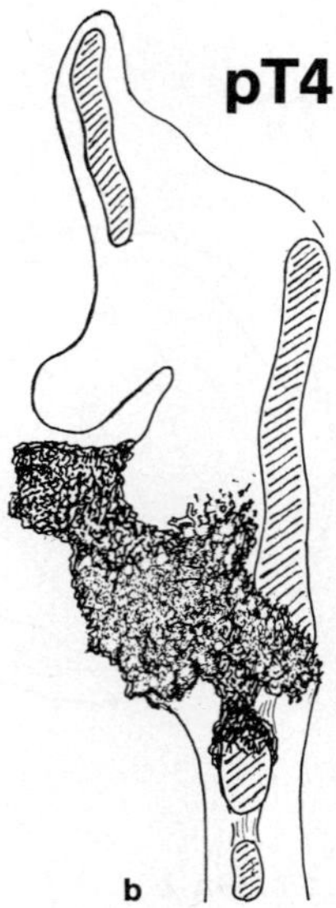

Fig. 61 a, b

N – Regional Lymph Nodes

See p. 5.

pTN Pathological Classification

The pT and pN categories correspond to the T and N categories.

Maxillary Sinus (ICD-O 160.2)

Rules for Classification

The classification applies only to carcinoma. There should be histological confirmation of the disease.

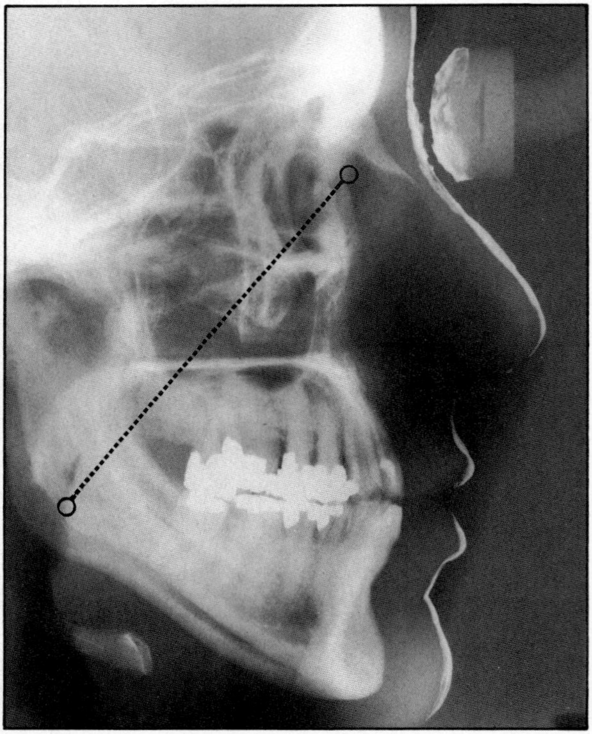

Fig. 62a. Ohngren's line

Anatomical Division (Figs. 62, 63)

Ohngren's line is defined as the plane which passes through the inner canthus and the mandibular angle and which divides the upper jaw into the superoposterior structure *(suprastructure)* and the inferoanterior structure *(infrastructure)*. The suprastructure includes the posterior bony wall and the posterior half of the superior bony wall. The other bony walls belong to the infrastructure.

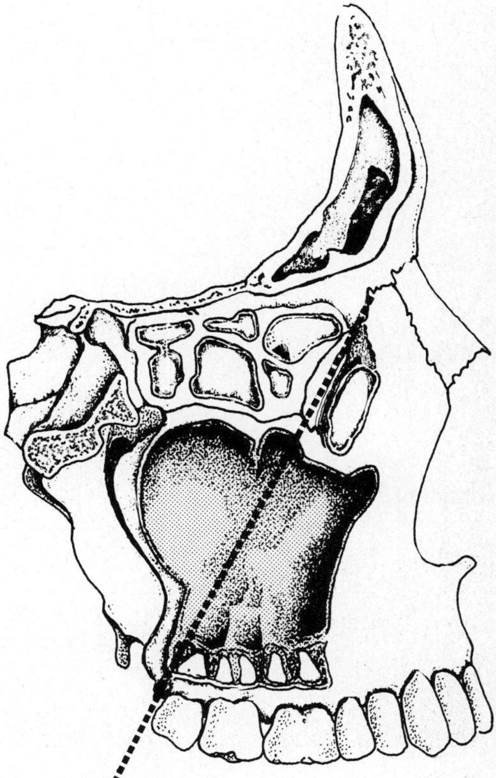

Fig. 62 b. Ohngren's line

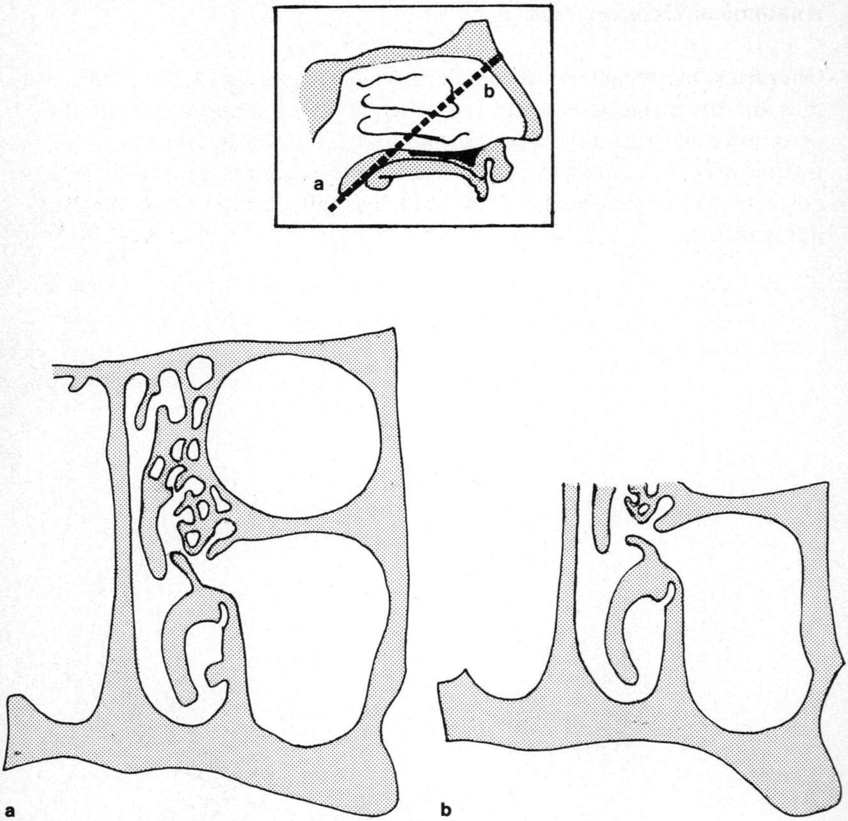

Fig. 63. **a** Suprastructure; **b** Infrastructure

Regional Lymph Nodes

See p. 5

TN Clinical Classification

T- Primary Tumour

TX Primary tumour cannot be assessed
T0 No evidence of primary tumour
Tis Carcinoma in situ
T1 Tumour limited to the antral mucosa with no erosion or destruction of bone (Fig. 64)
T2 Tumour with erosion or destruction of the infrastructure (see Anatomical Division, p. 46) including the hard palate and/or the middle nasal meatus (Fig. 65)

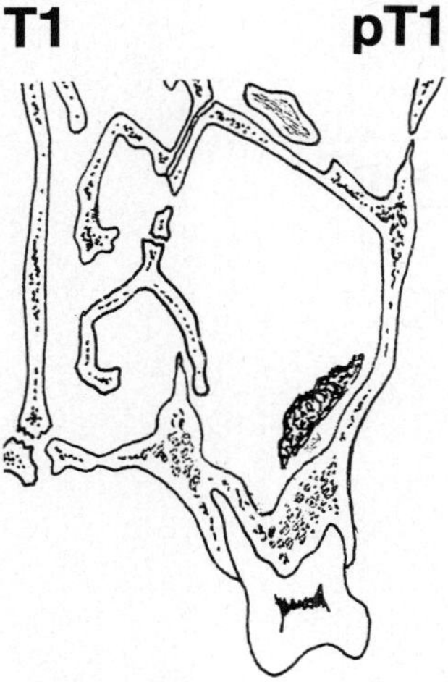

Fig. 64

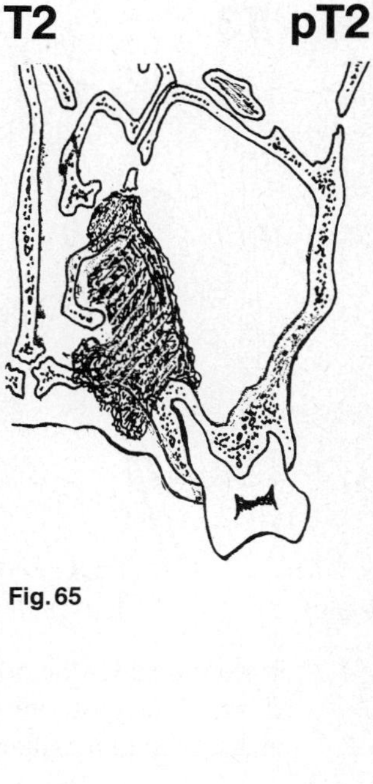

Fig. 65

T3 Tumour invades any of the following: skin of cheek, posterior wall of the maxillary sinus, floor or medial wall of orbit, anterior ethmoid sinus (Figs. 66, 67)

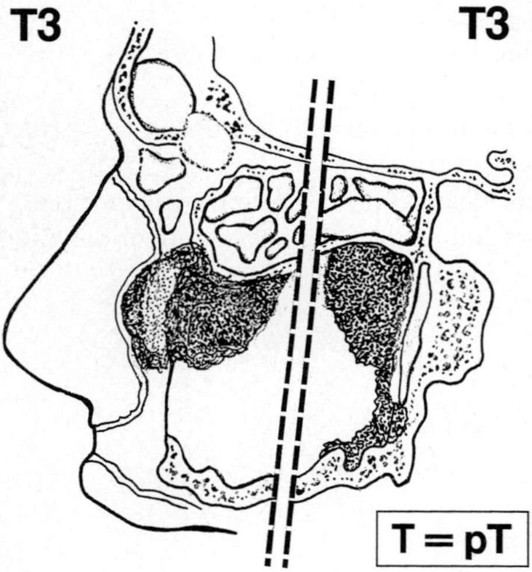

Fig. 66

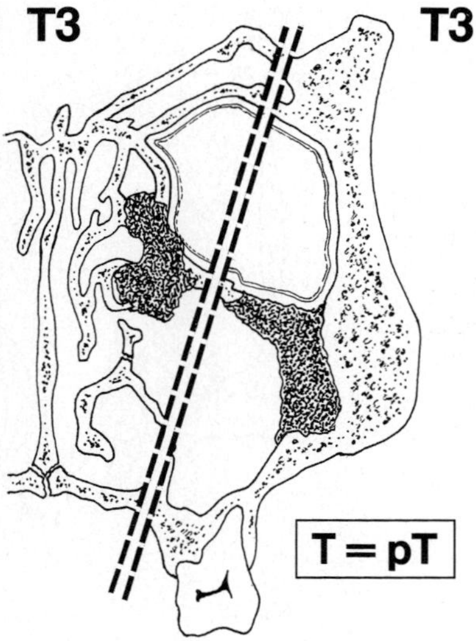

Fig. 67

T4 Tumour invades the orbital contents and/or any of the following: cribriform plate, posterior ethmoid or sphenoid sinuses, nasopharynx, soft palate, pterygomaxillary or temporal fossae, base of skull (Figs. 68–70)

T4 pT4

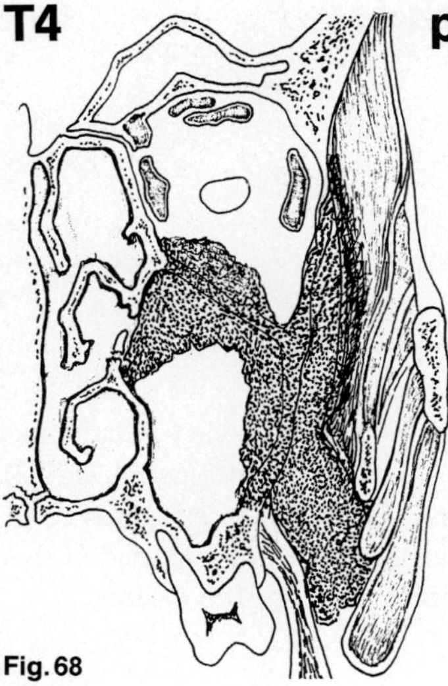

Fig. 68

T4 pT4

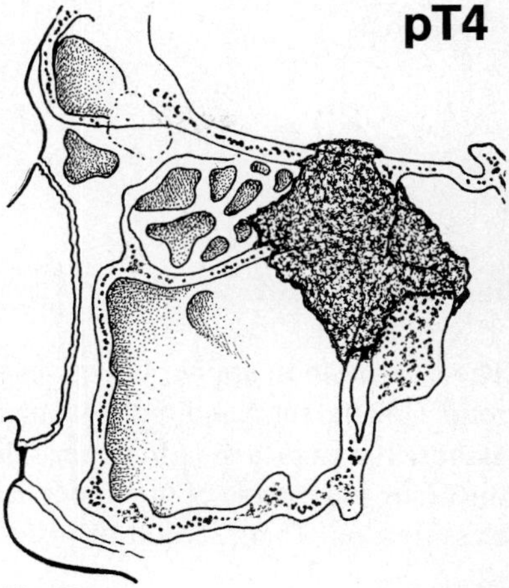

Fig. 69

T4 pT4

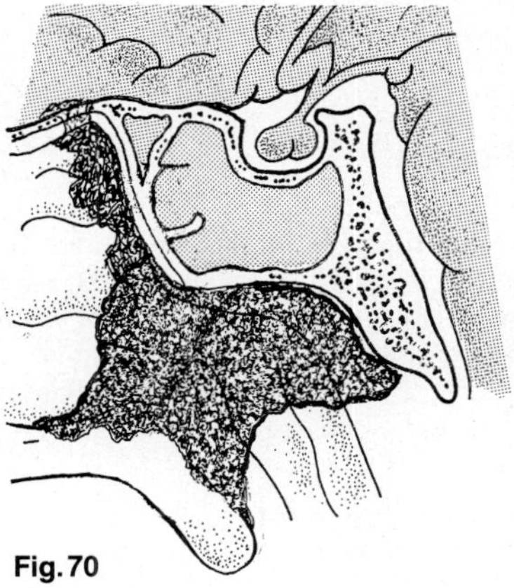

Fig. 70

N – Regional Lymph Nodes

See p. 5

pTN Pathological Classification

The pT and pN categories correspond to the T and N categories.

Salivary Glands (ICD-O 142)

Rules for Classification

The classification applies only to carcinoma of the major salivary glands: parotid (142.0), submandibular (submaxillary) (142.1), and sublingual (142.2) glands. Tumours arising in minor salivary glands (mucous-secreting glands in the lining membrane of the upper aerodigestive tract) are not included in this classification. There should be histological confirmation of the disease.

Regional Lymph Nodes

See p. 5

TN Clinical Classification

Note: All categories are subdivided: (a) no local extension (Figs. 71, 73, 75, 77); (b) local extension (Figs. 72, 74, 76, 78). Local extension is clinical or macroscopic evidence of invasion of skin, soft tissues, bone or nerve. Microscopic evidence alone is not local extension for classification purposes.

T – Primary Tumour

TX Primary tumour cannot be assessed
T0 No evidence of primary tumour

T1 Tumour 2 cm or less in greatest dimension (Figs. 71, 72)

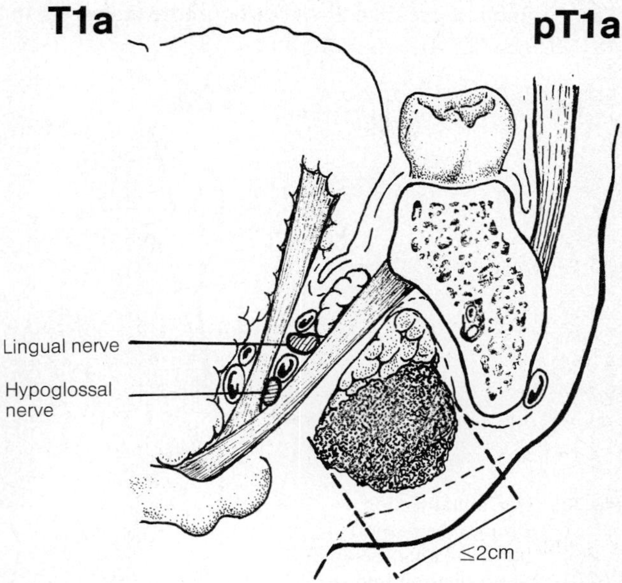

Fig. 71. Classification determined clinically on the basis of absence of paralysis or macroscopically on the basis of no local extension (a). Frontal section through the premolar region

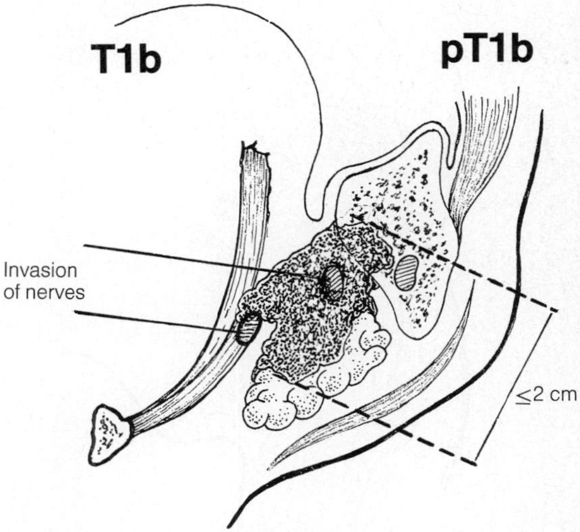

Fig. 72. Clinical or macroscopic evidence of local extension (b). Frontal section through the retromolar region

T2 Tumour more than 2 cm but not more than 4 cm in greatest dimension (Figs. 73, 74)

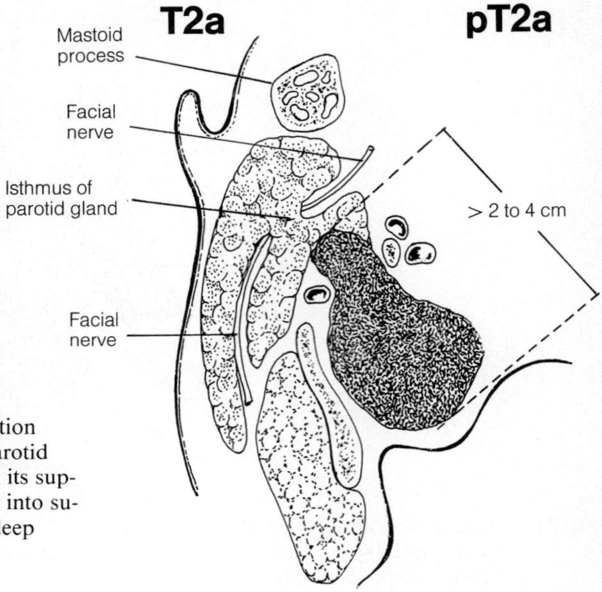

Fig. 73. Horizontal section through the parotid gland showing its supposed division into superficial and deep lobes

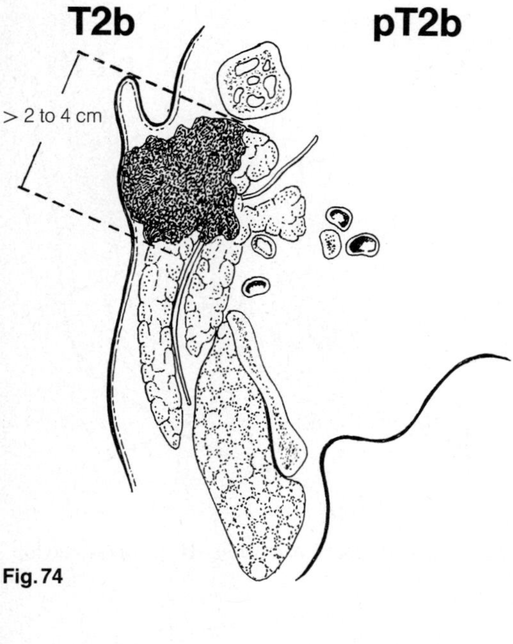

Fig. 74

T3 Tumour more than 4 cm but not more than 6 cm in greatest dimension (Figs. 75, 76)

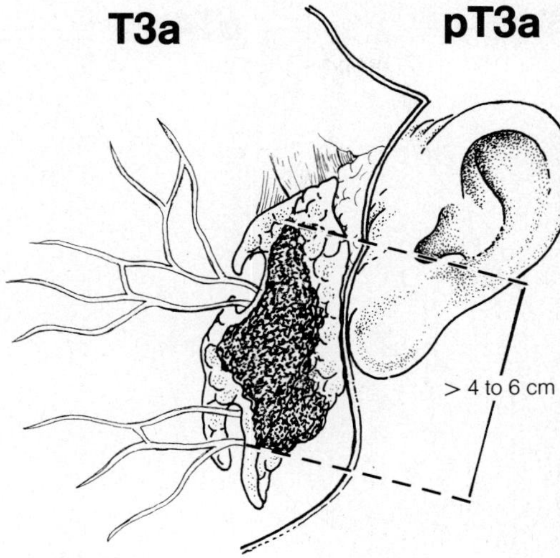

Fig. 75

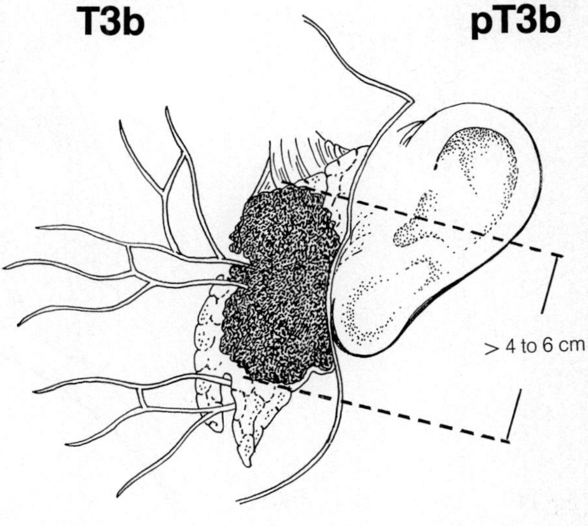

Fig. 76

T4 Tumour more than 6 cm in greatest dimension (Figs. 77, 78)

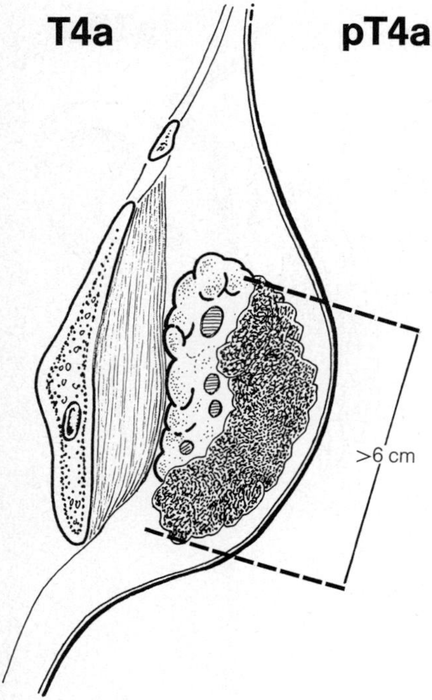

Fig. 77

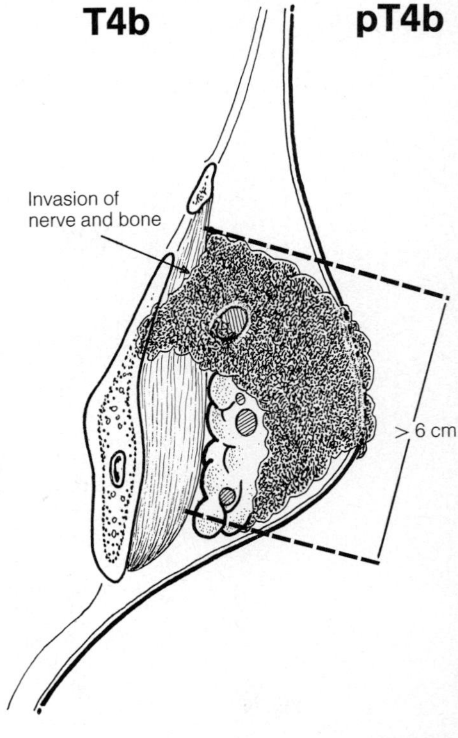

Fig. 78

N – Regional Lymph Nodes

See p. 5

pTN Pathological Classification

The pT and pN categories correspond to the T and N categories.

Thyroid Gland (ICD-O 193.9) (Fig. 79)

Rules for Classification

The classification applies only to carcinoma. There should be histological confirmation of the disease to permit division of cases by histological type.

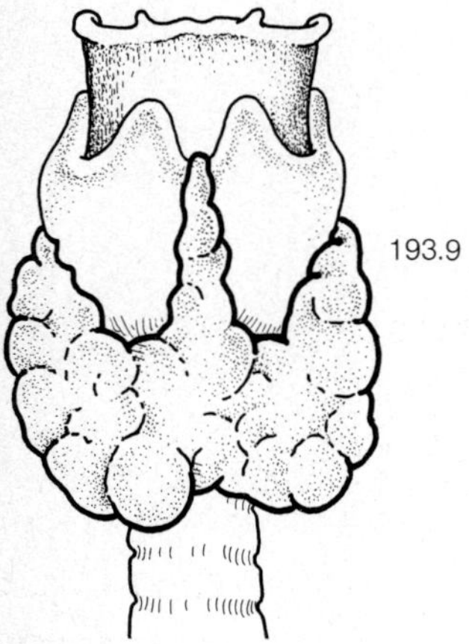

Fig. 79

Regional Lymph Nodes (Fig. 80)

The regional lymph nodes are the cervical *(1)* and upper mediastinal nodes *(2)*.

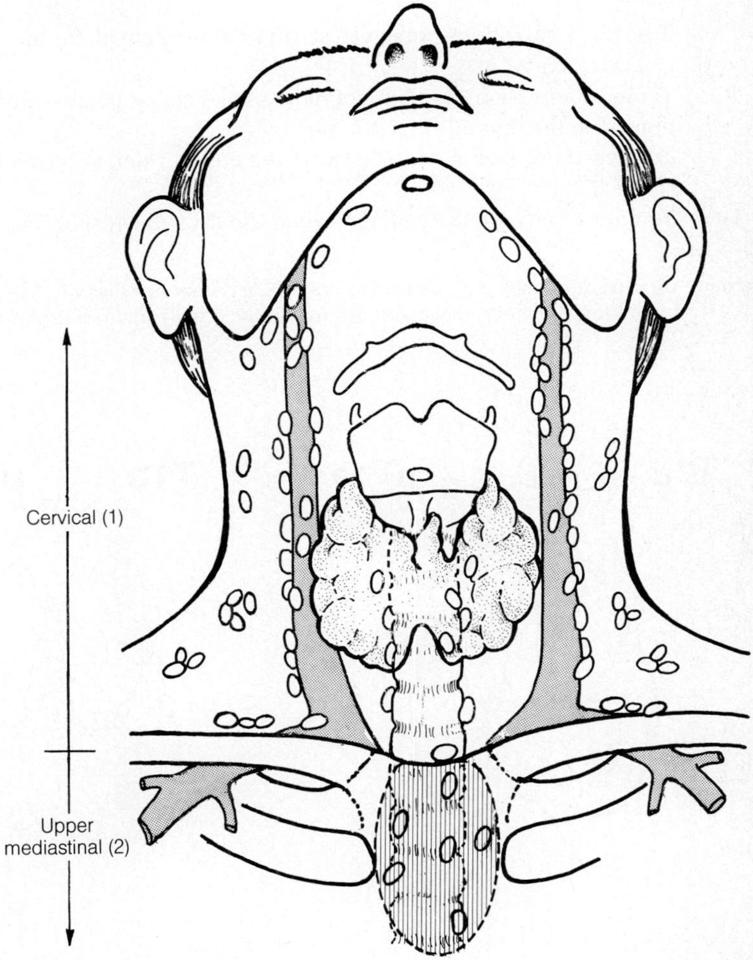

Fig. 80

TN Clinical Classification

T – Primary Tumour

TX Primary tumour cannot be assessed
T0 No evidence of primary tumour
T1 Tumour 1 cm or less in greatest dimension, limited to the thyroid (Figs. 81, 82)
T2 Tumour more than 1 cm but not more than 4 cm in greatest dimension, limited to the thyroid (Figs. 83, 84)
T3 Tumour more than 4 cm in greatest dimension, limited to the thyroid (Fig. 85)
T4 Tumour of any size extending beyond the thyroid capsule (Fig. 86)

Note: All categories may be subdivided: (a) solitary tumour (Figs. 81, 83, 85, 86); (b) multifocal tumour (the largest determines the classification) (Figs. 82, 84).

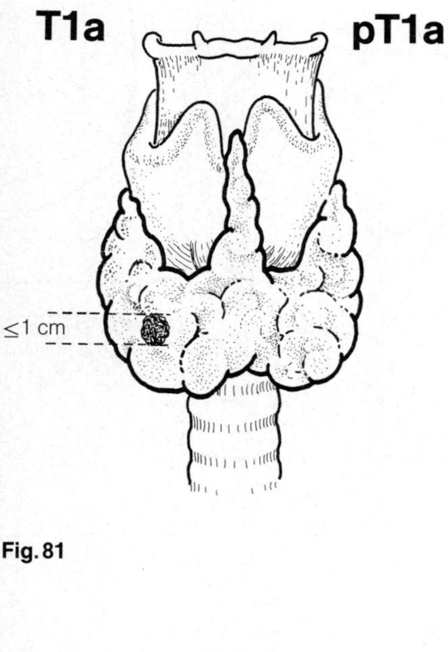

Fig. 81

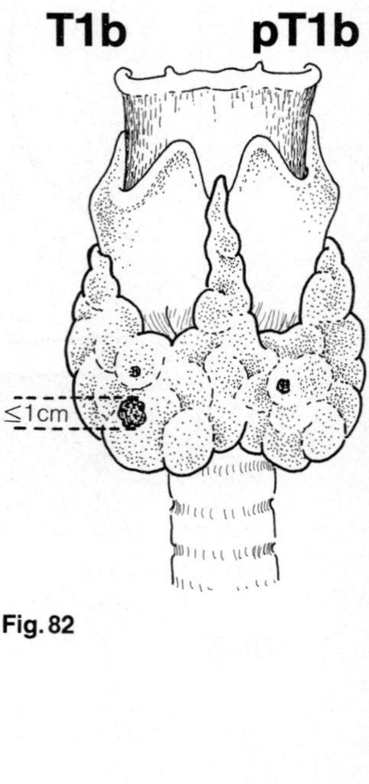

Fig. 82

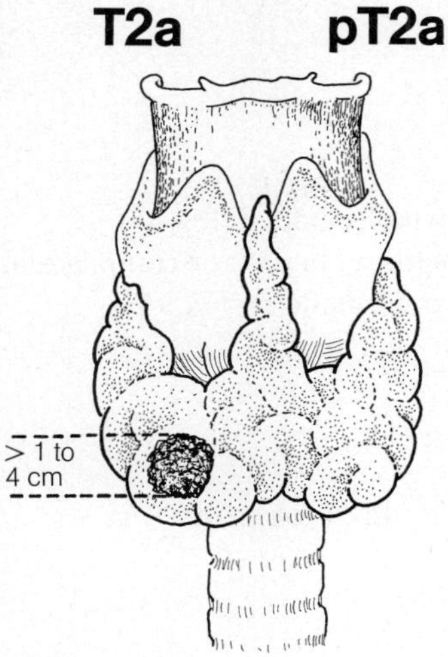

Fig. 83

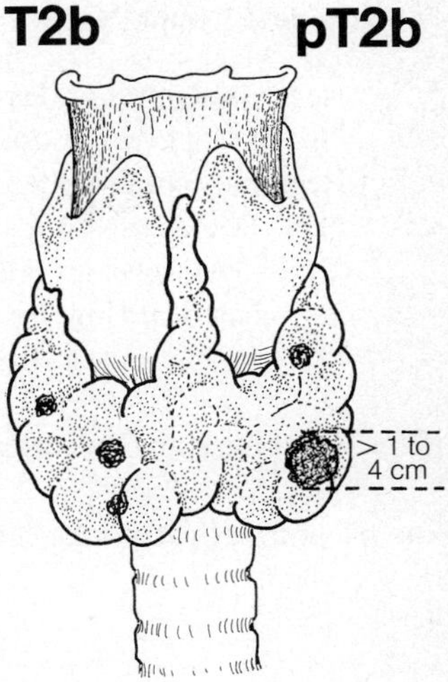

Fig. 84

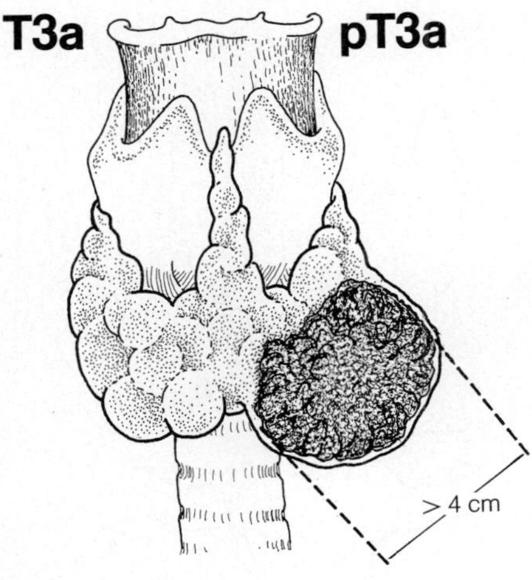

Fig. 85

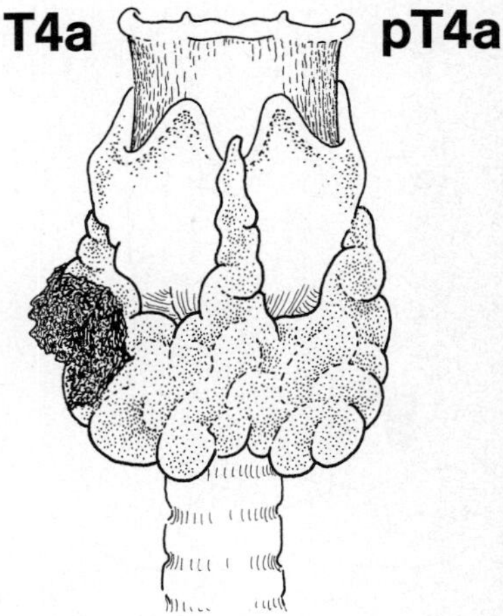

Fig. 86

N – Regional Lymph Nodes

NX Regional lymph nodes cannot be assessed
N0 No regional lymph node metastasis
N1 Regional lymph node metastasis
- N1a Metastasis in ipsilateral cervical lymph node(s) (Fig. 87)
- N1b Metastasis in bilateral (Fig. 88), midline (Fig. 89) or contralateral cervical (Fig. 90) or mediastinal lymph node(s) (Fig. 91)

pTN Pathological Classification

The pT and pN categories correspond to the T and N categories.

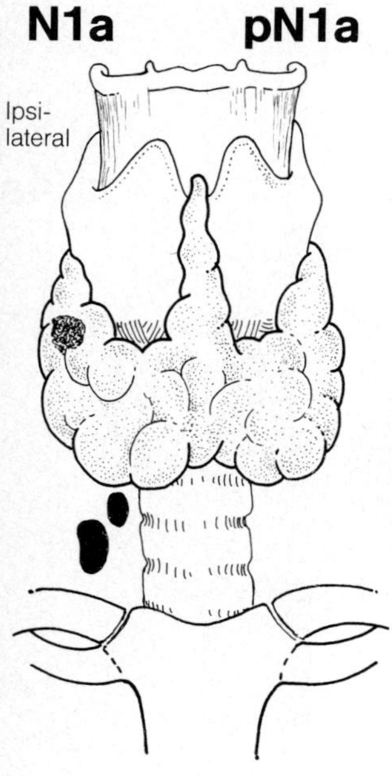

Fig. 87

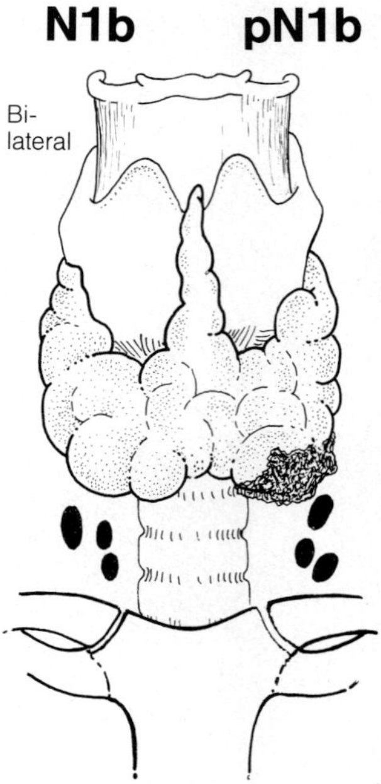

Fig. 88

N1b pN1b

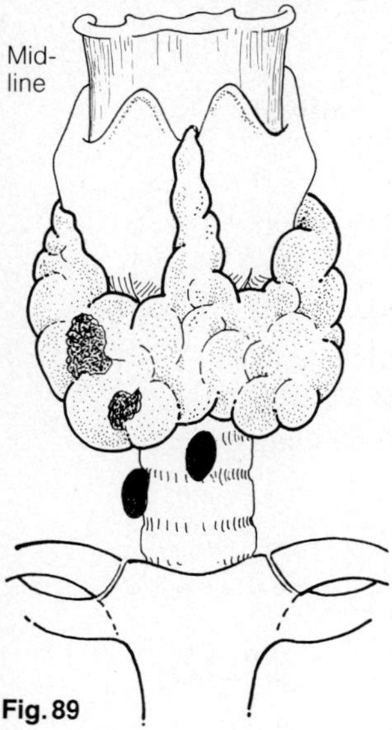

Fig. 89

N1b pN1b

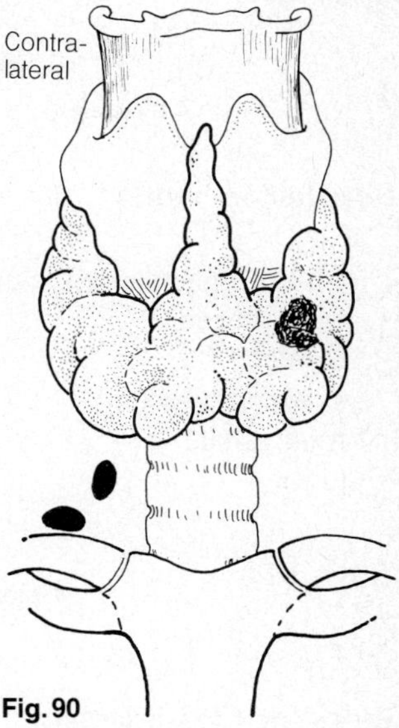

Fig. 90

N1b pN1b

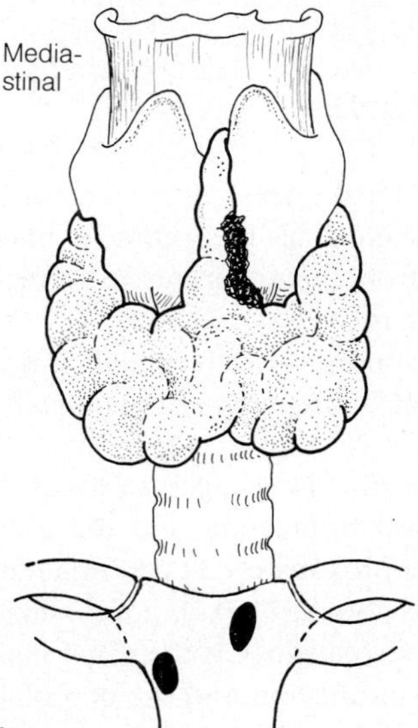

Fig. 91

DIGESTIVE SYSTEM TUMOURS

Introductory Notes

The following sites are included:

- Oesophagus
- Stomach
- Colon and rectum
- Anal canal
- Liver
- Gall bladder
- Extrahepatic bile ducts
- Ampulla of Vater
- Pancreas (excluding endocrine)

Oesophagus (ICD-O 150)

Rules for Classification

The classification applies only to carcinoma. There should be histological confirmation of the disease.

Anatomical Subsites (Fig. 92)

1. Cervical oesophagus (150.0): This commences at the lower border of the cricoid cartilage and ends at the thoracic inlet (suprasternal notch), approximately 18 cm from the upper incisor teeth
2. Intrathoracic oesophagus
   i) The upper thoracic portion (150.3) extends from the thoracic inlet to the level of the tracheal bifurcation, approximately 24 cm from the upper incisor teeth
   ii) The mid-thoracic portion (150.4) is the proximal half of the oesophagus between the tracheal bifurcation and the oesophagogastric junction. The lower level is approximately 32 cm from the upper incisor teeth
   iii) The lower thoracic portion (150.5), approximately 8 cm in length (includes abdominal oesophagus), is the distal half of the oesophagus between the tracheal bifurcation and the oesophagogastric junction. The lower level is approximately 40 cm from the upper incisor teeth

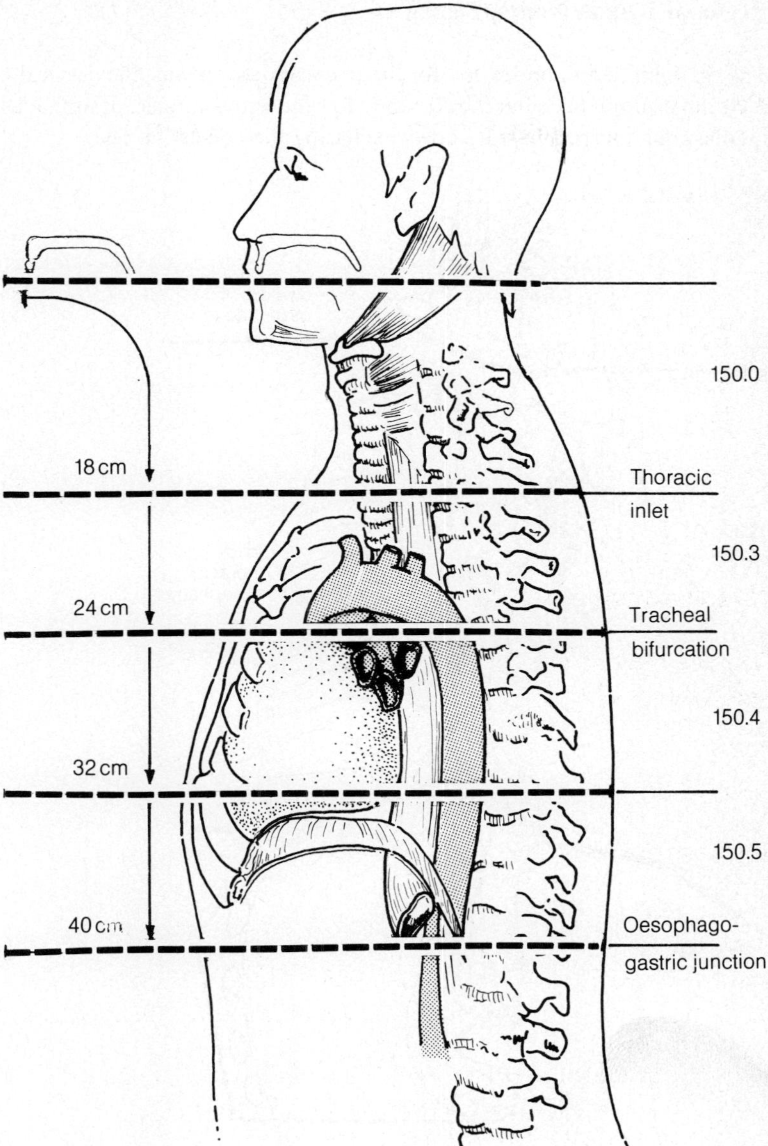
150.0
18 cm
Thoracic
inlet
150.3
24 cm
Tracheal
bifurcation
150.4
32 cm
150.5
40 cm
Oesophago-
gastric junction

Fig. 92

Regional Lymph Nodes (Fig. 93)

The regional lymph nodes are, for the cervical oesophagus, the cervical nodes including supraclavicular nodes and, for the intrathoracic oesophagus, the mediastinal and perigastric nodes, excluding the coeliac nodes.

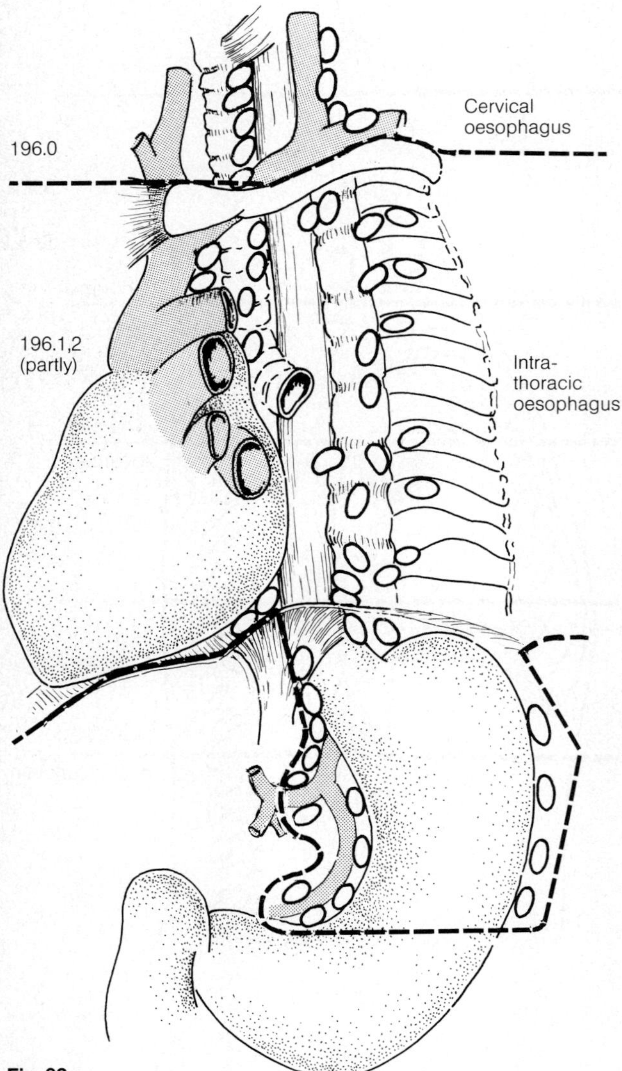

Fig. 93

TNM Clinical Classification

T – Primary Tumour

TX Primary tumour cannot be assessed
T0 No evidence of primary tumour
Tis Carcinoma in situ

T1 Tumour invades lamina propria or submucosa (Fig. 94)
T2 Tumour invades muscularis propria (Fig. 95)

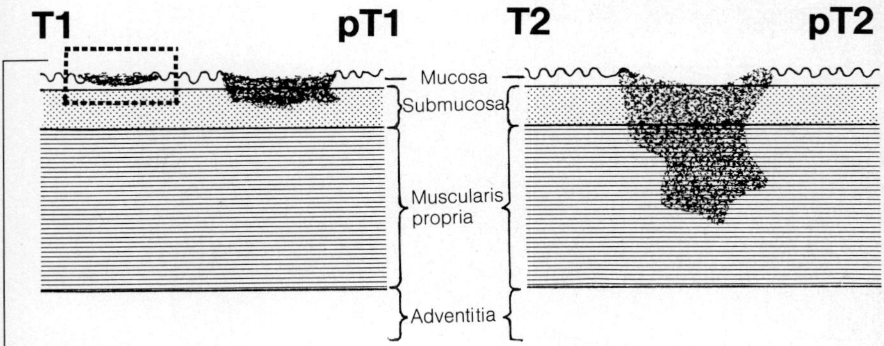

Fig. 94 **Fig. 95**

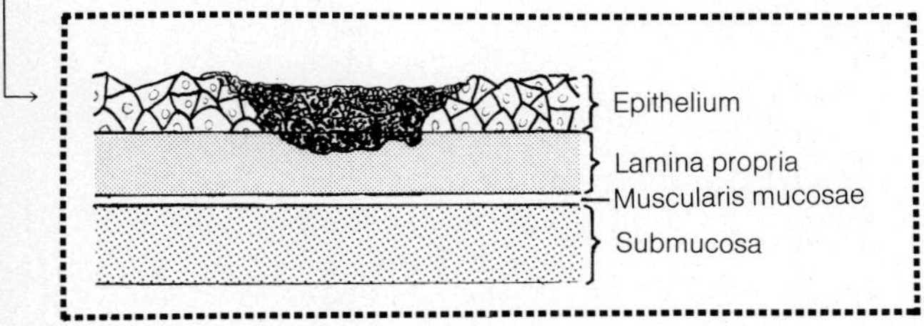

T3 Tumour invades adventitia (Fig. 96)
T4 Tumour invades adjacent structures (Fig. 97)

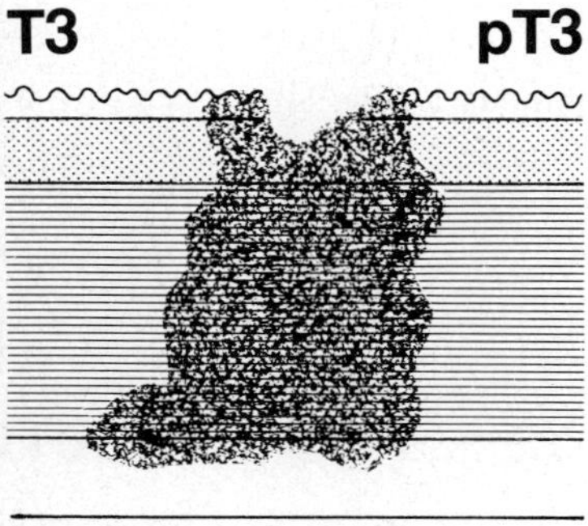

Fig. 96

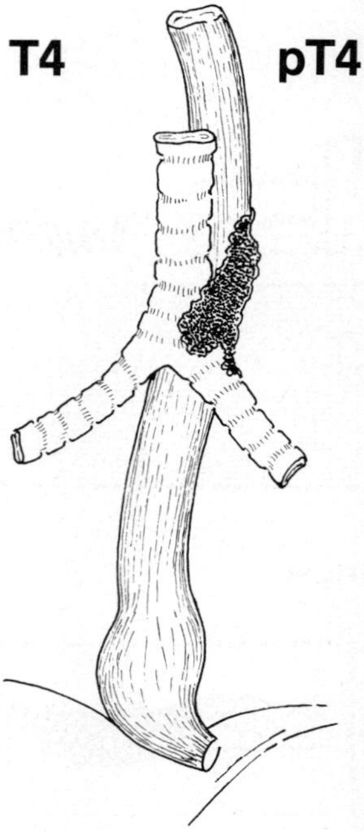

Fig. 97

N – Regional Lymph Nodes

NX Regional lymph nodes cannot be assessed
N0 No regional lymph node metastasis
N1 Regional lymph node metastasis (Figs. 98–101)

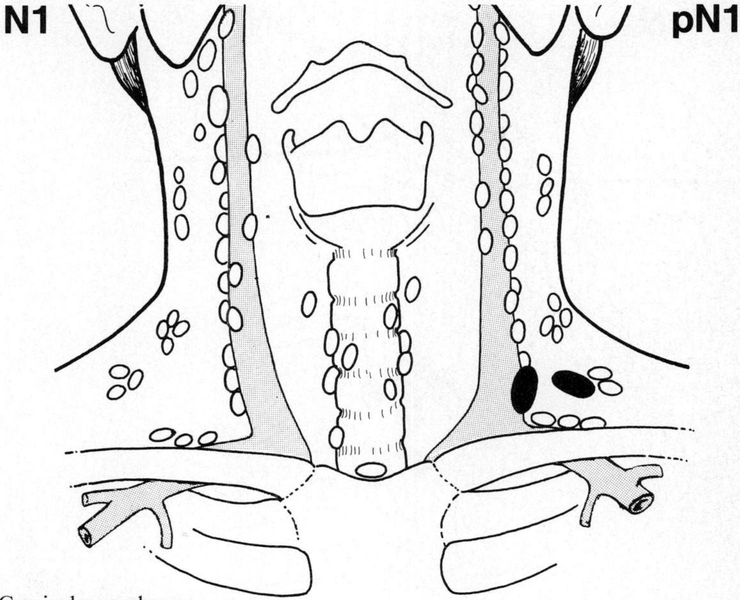

Fig. 98. Cervical oesophagus

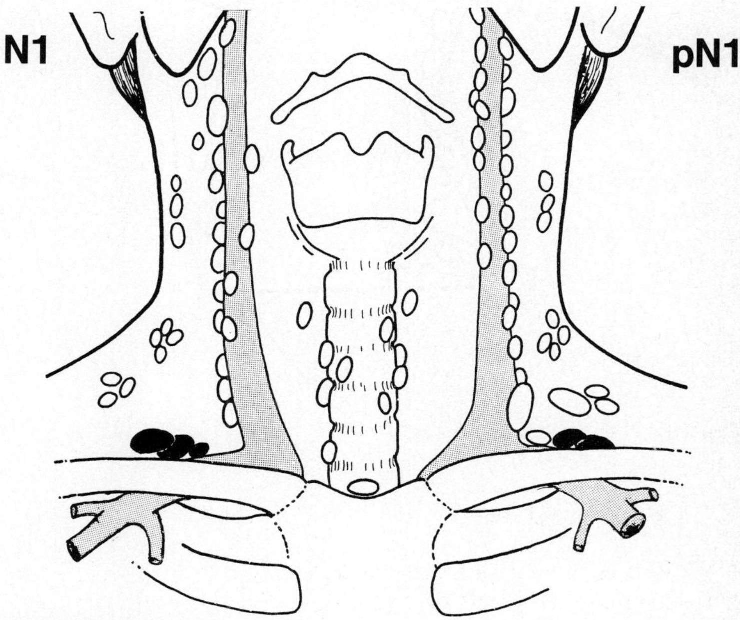

Fig. 99. Cervical oesophagus

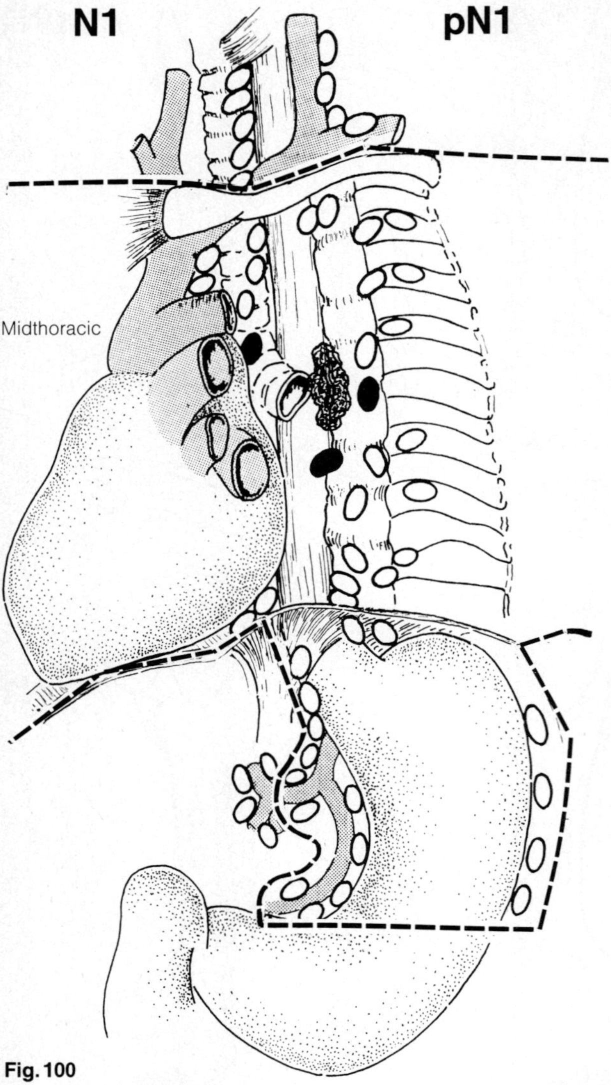

Fig. 100

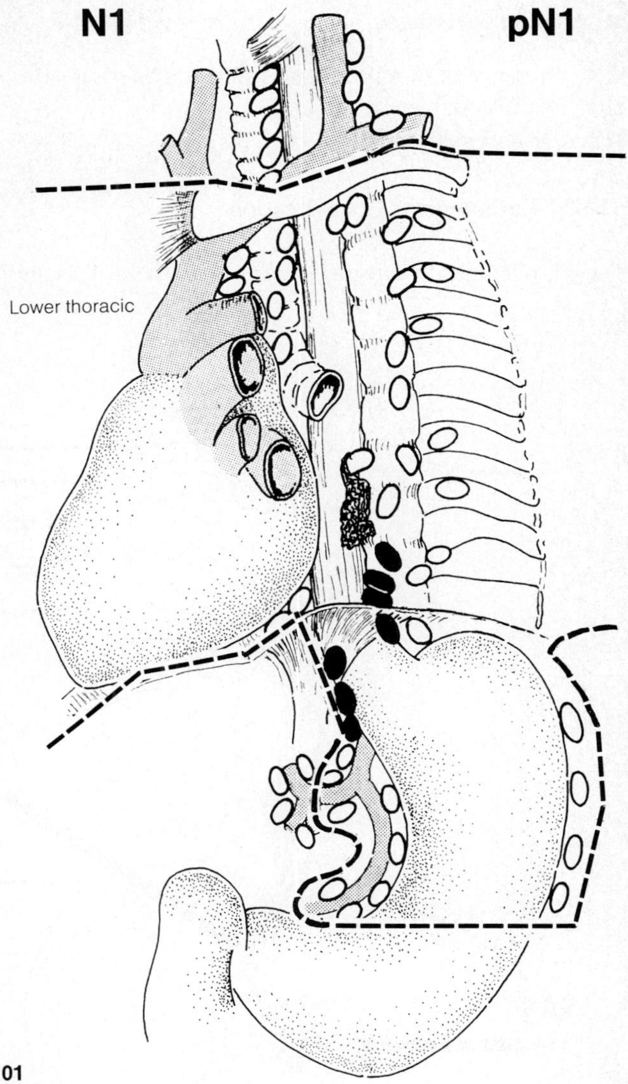

Fig. 101

M - Distant Metastasis

MX Presence of distant metastasis cannot be assessed
M0 No distant metastasis
M1 Distant metastasis (Fig. 102)

pTNM Pathological Classification

The pT, pN and pM categories correspond to the T, N and M categories.

Lower thoracic

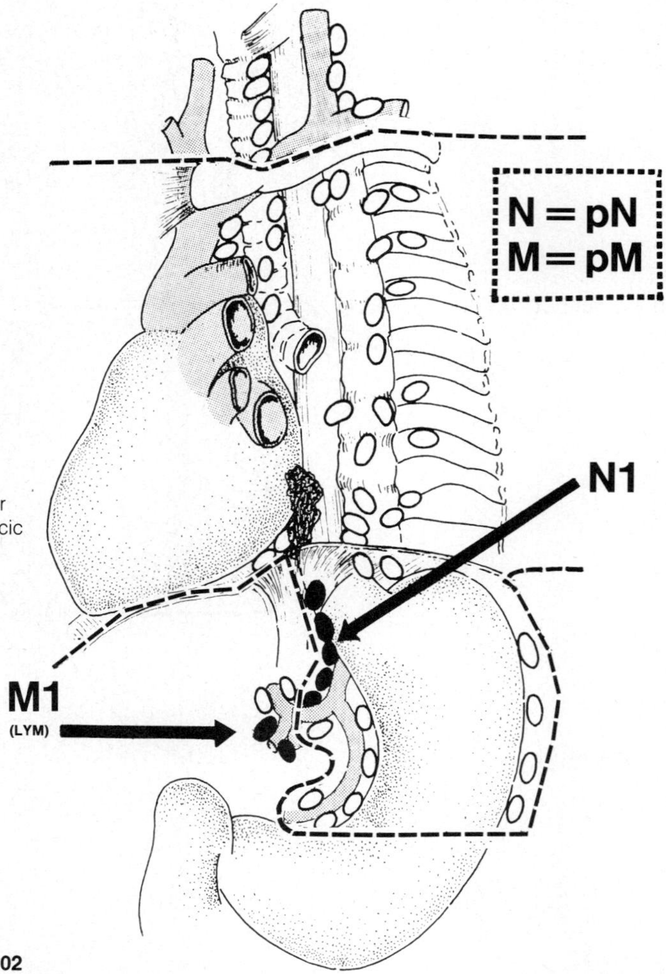

Fig. 102

Stomach (ICD-O 151)

Rules for Classification

The classification applies only to carcinoma. There should be histological confirmation of the disease.

Anatomical Subsites (Fig. 103)

1. Upper third: includes the cardiac area (151.0) and fundus (151.3)
2. Middle third: includes the bulk of the corpus (151.4)
3. Lower third: includes the pylorus (151.1) and antral area (151.2)

To delimit these subsites, the lesser and greater curvatures are divided at two equidistant points and these are joined. The tumour is assigned to the region in which the bulk of it is situated.

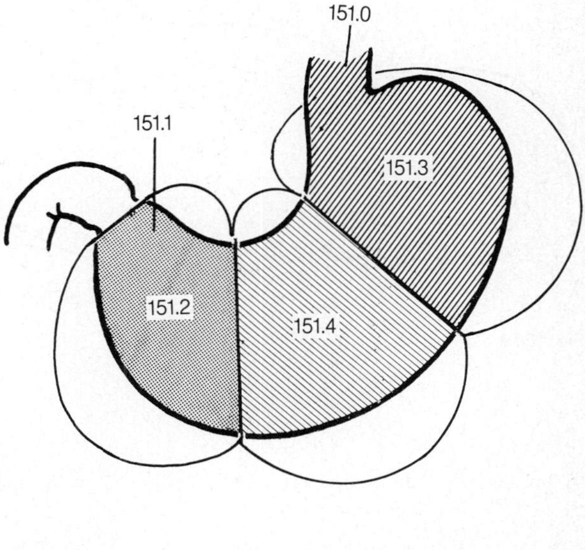

Fig. 103

Regional Lymph Nodes (Fig. 104)

The regional lymph nodes are the perigastric nodes along the lesser *(1, 3, 5)* and greater *(2, 4a, 4b, 6)* curvatures and the nodes located along the left gastric *(7)*, common hepatic *(8)*, splenic *(10, 11)* and coeliac arteries *(9)*. Involvement of other intra-abdominal lymph nodes, such as the hepatoduodenal *(12)*, retropancreatic, mesenteric and para-aortic, is classified as distant metastasis.

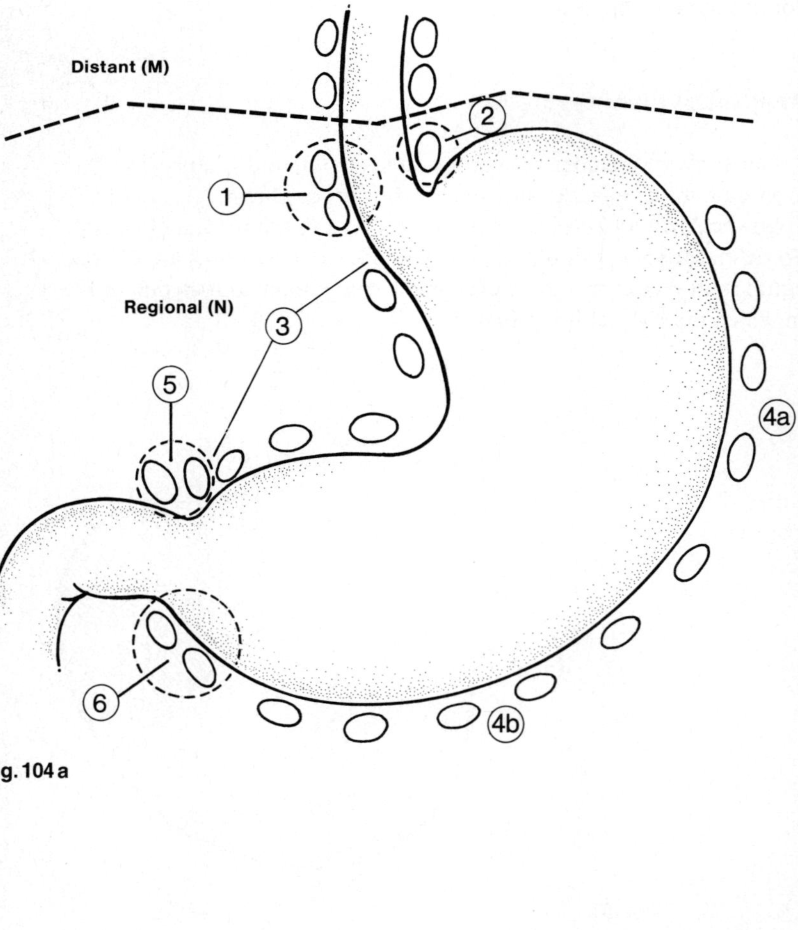

Fig. 104 a

Note: The numerical order corresponds to the proposals of the Japanese Research Society for Gastric Cancer [(1982) *General Rules for the Gastric Cancer Study in Surgery and Pathology.* Japanese Journal of Surgery, Tokyo 11: 127–145]

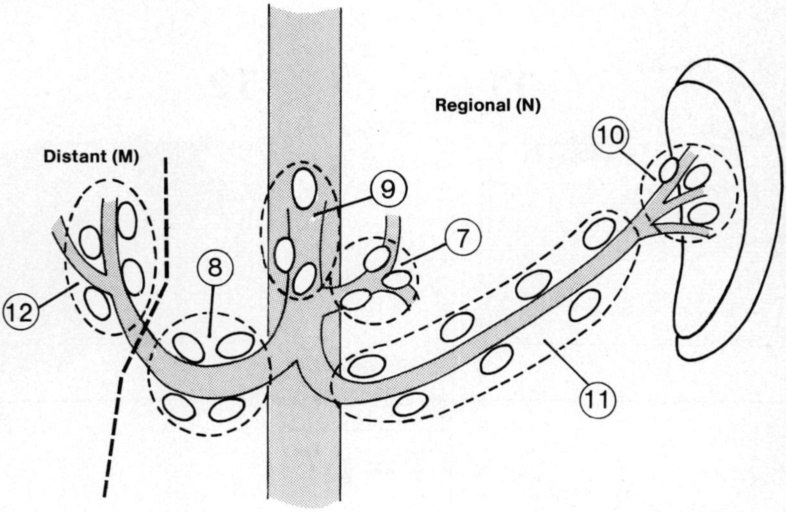

Fig. 104 b

TNM Clinical Classification

T - Primary Tumour

TX Primary tumour cannot be assessed
T0 No evidence of primary tumour
Tis Carcinoma in situ: intraepithelial tumour without invasion of lamina propria
T1 Tumour invades lamina propria or submucosa (Fig. 105)
T2 Tumour invades muscularis propria or subserosa[1] (Figs. 106, 107)

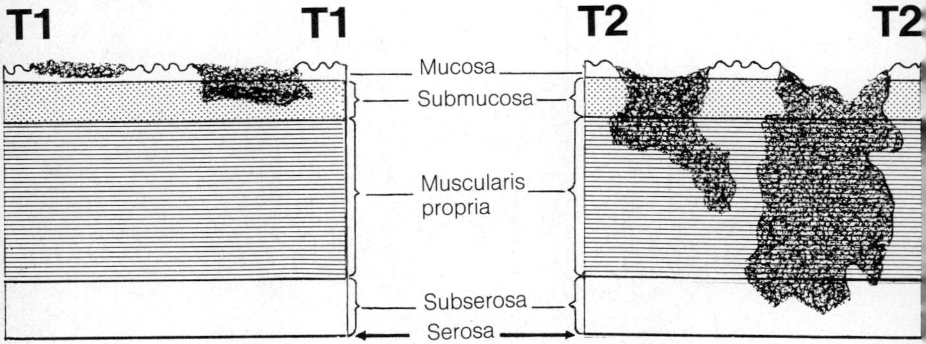

T = pT

Fig. 105

Fig. 106

[1] Note see p. 77

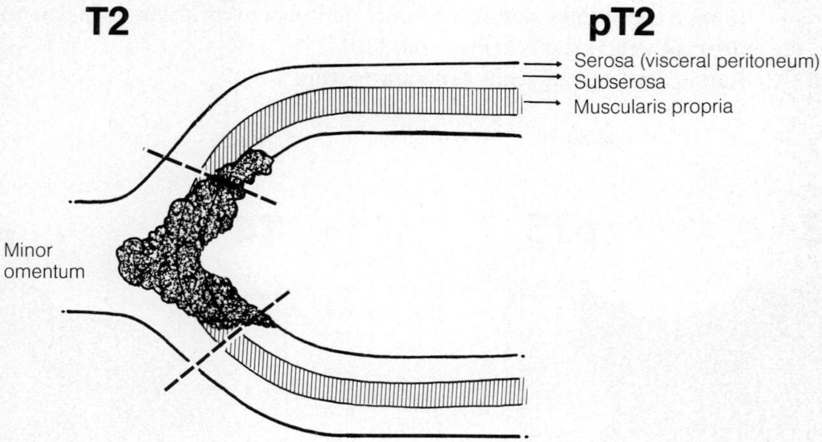
T2
pT2
Serosa (visceral peritoneum)
Subserosa
Muscularis propria
Minor
omentum

Fig. 107

T3 Tumour penetrates serosa (visceral peritoneum) without invasion of adjacent structures[1, 2, 3] (Figs. 108, 110)

T4 Tumour invades adjacent structures[2, 3] (Fig. 109)

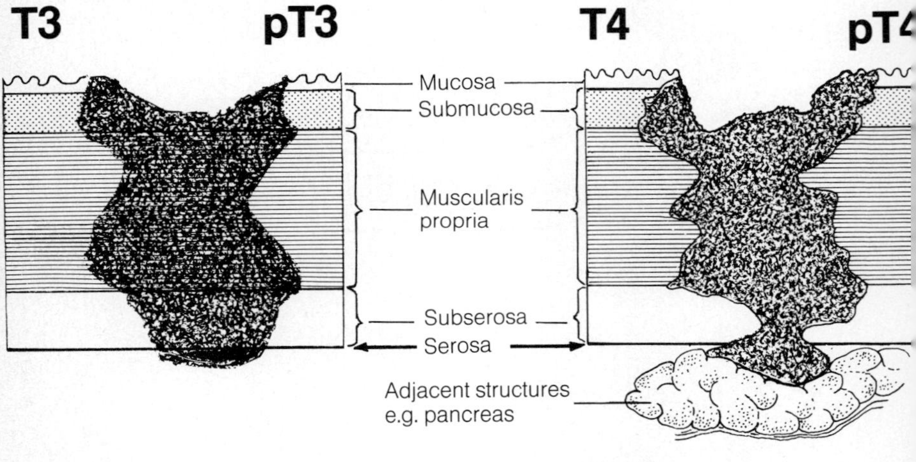

Fig. 108

Fig. 109

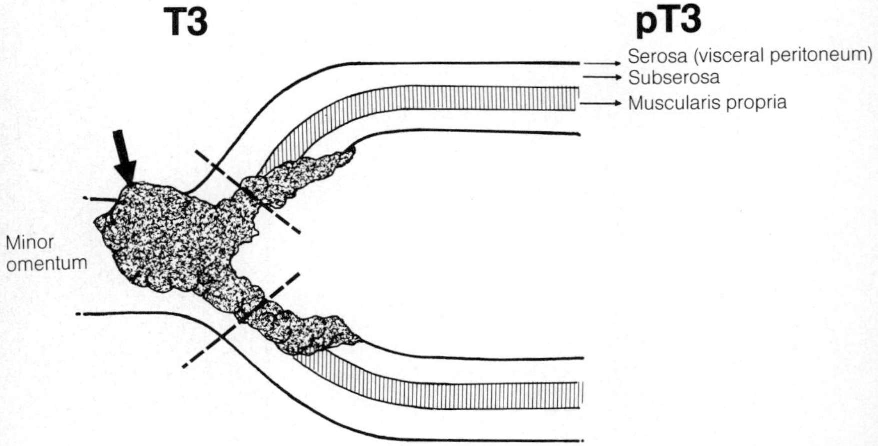

Fig. 110

Notes: [1] A tumour may penetrate the muscularis propria with extension into the gastrocolic or gastrohepatic ligaments or the greater or lesser omentum without perforation of the visceral peritoneum covering these structures. In this case, the tumour is classified T2 (Fig. 107). If there is perforation of the visceral peritoneum covering the gastric ligaments or omenta, the tumour is classified T3 (Fig. 110).

[2] The adjacent structures of the stomach are the spleen, transverse colon, liver, diaphragm, pancreas, abdominal wall, adrenal gland, kidney, small intestine and retroperitoneum.

[3] Intramural extension to the duodenum or oesophagus is classified by the depth of greatest invasion in any of these sites including stomach (Figs. 111, 112).

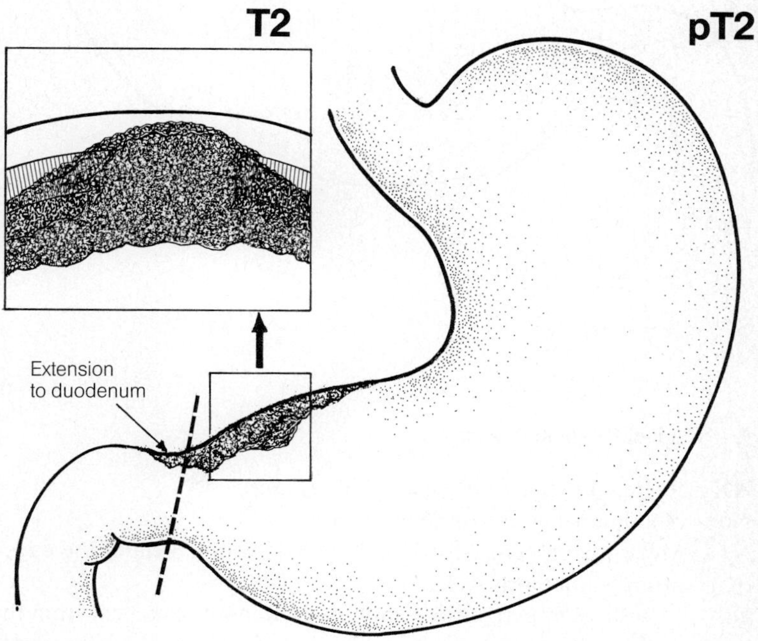

Fig. 111

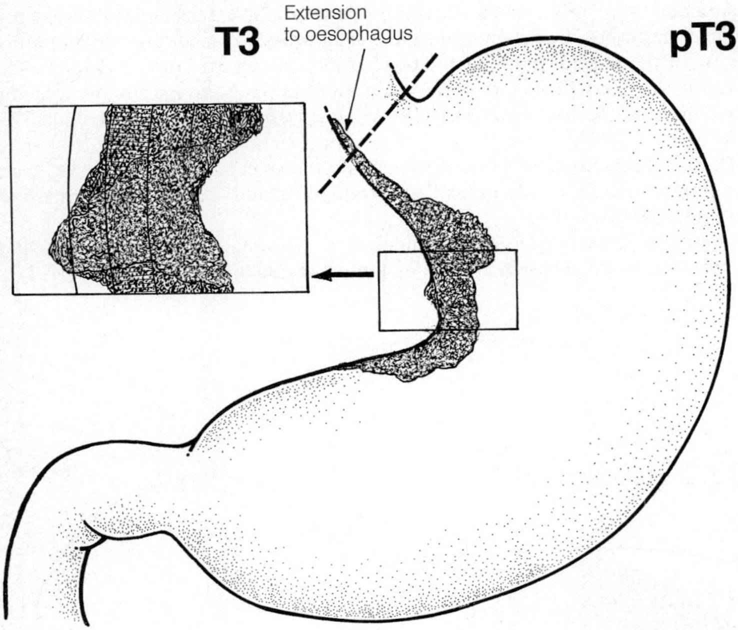

Fig. 112

N - Regional Lymph Nodes

NX Regional lymph nodes cannot be assessed

N0 No regional lymph node metastasis

N1 Metastasis in perigastric lymph node(s) within 3 cm of the edge of the primary tumour (Fig. 113)

N2 Metastasis in perigastric lymph node(s) more than 3 cm from the edge of the primary tumour or in lymph nodes along the left gastric, common hepatic, splenic or coeliac arteries (Fig. 114)

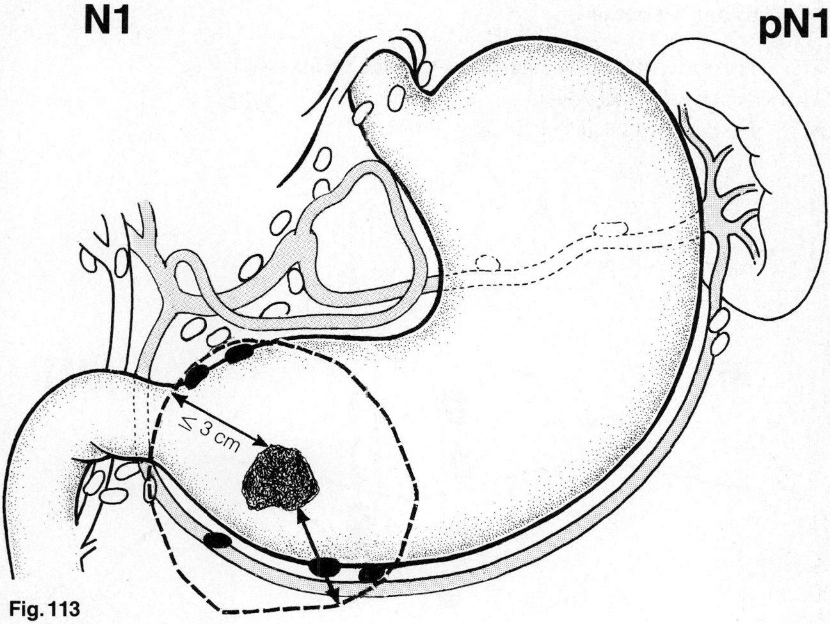

Fig. 113

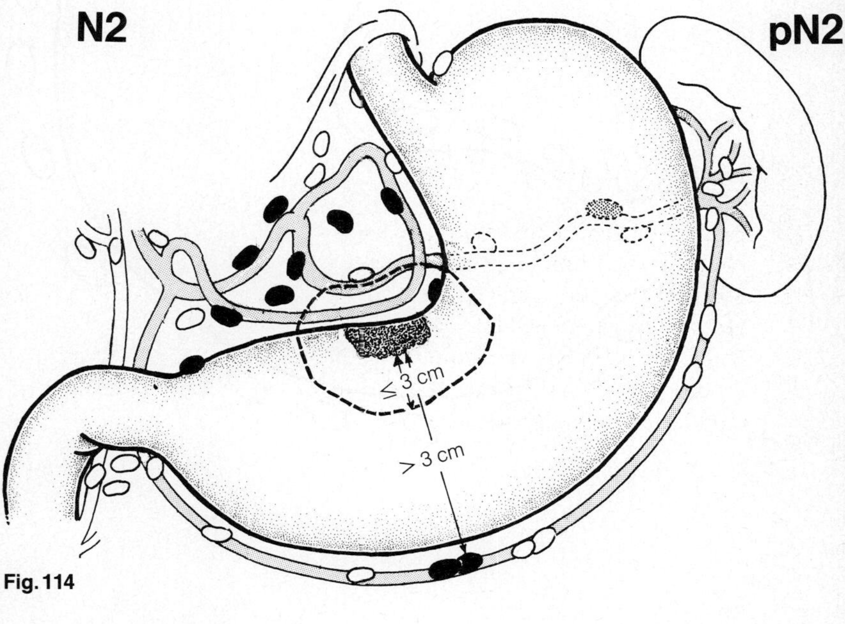

Fig. 114

M – Distant Metastasis

MX Presence of distant metastasis cannot be assessed
M0 No distant metastasis
M1 Distant metastasis (Figs. 115, 116)

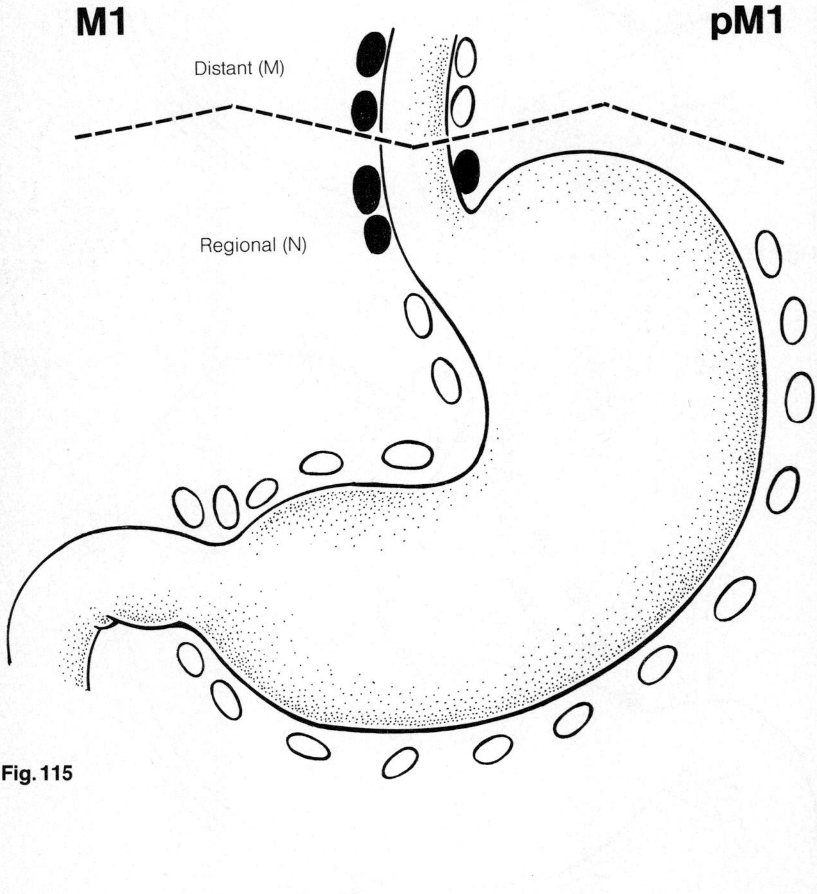

Fig. 115

pTNM Pathological Classification

The pT, pN and pM categories correspond to the T, N and M categories.

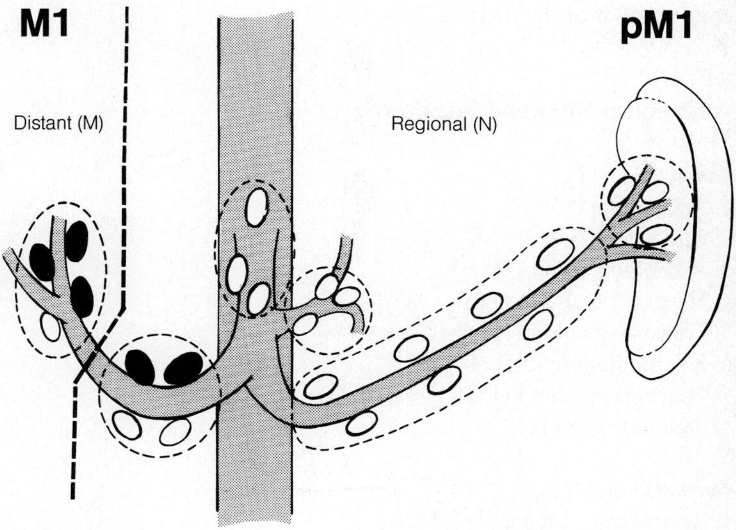

Fig. 116

Colon and Rectum (ICD-O 153, 154.0,1)

Rules for Classification

The classification applies only to carcinoma. There should be histological confirmation of the disease.

Anatomical Sites and Subsites

Colon (Fig. 117)
1. Appendix (153.5)
2. Caecum (153.4)
3. Ascending colon (153.6)
4. Hepatic flexure (153.0)
5. Transverse colon (153.1)
6. Splenic flexure (153.7)
7. Descending colon (153.2)
8. Sigmoid colon (153.3)

Rectum (Fig. 118)
1. Rectosigmoid junction (154.0)
2. Rectum (154.1)

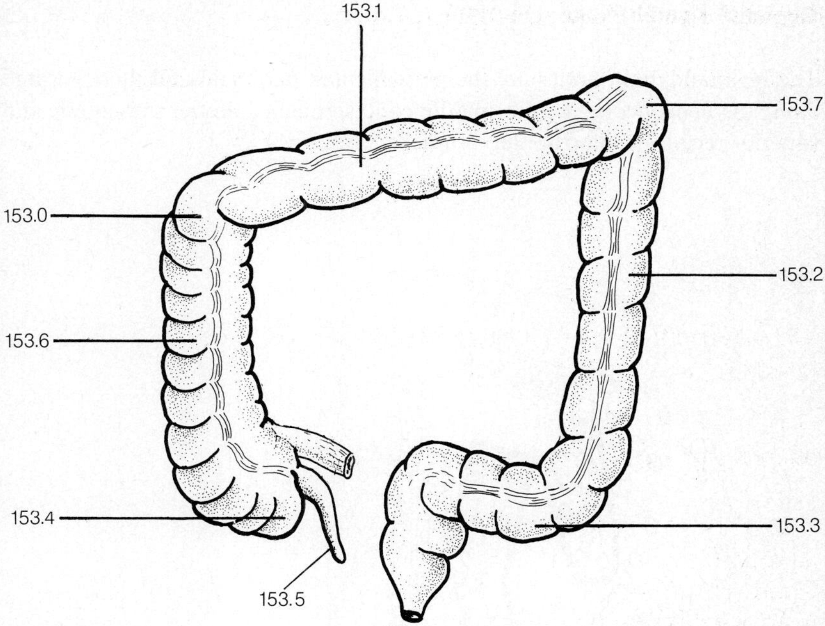

Fig. 117

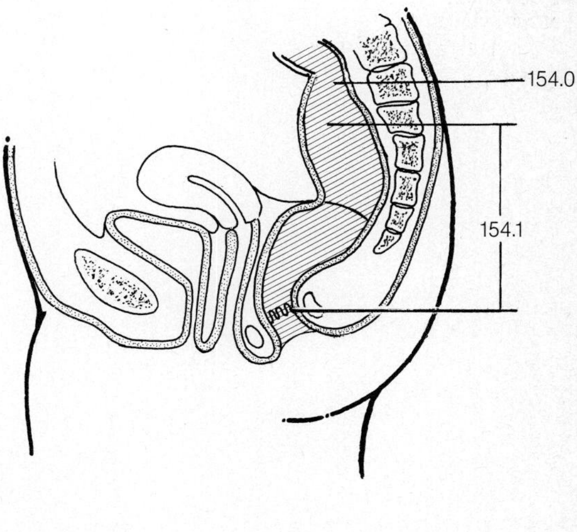

Fig. 118

Regional Lymph Nodes (Fig. 119)

The regional lymph nodes are the pericolic and perirectal and those located along the ileocolic, right colic, middle colic, left colic, inferior mesenteric and superior rectal (haemorrhoidal) arteries.

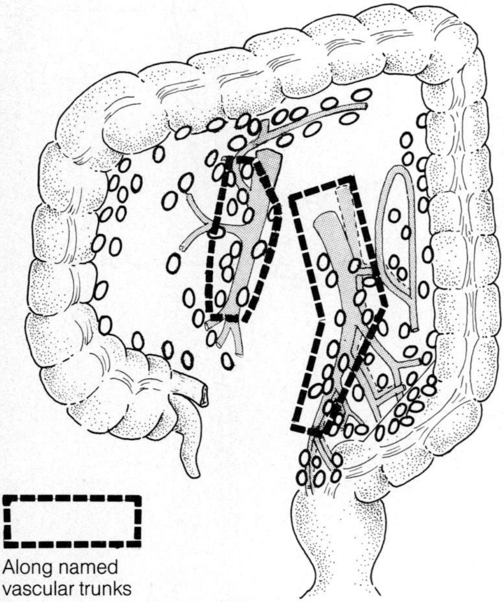

Fig. 119

TN Clinical Classification

T – Primary Tumour

TX Primary tumour cannot be assessed
T0 No evidence of primary tumour
Tis Carcinoma in situ

T1 Tumour invades submucosa (Fig. 120)
T2 Tumour invades muscularis propria (Fig. 121)

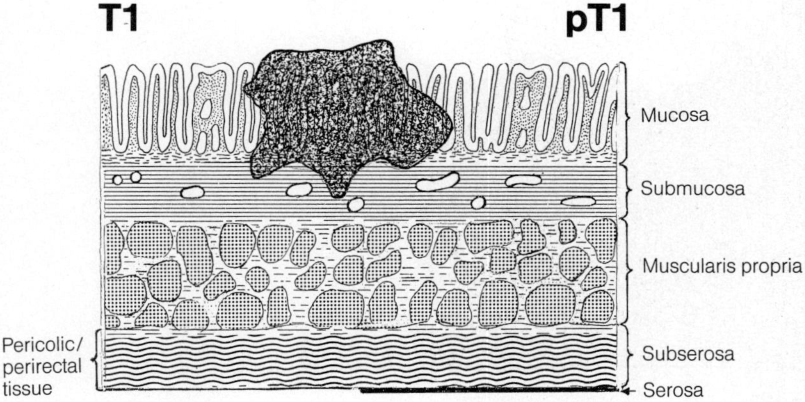

Fig. 120

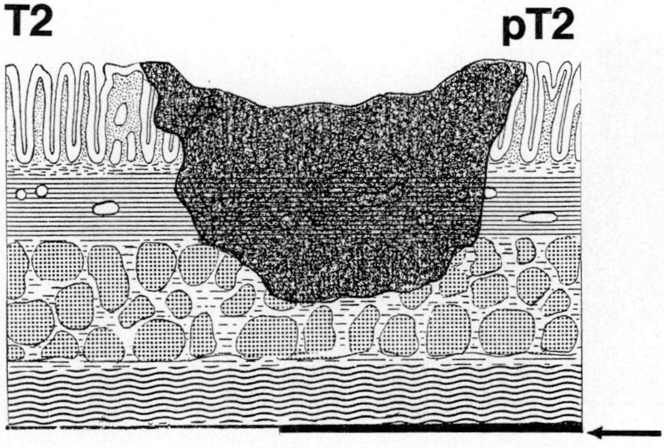

Fig. 121

T3 Tumour invades through muscularis propria into subserosa or into non-peritonealized pericolic or perirectal tissues (Fig. 122)

T4 Tumour perforates the visceral peritoneum or directly invades other organs or structures (Figs. 123–125)

Note: Direct invasion in T4 includes invasion of other segments of the colorectum by way of the serosa, e.g. invasion of the sigmoid colon by a carcinoma of the caecum.

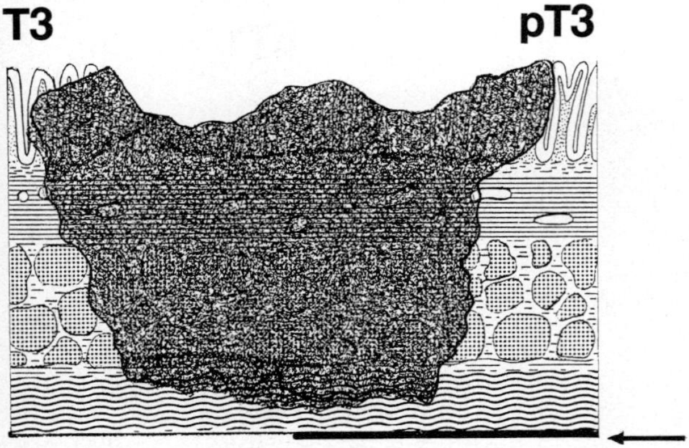

Fig. 122

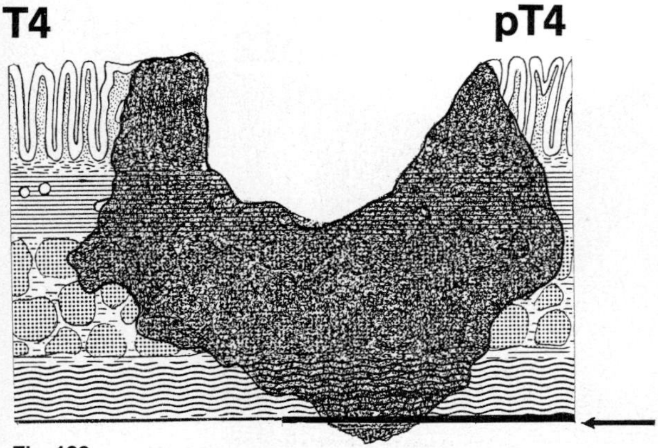

Fig. 123

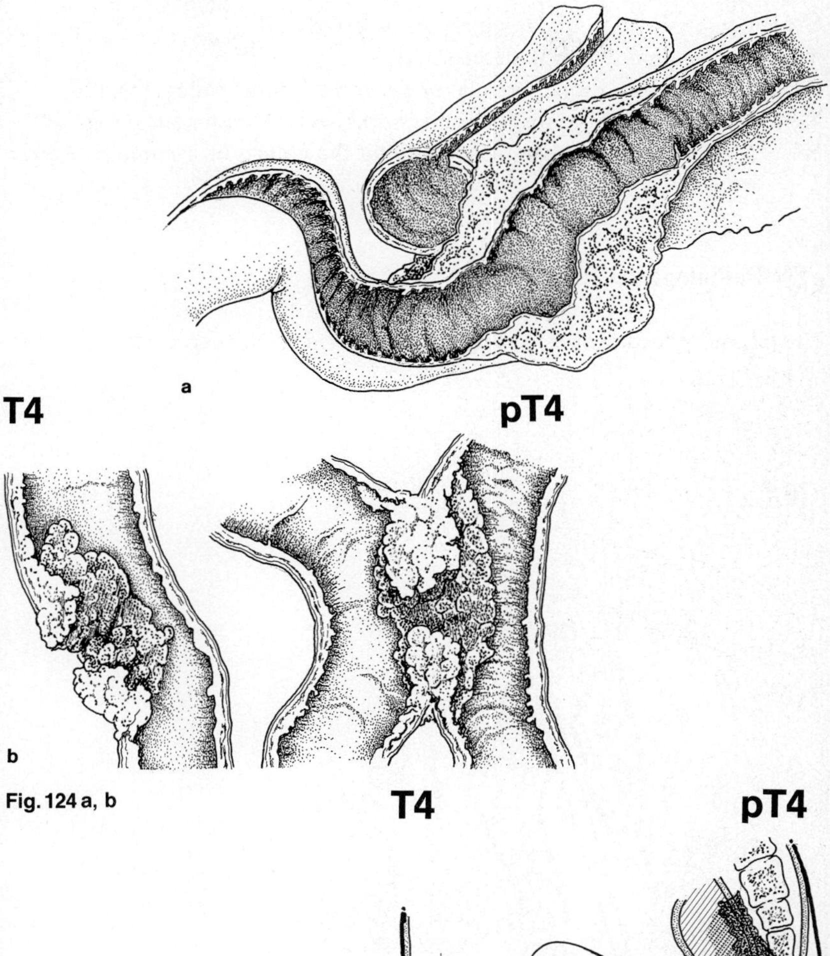

Fig. 124 a, b

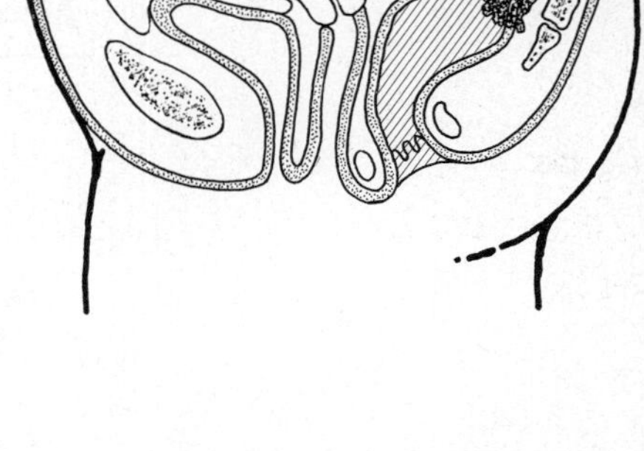

Fig. 125

N - Regional Lymph Nodes

NX Regional lymph nodes cannot be assessed
N0 No regional lymph node metastasis
N1 Metastasis in 1 to 3 pericolic or perirectal lymph nodes (Fig. 126)
N2 Metastasis in 4 or more pericolic or perirectal lymph nodes (Fig. 127)
N3 Metastasis in any lymph node along the course of a named vascular trunk (Fig. 128)

pTN Pathological Classification

The pT and pN categories correspond to the T and N categories.

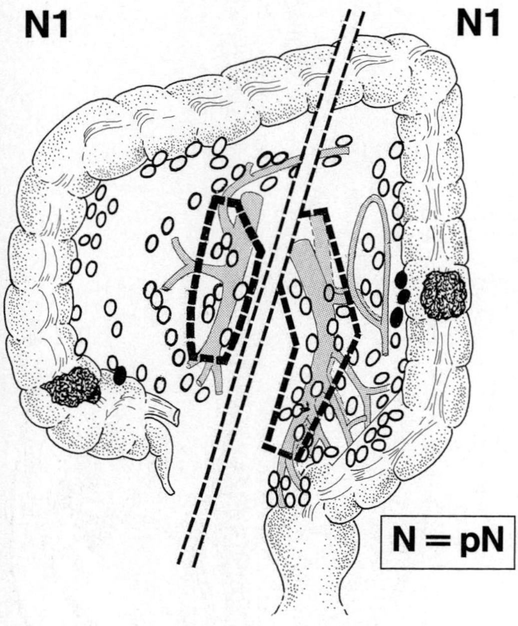

Fig. 126

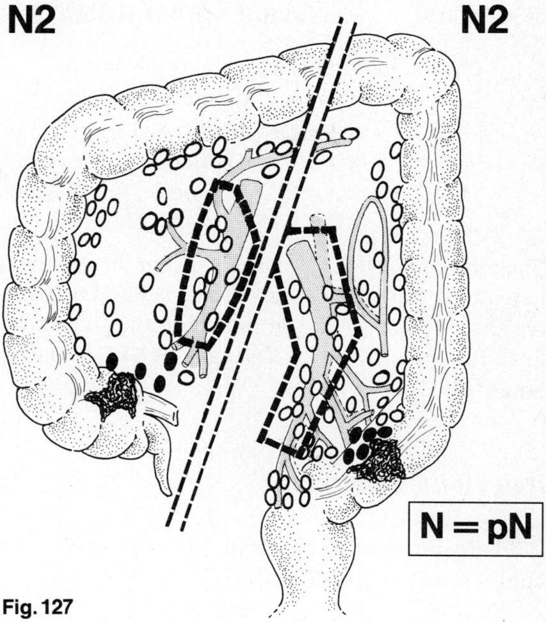

Fig. 127

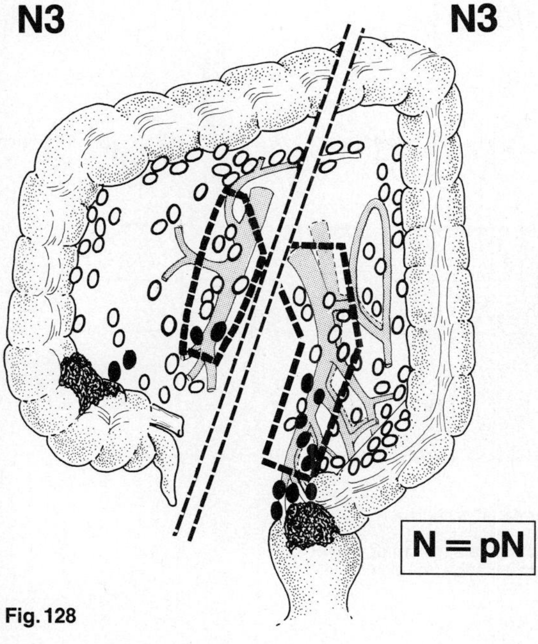

Fig. 128

Anal Canal (ICD-O 154.2)

The anal canal (Fig. 129) extends from the rectum to the perianal skin (to the junction with hair-bearing skin). It is lined by the mucous membrane overlying the internal sphincter, including the transitional epithelium and dentate line. Tumours of the anal margin (ICD-O 173.5) are classified with skin tumours (p. 151).

Rules for Classification

The classification applies only to carcinoma. There should be histological confirmation of the disease.

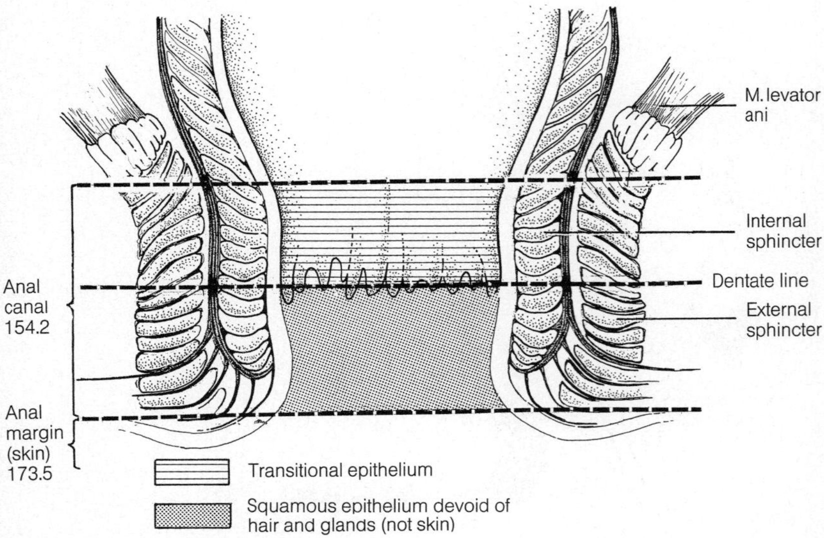

Fig. 129

Regional Lymph Nodes (Fig. 130)

The regional lymph nodes are the perirectal *(1)*, the internal iliac *(2)* and the inguinal lymph nodes *(3)*.

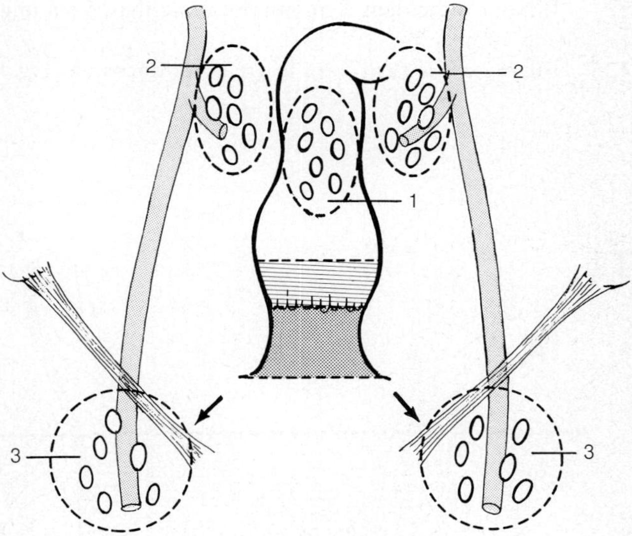

Fig. 130

TN Clinical Classification

T – Primary Tumour

TX	Primary tumour cannot be assessed
T0	No evidence of primary tumour
Tis	Carcinoma in situ
T1	Tumour 2 cm or less in greatest dimension (Fig. 131)
T2	Tumour more than 2 cm but not more than 5 cm in greatest dimension (Fig. 132)
T3	Tumour more than 5 cm in greatest dimension (Fig. 133)

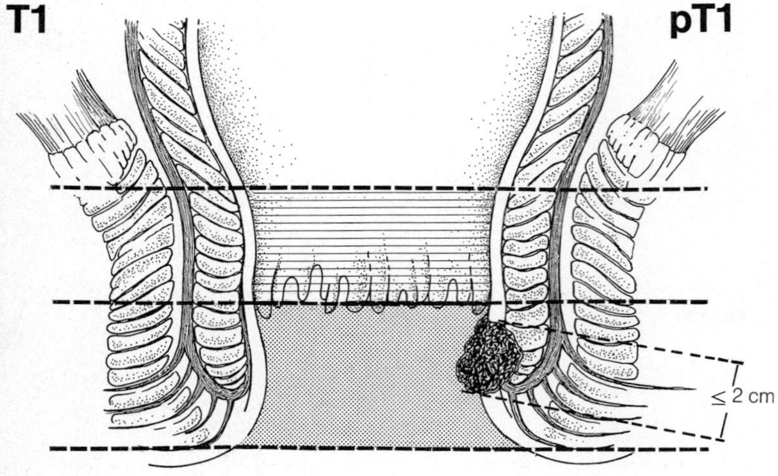

Fig. 131

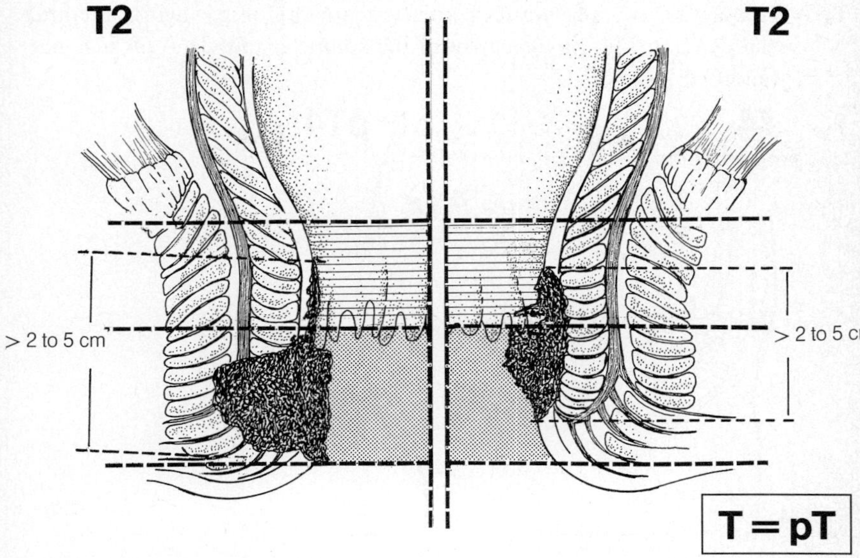

Fig. 132

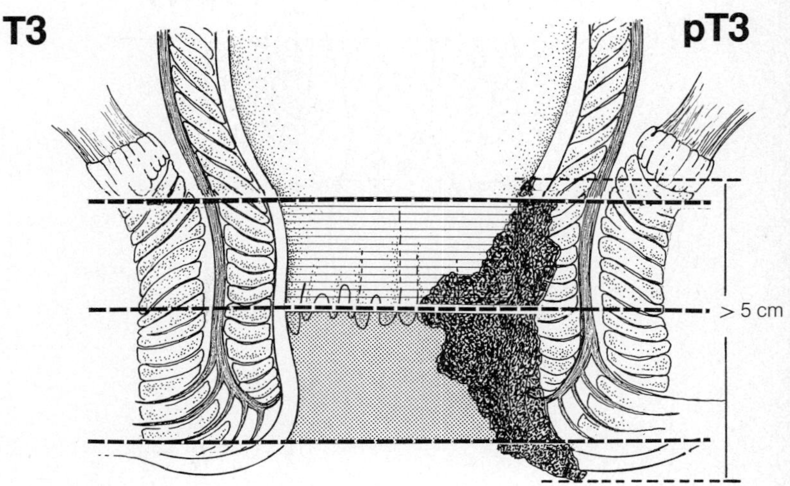

Fig. 133

T4 Tumour of any size invades adjacent organ(s), e.g. vagina, urethra, bladder (Fig. 134) (involvement of the sphincter muscle(s) *alone* is not classified T4)

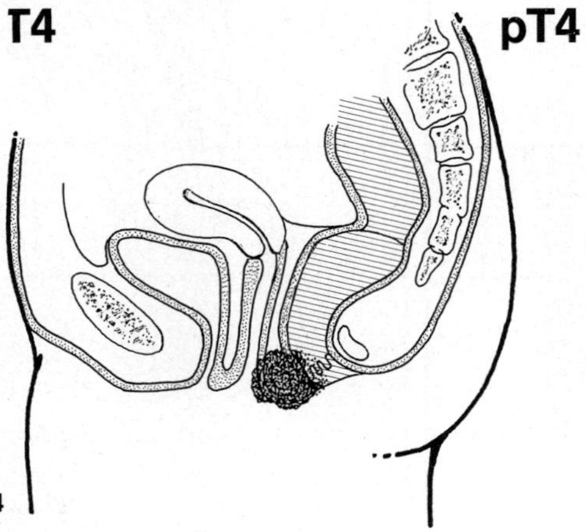

Fig. 134

N – Regional Lymph Nodes

NX Regional lymph nodes cannot be assessed
N0 No regional lymph node metastasis
N1 Metastasis in perirectal lymph node(s) (Fig. 135)

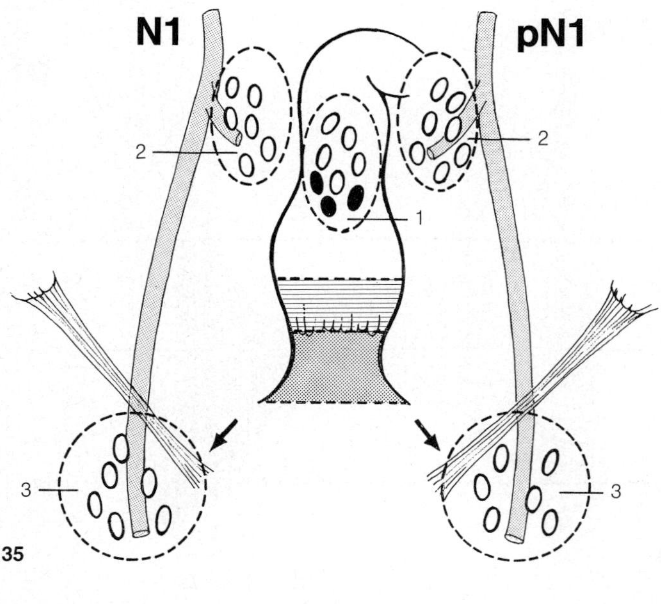

Fig. 135

N2 Metastasis in unilateral internal iliac and/or inguinal lymph node(s) (Figs. 136, 137)

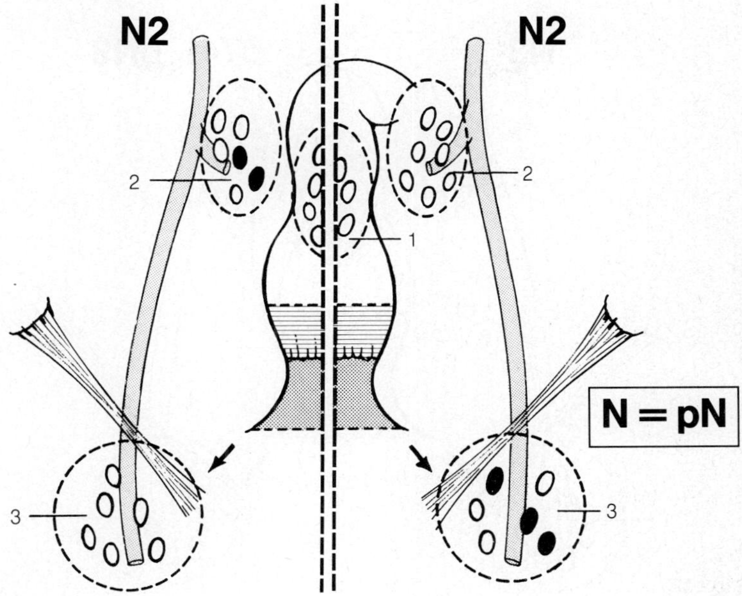

Fig. 136

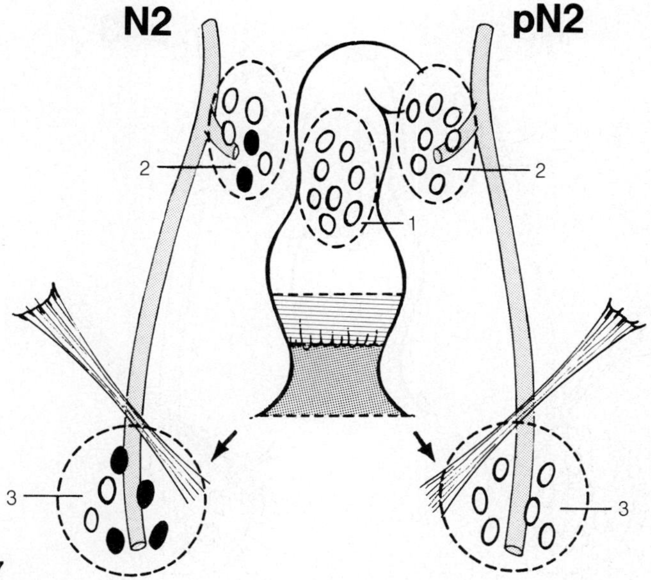

Fig. 137

N3 Metastasis in perirectal and inguinal lymph nodes and/or bilateral internal iliac and/or inguinal lymph nodes (Figs. 138–140)

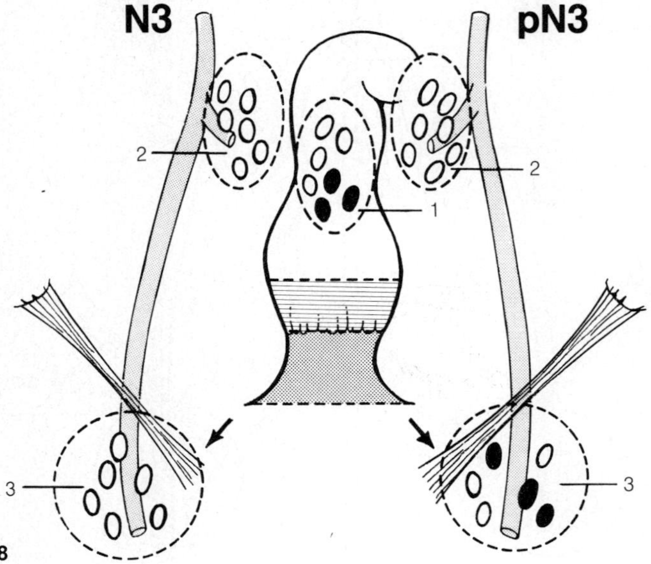

Fig. 138

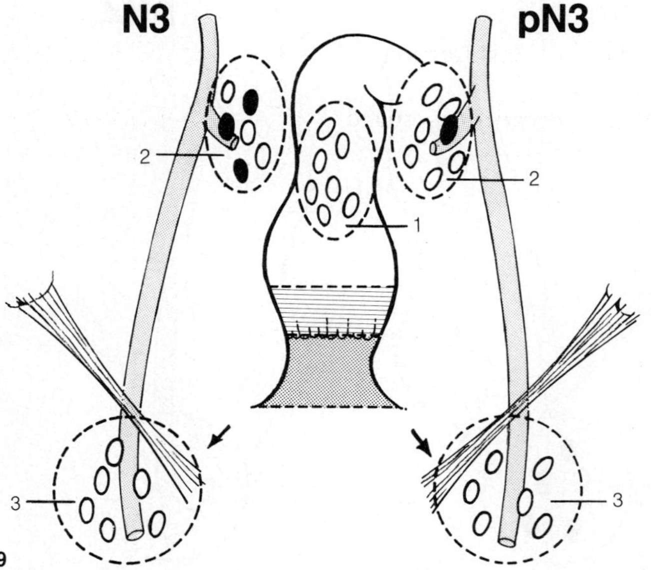

Fig. 139

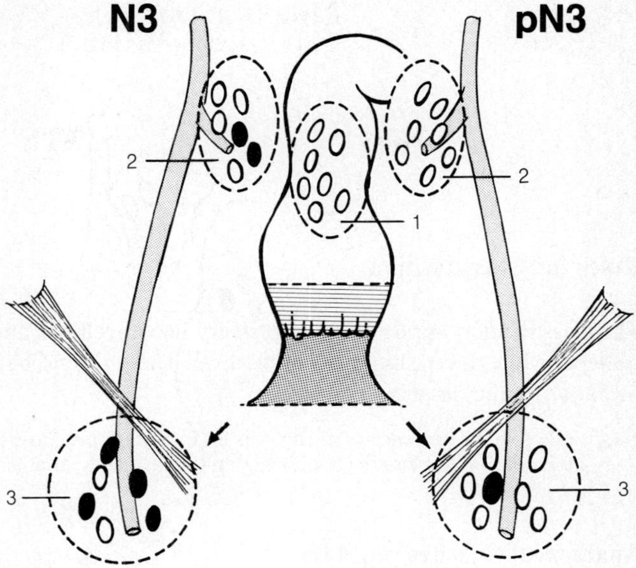

Fig. 140

pTN Pathological Classification

The pT and pN categories correspond to the T and N categories.

Liver (ICD-O 155)

Rules for Classification

The classification applies only to primary hepatocellular and cholangio- (intrahepatic bile duct) carcinoma of the liver. There should be histological confirmation of the disease.

Note: Although the presence of cirrhosis is an important prognostic factor, it does not affect the TNM classification, being an independent variable.

Anatomical Subsites (Fig. 141)

1. Liver (155.0)
2. Intrahepatic bile duct (155.1)

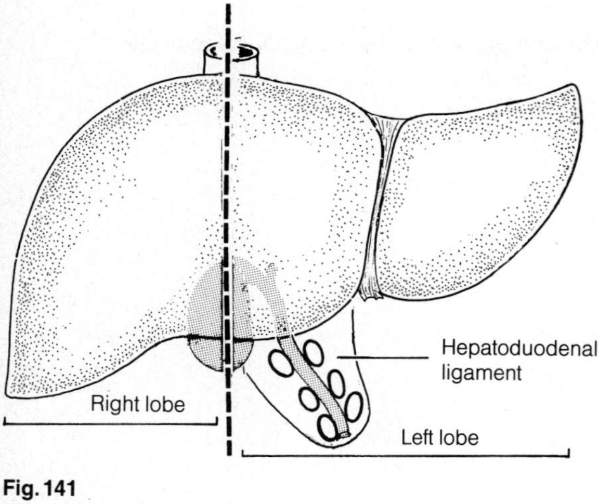

Fig. 141

Regional Lymph Nodes (Fig. 141)

The regional lymph nodes are the hilar nodes (i.e. those in the hepatoduodenal ligament).

TN Clinical Classification

T – Primary Tumour

TX Primary tumour cannot be assessed
T0 No evidence of primary tumour
T1 Solitary tumour 2 cm or less in greatest dimension without vascular invasion (Fig. 142)

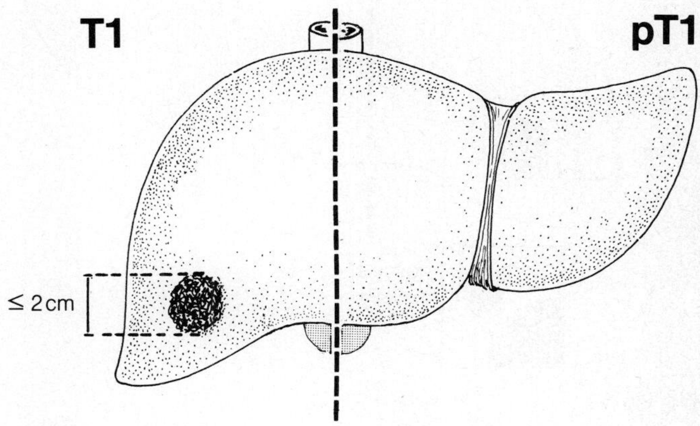

Fig. 142

T2 Solitary tumour 2 cm or less in greatest dimension with vascular invasion (Fig. 143);
or multiple tumours limited to one lobe, none more than 2 cm in greatest dimension without vascular invasion (Fig. 144);
or solitary tumour more than 2 cm in greatest dimension without vascular invasion (Fig. 145)

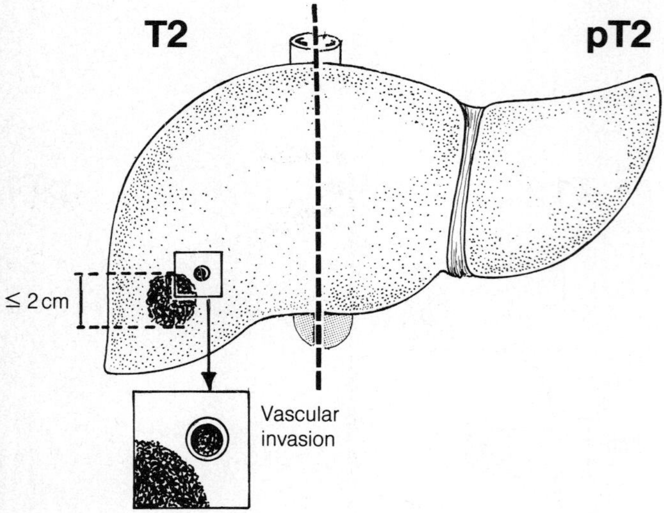

Fig. 143

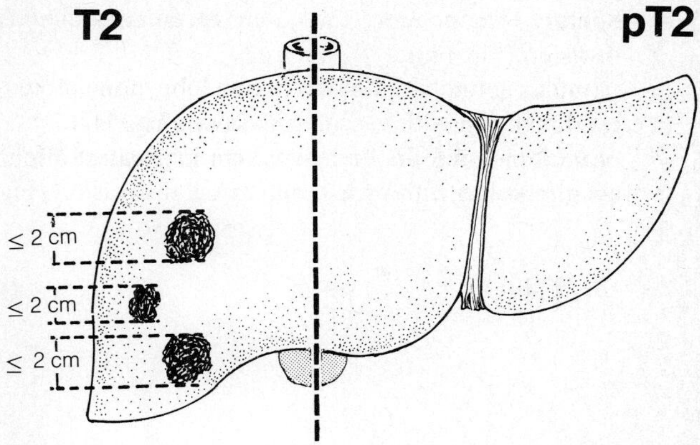

Fig. 144

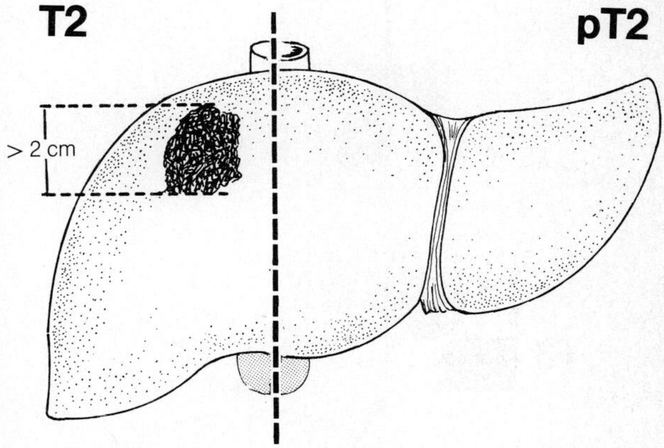

Fig. 145

T3 Solitary tumour more than 2 cm in greatest dimension with vascular invasion (Fig. 146);
or multiple tumours limited to one lobe, none more than 2 cm in greatest dimension with vascular invasion (Fig. 147);
or multiple tumours limited to one lobe, any more than 2 cm in greatest dimension with or without vascular invasion (Figs. 148, 149)

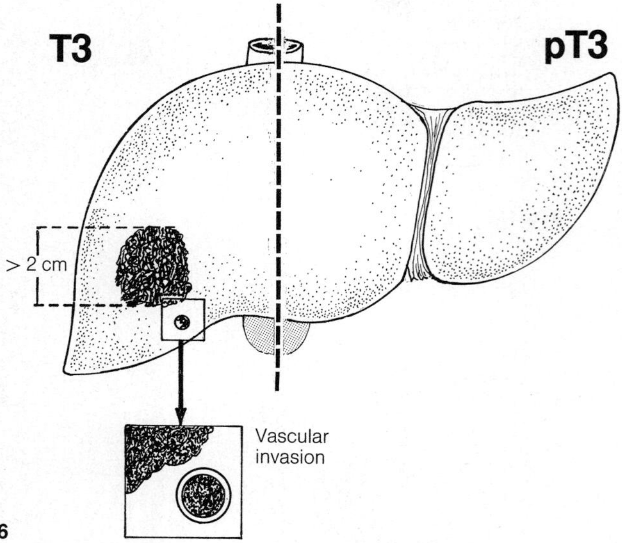

Fig. 146

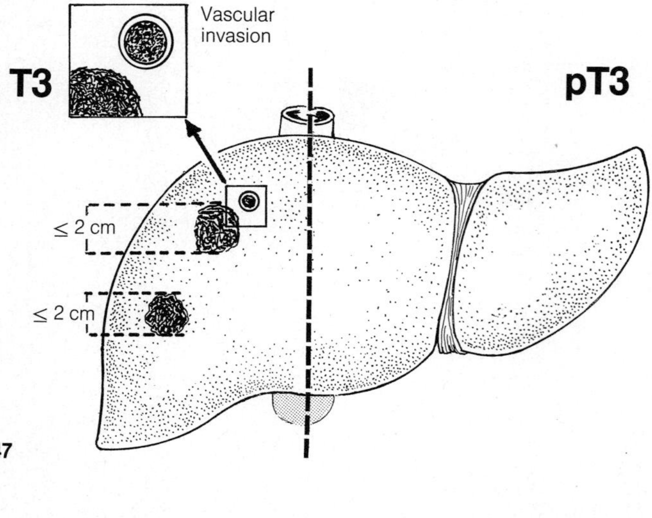

Fig. 147

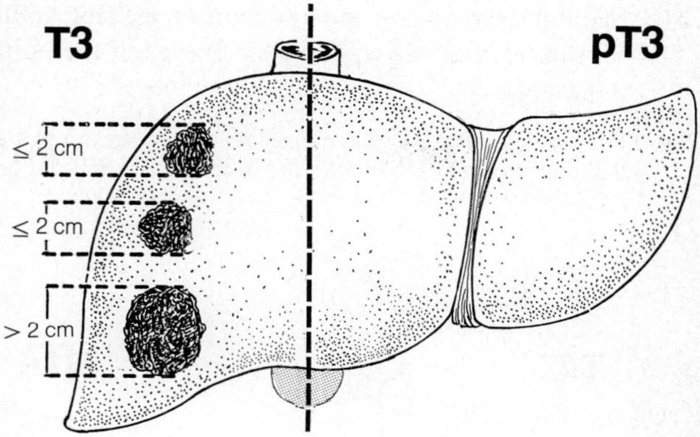

Fig. 148

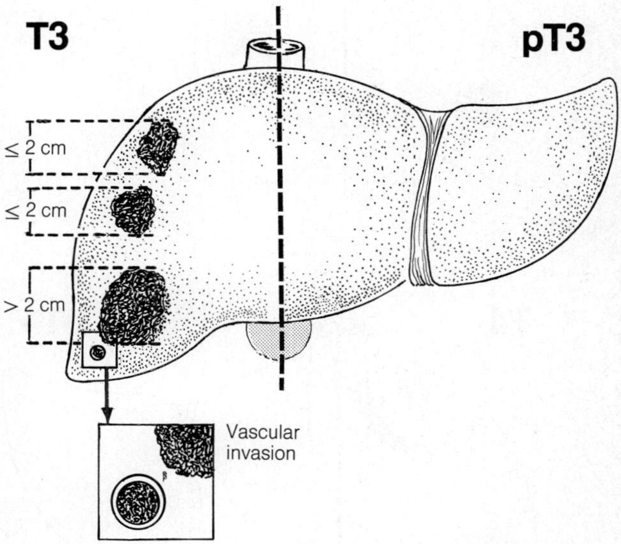

Fig. 149

T4 Multiple tumours in more than one lobe (Fig. 150),
or tumour(s) involve(s) a major branch of the portal or hepatic vein(s) (Fig. 151)

Note: For classification, the plane projecting between the bed of the gallbladder and the inferior vena cava divides the liver into two lobes (Fig. 141, p. 98).

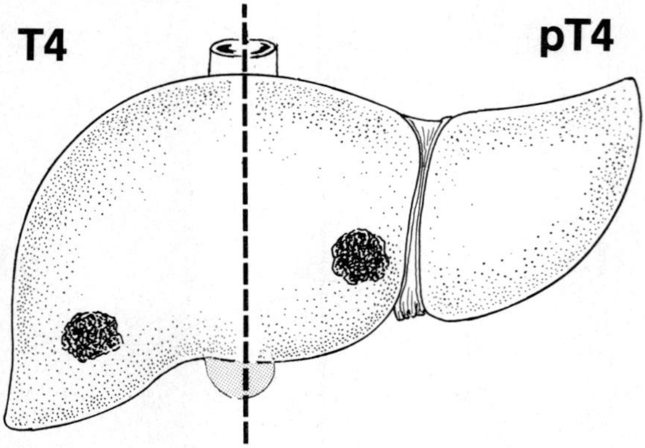

Fig. 150

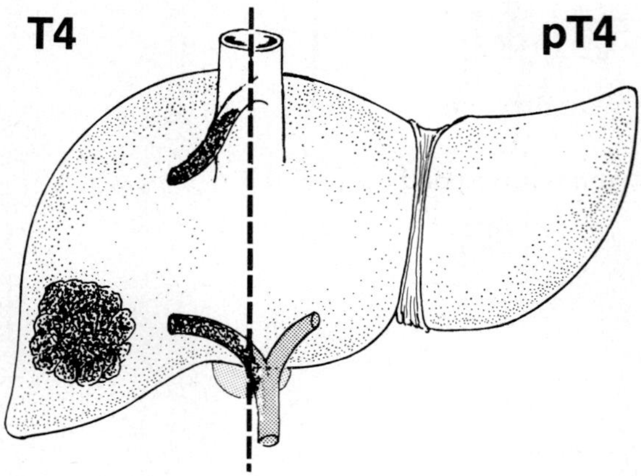

Fig. 151

N – Regional Lymph Nodes

NX Regional lymph nodes cannot be assessed
N0 No regional lymph node metastasis
N1 Regional lymph node metastasis (Fig. 152)

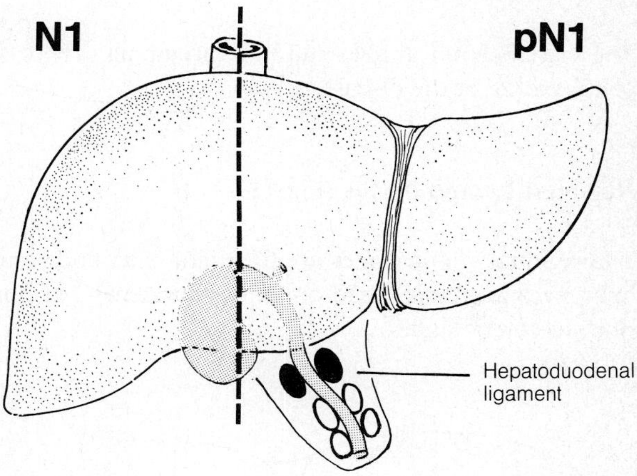

Fig. 152

pTN Pathological Classification

The pT and pN categories correspond to the T and N categories.

Gallbladder (ICD-O 156.0)

Rules for Classification

The classification applies only to carcinoma. There should be histological confirmation of the disease.

Regional Lymph Nodes (Fig. 153)

The regional lymph nodes are the cystic duct node and the pericholedochal, hilar, peripancreatic (head only), periduodenal, periportal, coeliac and superior mesenteric nodes.

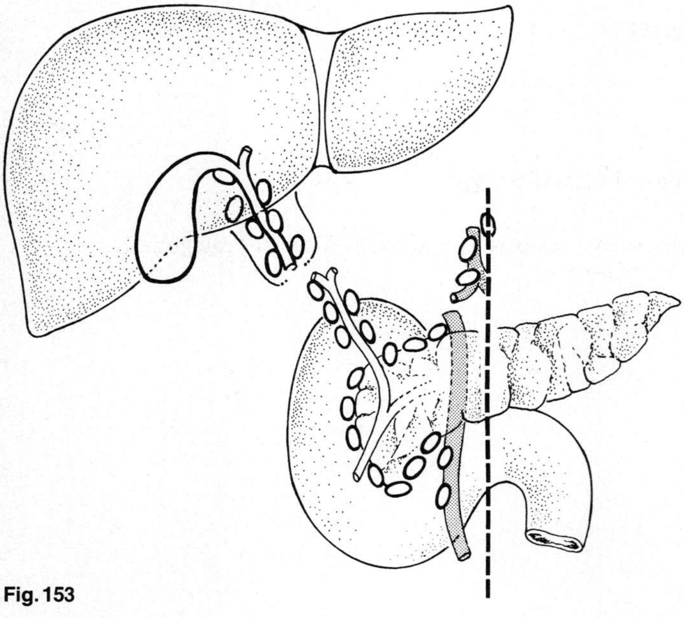

Fig. 153

TN Clinical Classification

T – Primary Tumour

TX Primary tumour cannot be assessed
T0 No evidence of primary tumour
Tis Carcinoma in situ

T1 Tumour invades mucosa or muscle layer (Fig. 154)
 T1a Tumour invades mucosa
 T1b Tumour invades muscle layer

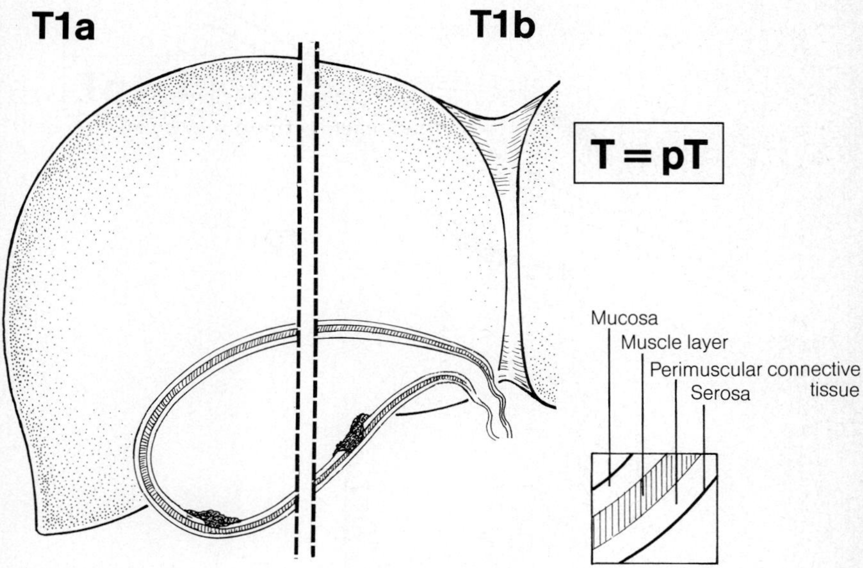

Fig. 154

T2 Tumour invades perimuscular connective tissue, no extension beyond serosa or into liver (Fig. 155)

T3 Tumour invades beyond serosa or into one adjacent organ or both (extension 2 cm or less into liver) (Figs. 156, 157)

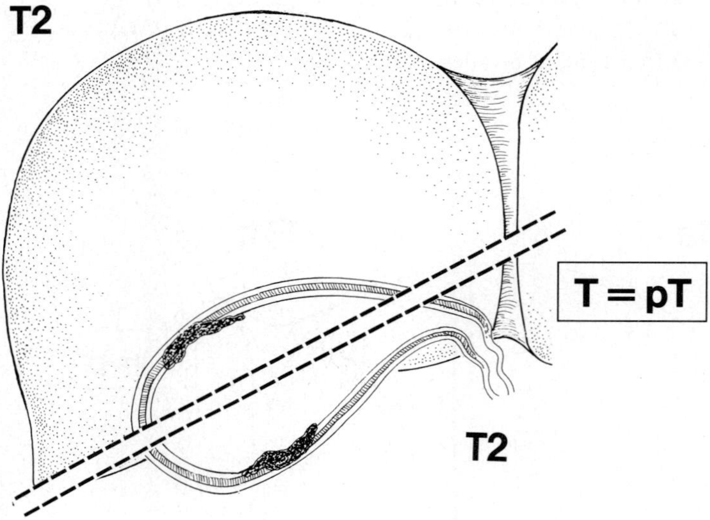

Fig. 155

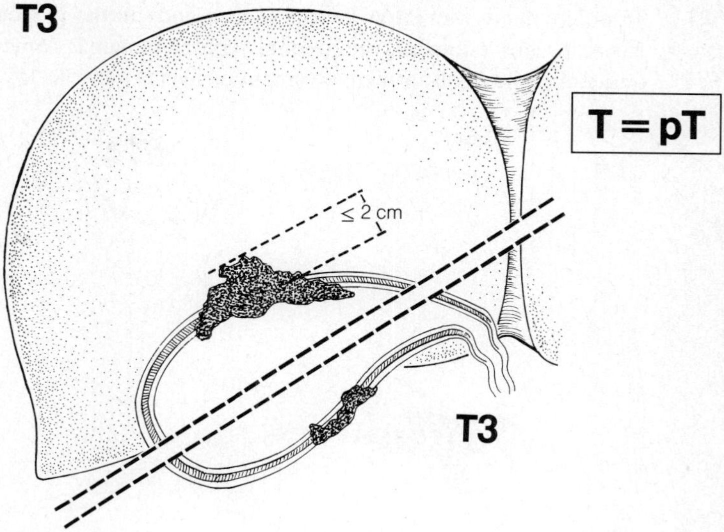

Fig. 156

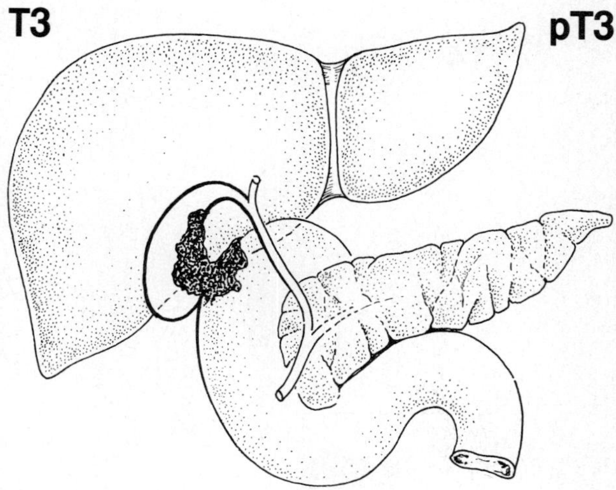

Fig. 157

T4 Tumour extends more than 2 cm into liver and/or into two or more adjacent organs (stomach, duodenum, colon, pancreas, omentum, extrahepatic bile ducts, any involvement of liver) (Fig. 158, 159)

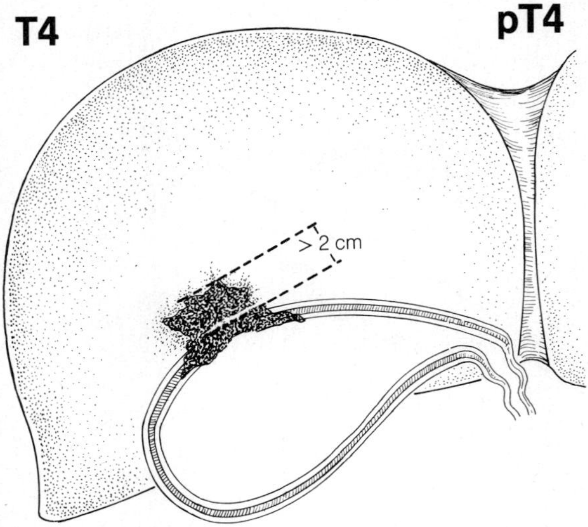

Fig. 158

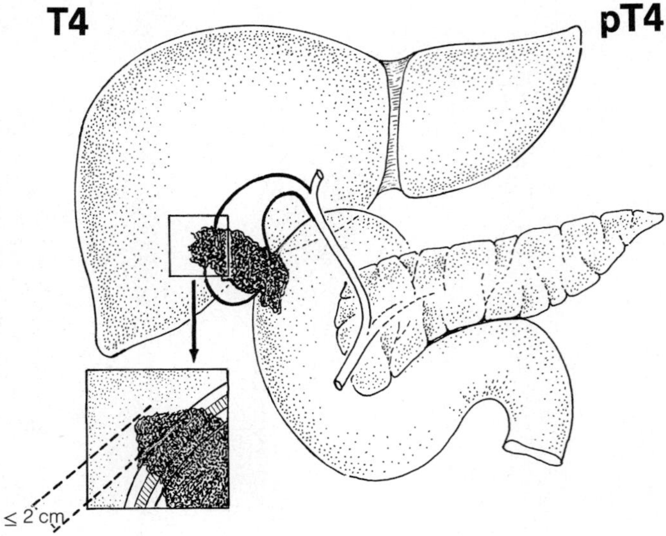

Fig. 159

N – Regional Lymph Nodes

NX Regional lymph nodes cannot be assessed
N0 No regional lymph node metastasis
N1 Regional lymph node metastasis
  N1a Metastasis in cystic duct, pericholedochal, and/or hilar lymph nodes (i.e. those in the hepatoduodenal ligament) (Figs. 160, 161)

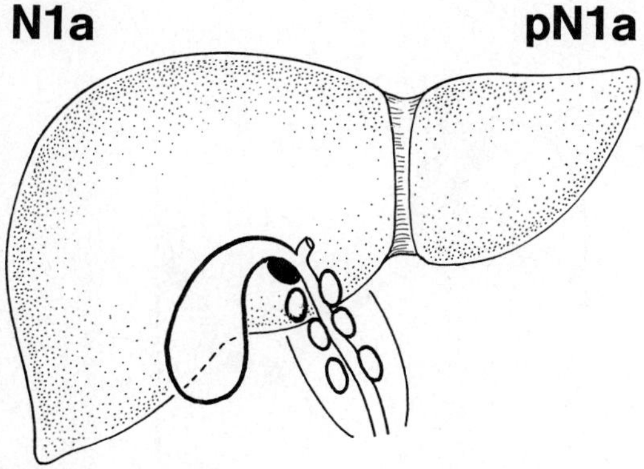

Fig. 160

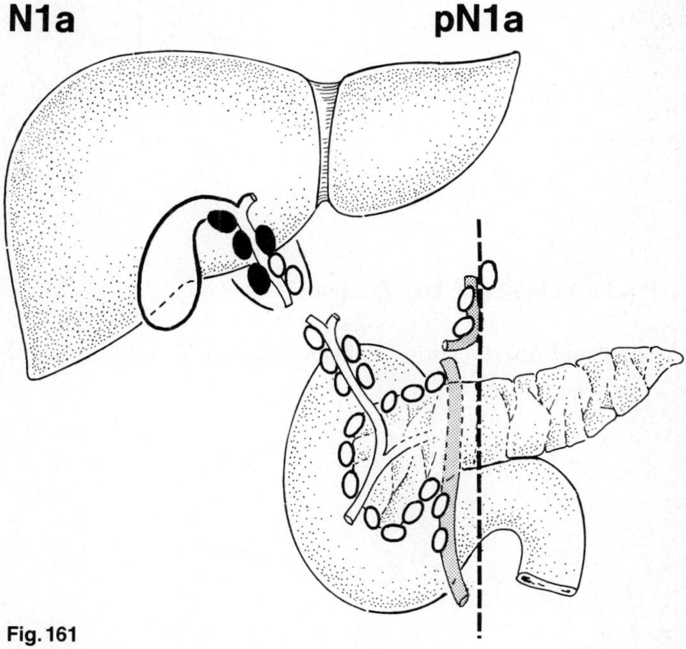

Fig. 161

N1b Metastasis in peripancreatic (head only), periduodenal, periportal, coeliac and/or superior mesenteric lymph nodes (Fig. 162)

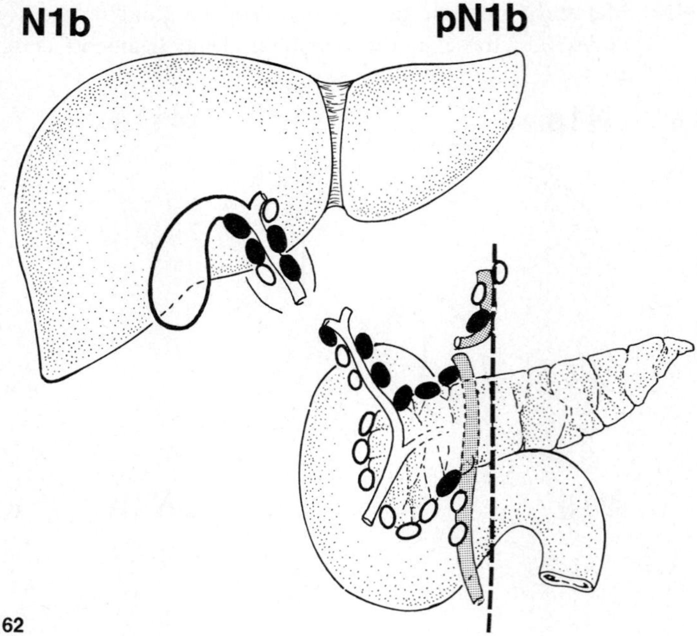

Fig. 162

pTN Pathological Classification

The pT and pN categories correspond to the T and N categories.

Extrahepatic Bile Ducts (ICD-O 156.1)

Rules for Classification

The classification applies only to carcinoma. There should be histological confirmation of the disease.

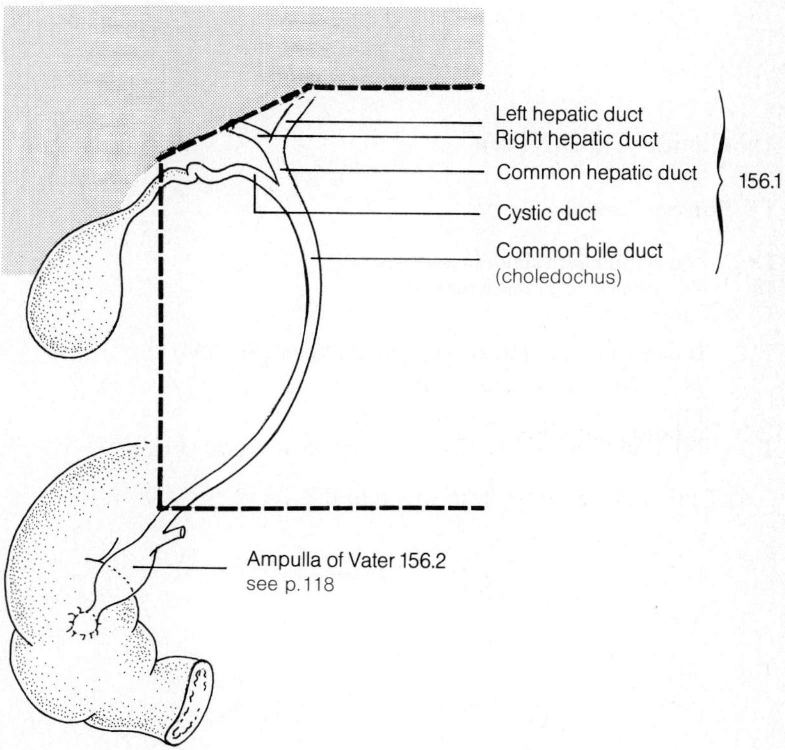

Fig. 163

Anatomical Subsites (Fig. 163)

1. Right hepatic duct
2. Left hepatic duct
3. Common hepatic duct
4. Cystic duct
5. Common bile duct (choledochus)

Regional Lymph Nodes (See Fig. 153, p. 106)

The regional lymph nodes are the cystic duct, pericholedochal, hilar, peripancreatic (head only), periduodenal, periportal, coeliac and superior mesenteric nodes.

TN Clinical Classification

T – Primary Tumour

TX Primary tumour cannot be assessed
T0 No evidence of primary tumour
Tis Carcinoma in situ

T1 Tumour invades mucosa or muscle layer (Fig. 164)
- T1a Tumour invades mucosa
- T1b Tumour invades muscle layer

T2 Tumour invades perimuscular connective tissue (Fig. 165)

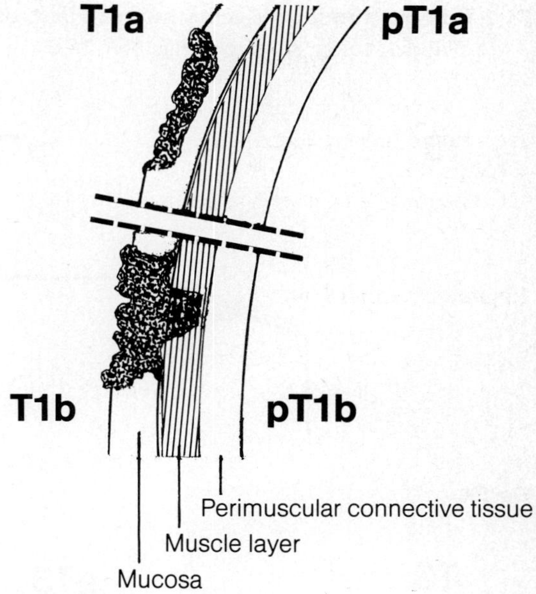

Fig. 164

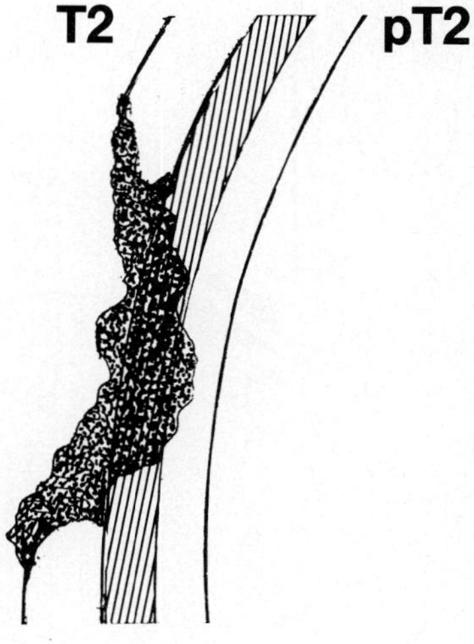

Fig. 165

T3 Tumour invades adjacent structures: liver, pancreas, duodenum, gallbladder, colon, stomach (Figs. 166, 167)

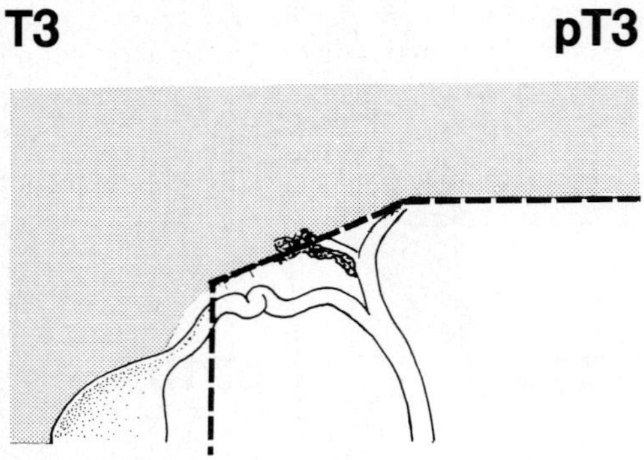

Fig. 166

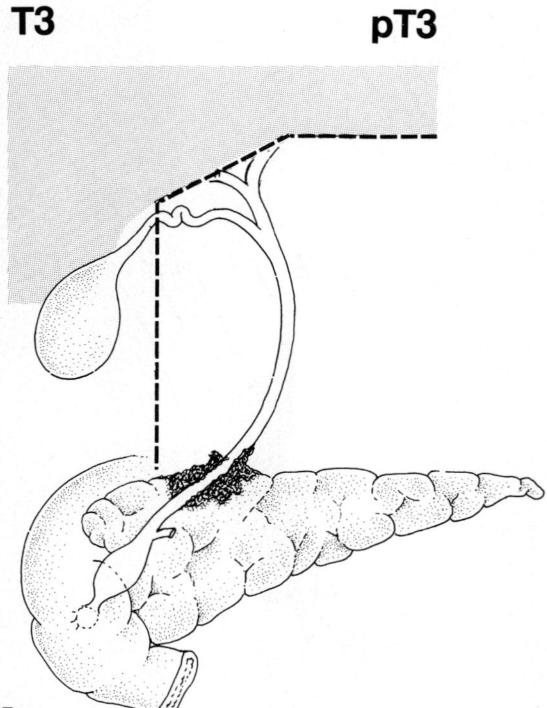

Fig. 167

N – Regional Lymph Nodes

- NX Regional lymph nodes cannot be assessed
- N0 No regional lymph node metastasis
- N1 Regional lymph node metastasis
  - N1a Metastasis in cystic duct, pericholedochal and/or hilar lymph nodes (i.e. those in the hepatoduodenal ligament) (see Figs. 160, 161, p. 111)
  - N1b Metastasis in peripancreatic (head only), periduodenal, periportal, coeliac and/or superior mesenteric lymph nodes (see Fig. 162, p. 112)

pTN Pathological Classification

The pT and pN categories correspond to the T and N categories.

Ampulla of Vater (ICD-O 156.2) (Fig. 168)

Rules for Classification

The classification applies only to carcinoma. There should be histological confirmation of the disease.

Regional Lymph Nodes (Fig. 169)

The regional lymph nodes are:

Superior	Superior to head *(1)* and body *(2)* of the pancreas
Inferior	Inferior to head *(3)* and body *(4)* of the pancreas

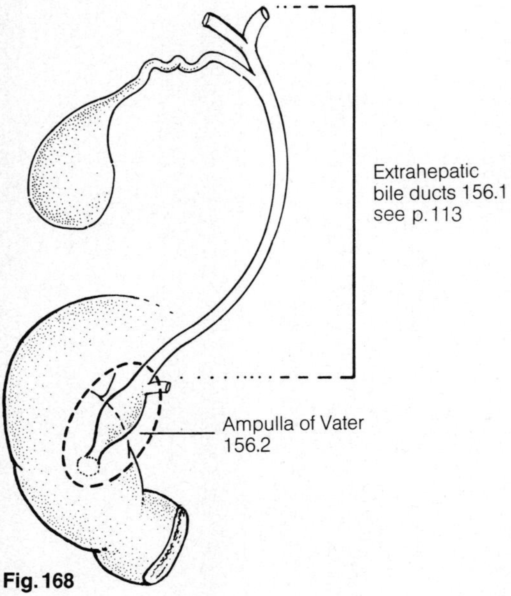

Fig. 168

Anterior	Anterior pancreaticoduodenal *(5)*, pyloric (*6*, not shown in Fig. 169), and proximal mesenteric *(7)*
Posterior	Posterior pancreaticoduodenal *(8)*, common bile duct *(9)* and proximal mesenteric *(7)*

Note: The splenic lymph nodes and those at the tail of the pancreas are *not* regional; metastases to these lymph nodes are coded M1.

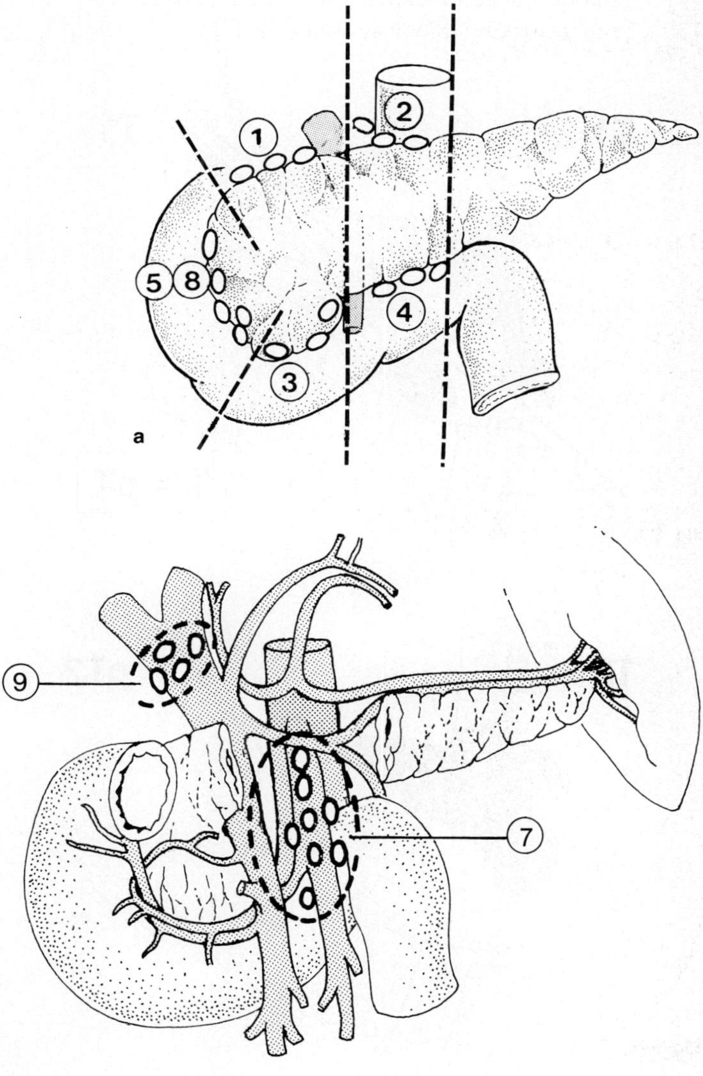

a

b

Fig. 169 a, b

TNM Clinical Classification

T – Primary Tumour

TX Primary tumour cannot be assessed
T0 No evidence of primary tumour
Tis Carcinoma in situ

T1 Tumour limited to ampulla of Vater (Fig. 170)
T2 Tumour invades duodenal wall (Fig. 171)

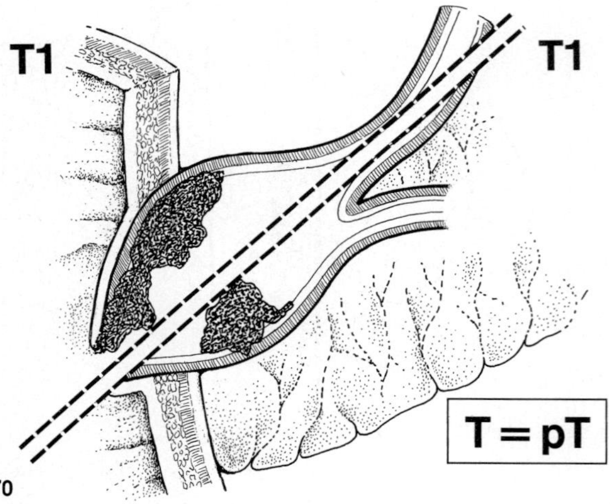

Fig. 170

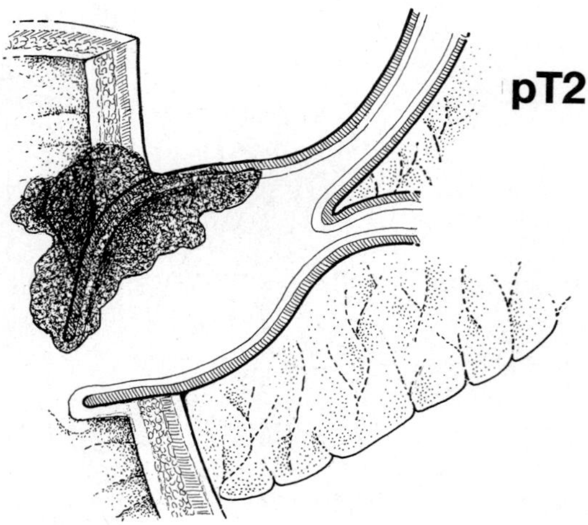

Fig. 171

T3 Tumour invades 2 cm or less into pancreas (Fig. 172)

T4 Tumour invades more than 2 cm into pancreas and/or into other adjacent organs (Fig. 173)

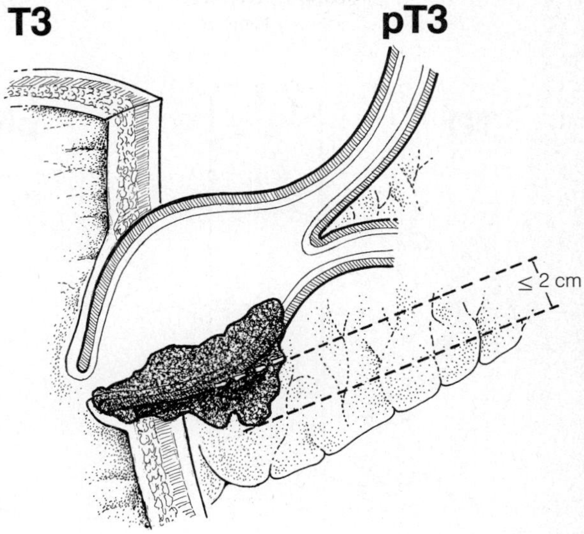

Fig. 172

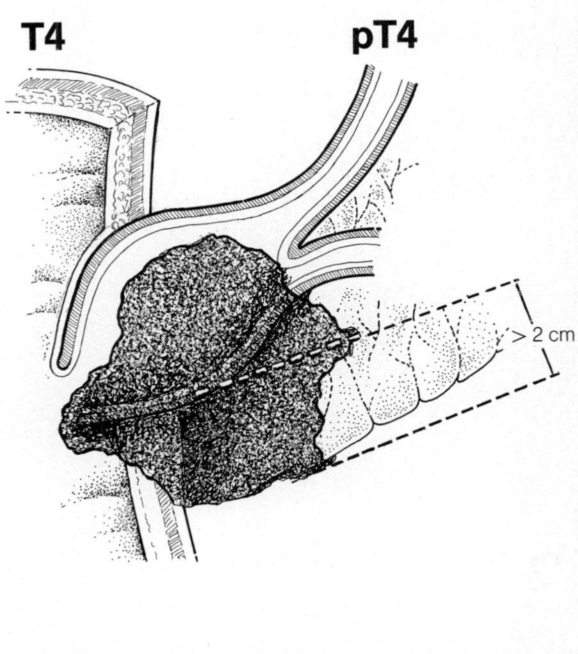

Fig. 173

N – Regional Lymph Nodes

NX Regional lymph nodes cannot be assessed
N0 No regional lymph node metastasis
N1 Regional lymph node metastasis (Figs. 174, 175)

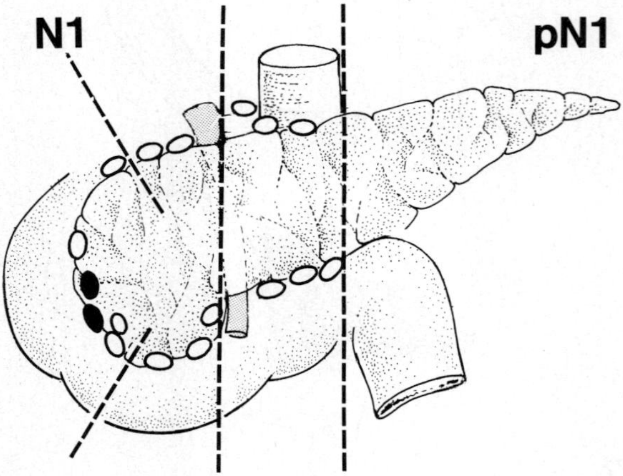

Fig. 174

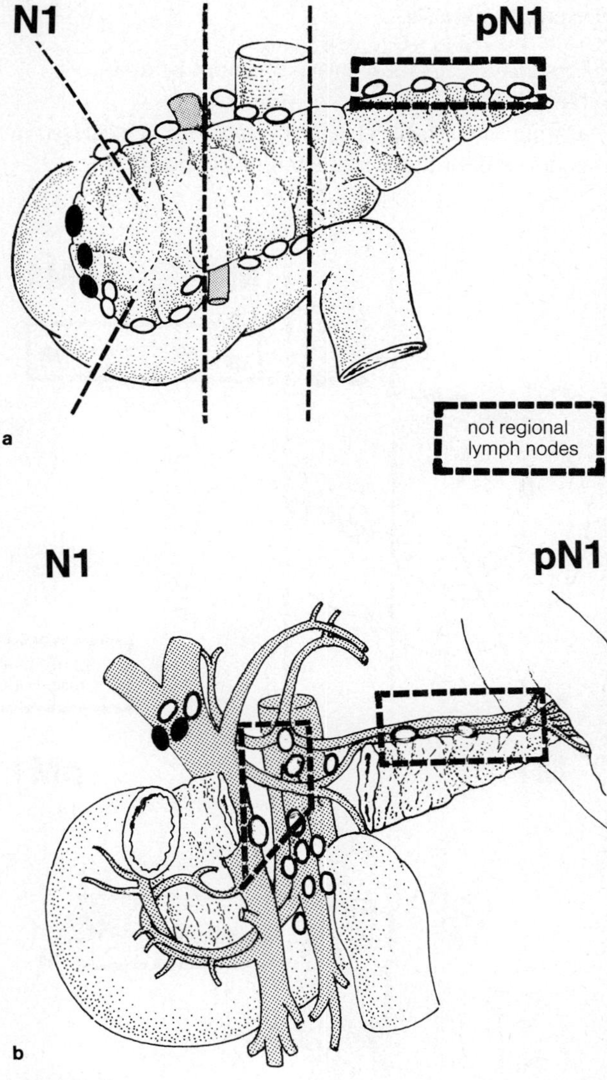

Fig. 175 a, b

M – Distant Metastasis

MX Presence of distant metastasis cannot be assessed
M0 No distant metastasis
M1 Distant metastasis (Fig. 176) (includes metastasis in splenic lymph nodes and/or those at the tail of the pancreas)

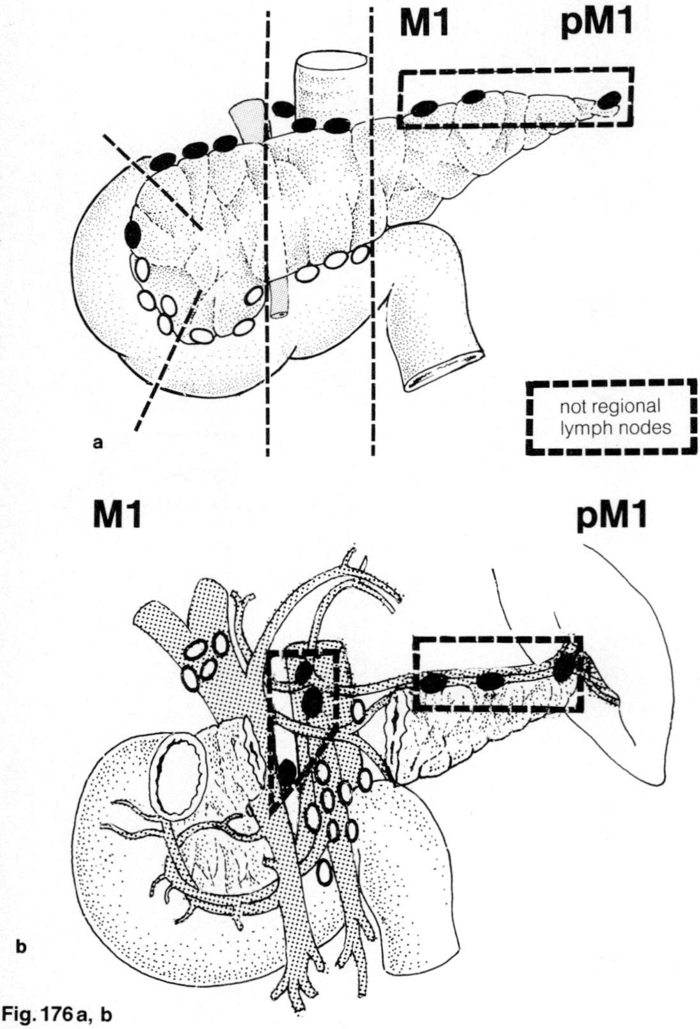

Fig. 176 a, b

pTNM Pathological Classification

The pT, pN and pM categories correspond to the T, N and M categories.

Pancreas (ICD-O 157.0–2,8)

Rules for Classification

The classification applies only to carcinoma of the exocrine pancreas. There should be histological or cytological confirmation of the disease.

Anatomical Subsites (Fig. 177)

1. Head of pancreas[1] (157.0)
2. Body of pancreas[2] (157.1)
3. Tail of pancreas[3] (157.2)
4. Entire pancreas (157.8)

Notes: [1] Tumours of the head of the pancreas are those arising to the right of the left border of the superior mesenteric vein. The uncinate process is considered as part of the head.

[2] Tumours of the body are those arising between the left border of the superior mesenteric vein and the left border of the aorta.

[3] Tumours of the tail are those arising between the left border of the aorta and the hilum of the spleen.

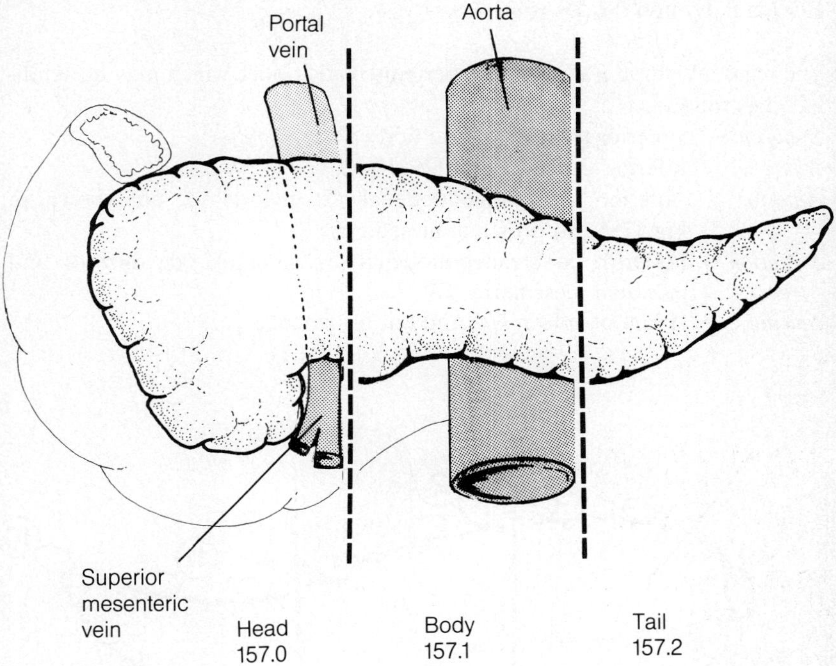
Portal vein
Aorta
Superior mesenteric vein
Head 157.0
Body 157.1
Tail 157.2

Fig. 177

Regional Lymph Nodes (Fig. 178)

The regional lymph nodes are the peripancreatic nodes which may be subdivided as follows:

Superior	Superior to head *(1)* and body *(2)*
Inferior	Inferior to head *(3)* and body *(4)*
Anterior	Anterior pancreaticoduodenal *(5)*, pyloric (*6*, not shown in Fig. 178) and proximal mesenteric *(7)*
Posterior	Posterior pancreaticoduodenal *(8)*, common bile duct *(9)* and proximal mesenteric *(7)*
Splenic	Hilum of spleen *(10)* and tail of pancreas *(11)*

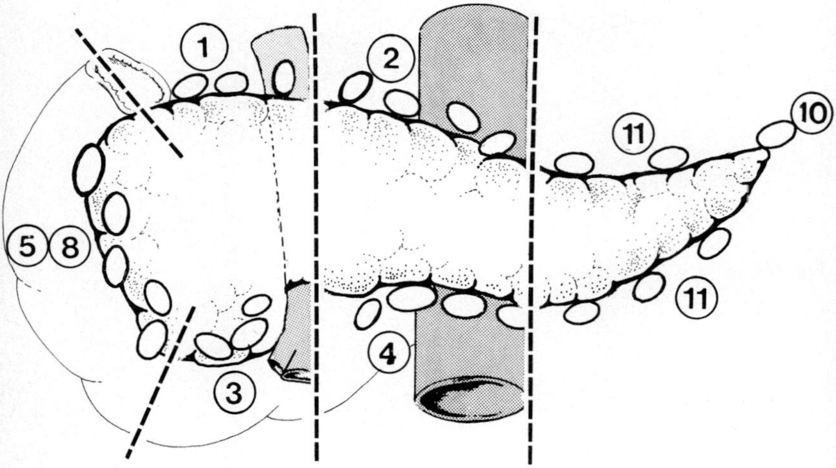

Fig. 178 a

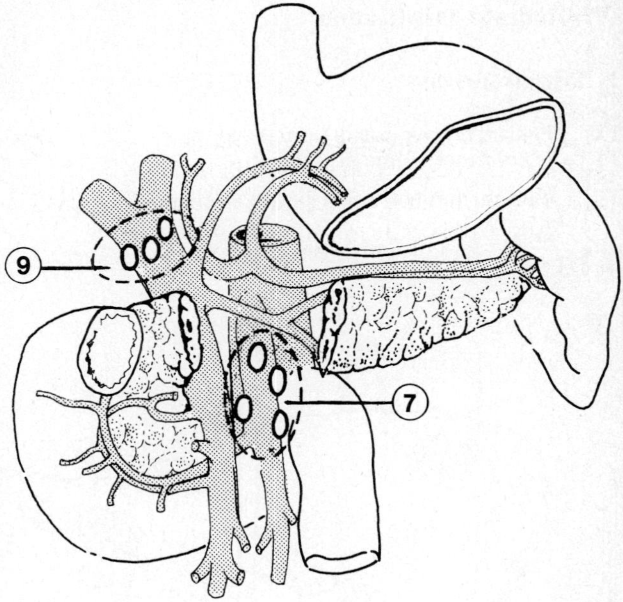

Fig. 178 b

TN Clinical Classification

T– Primary Tumour

TX Primary tumour cannot be assessed
T0 No evidence of primary tumour

T1 Tumour limited to the pancreas (Fig. 179)

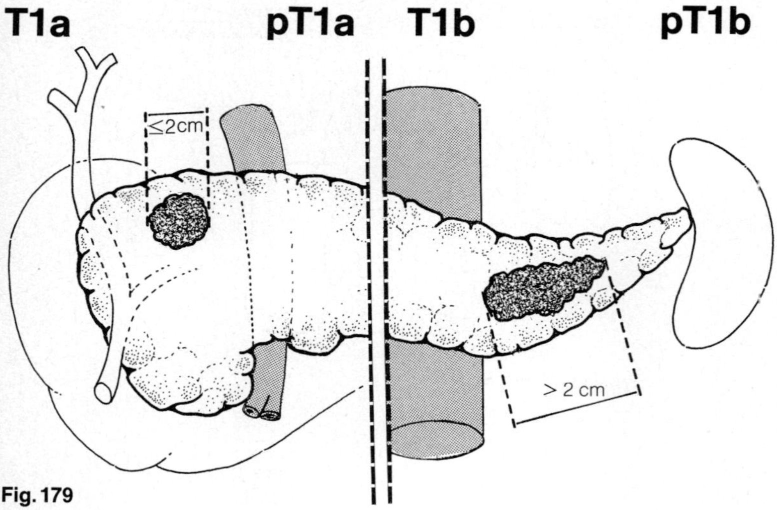

Fig. 179

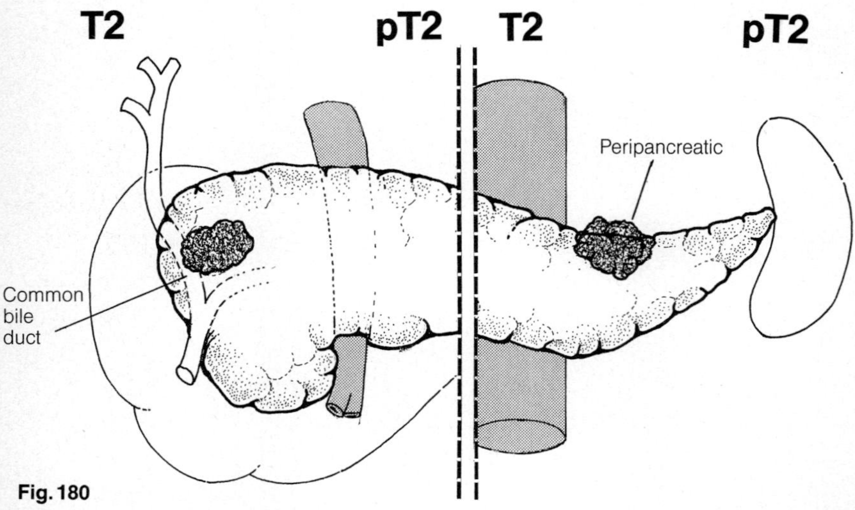

Fig. 180

T1a Tumour 2 cm or less in greatest dimension

T1b Tumour more than 2 cm in greatest dimension

T2 Tumour extends directly to any of the following: duodenum, bile duct, peripancreatic tissues (Figs. 180, 181)

T3 Tumour extends directly to any of the following: stomach, spleen, colon, adjacent large vessels (Fig. 182)

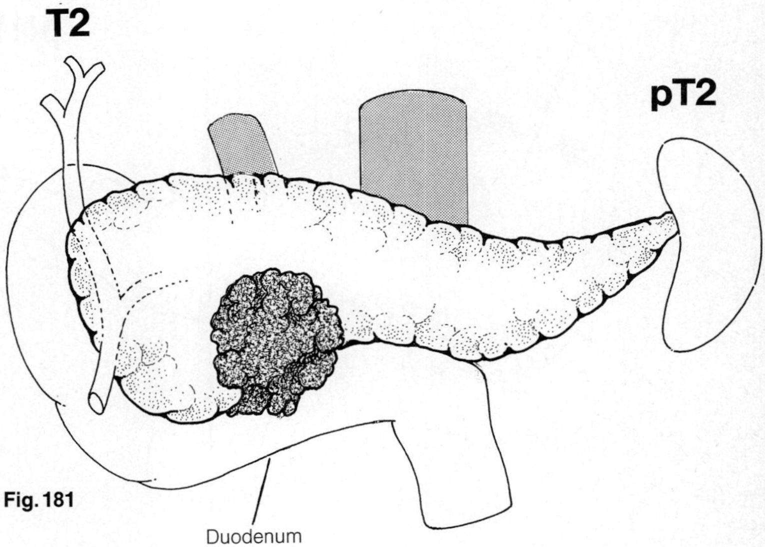

Fig. 181

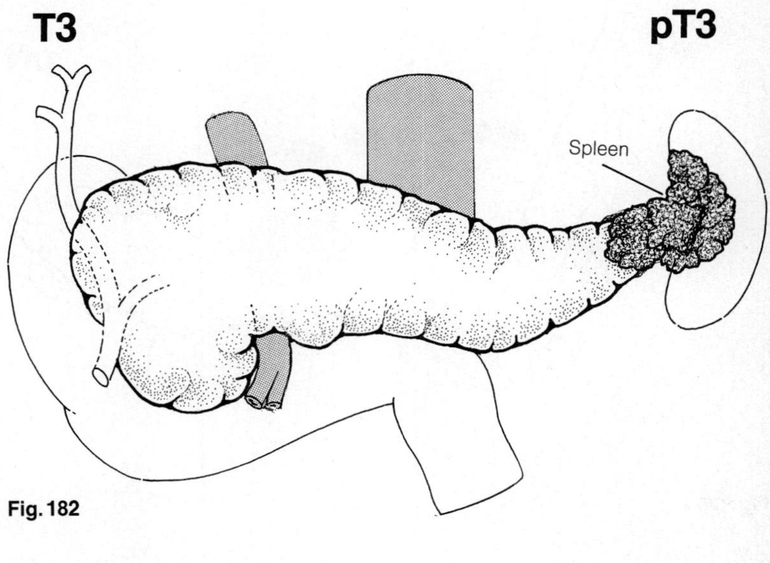

Fig. 182

N - Regional Lymph Nodes

NX Regional lymph nodes cannot be assessed
N0 No regional lymph node metastasis
N1 Regional lymph node metastasis (Figs. 183–185)

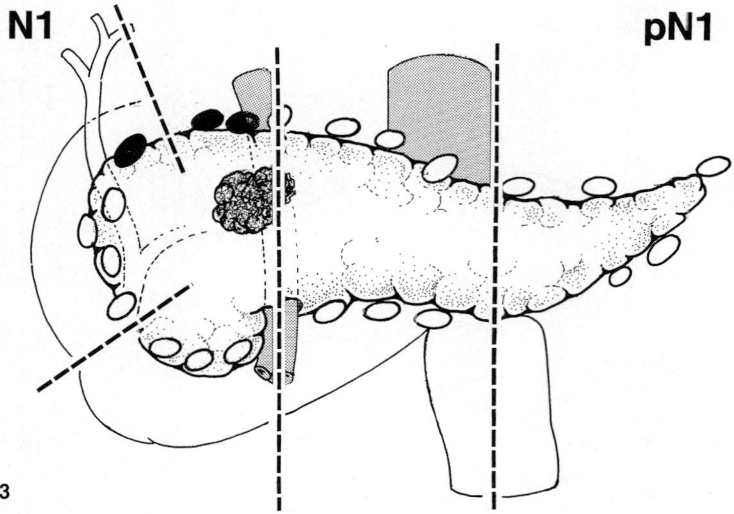

Fig. 183

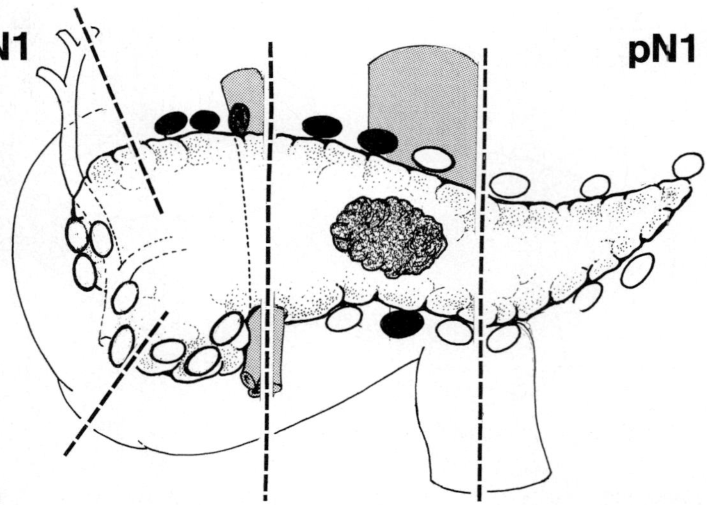

Fig. 184 a

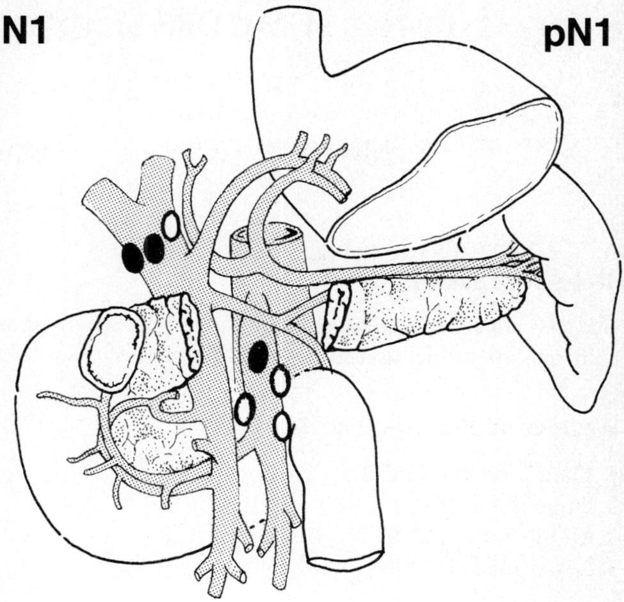

Fig. 184 b

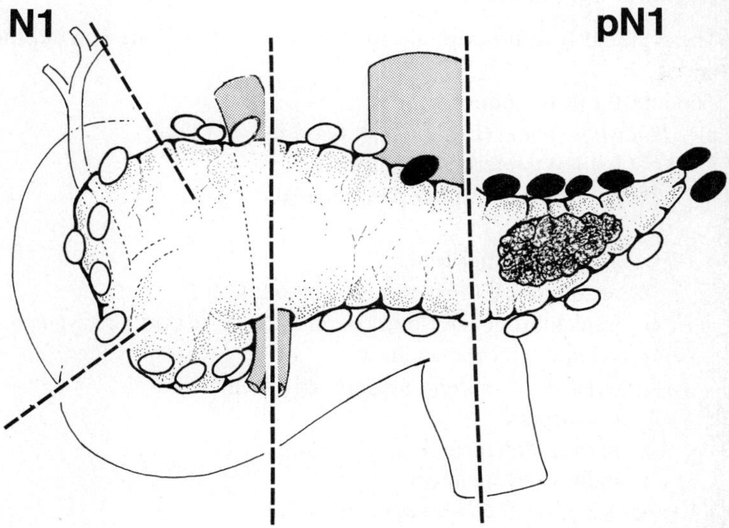

Fig. 185

pTN Pathological Classification

The pT and pN categories correspond to the T and N categories.

LUNG TUMOURS (ICD-O 162.2–9)

Rules for Classification

The classification applies only to carcinoma. There should be histological confirmation of the disease to permit division of cases by histological type.

Anatomical Subsites (Fig. 186)

1. Main bronchus (162.2)
2. Upper lobe (162.3)
3. Middle lobe (162.4)
4. Lower lobe (162.5)

Regional Lymph Nodes (Fig. 187)

The regional lymph nodes are the intrathoracic, scalene and supraclavicular nodes.

The intrathoracic nodes include:

a) *Mediastinal nodes* (Fig. 187b, c; *black* in Fig. 187a):
   - *(1)* highest (superior) mediastinal
   - *(2)* paratracheal (upper paratracheal)
   - *(3)* pretracheal
   - *(3a)* anterior mediastinal
   - *(3b)* retrotracheal (posterior mediastinal)
   - *(4)* tracheobronchial (lower paratracheal) (including azygos nodes)
   - *(5)* subaortic (aortic window)
   - *(6)* para-aortic (ascending aorta or phrenic)
   - *(7)* subcarinal
   - *(8)* paraoesophageal (below carina)
   - *(9)* pulmonary ligament

b) *Peribronchial and hilar nodes* (Fig. 187a):
   - *(10)* hilar (main bronchus)
   - *(11)* interlobar
   - *(12)* lobar
   - *(13)* segmental

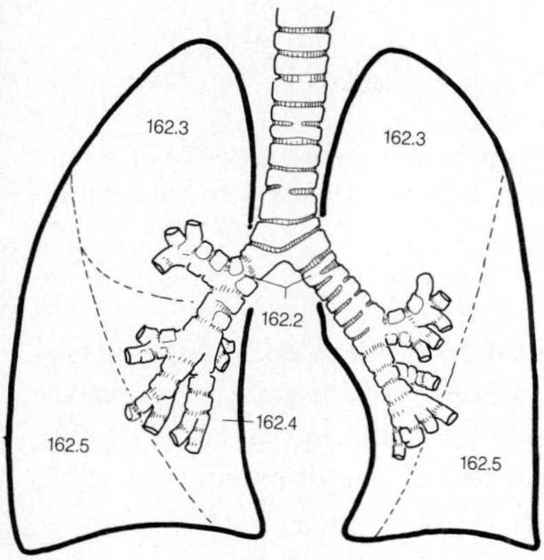

Fig. 186

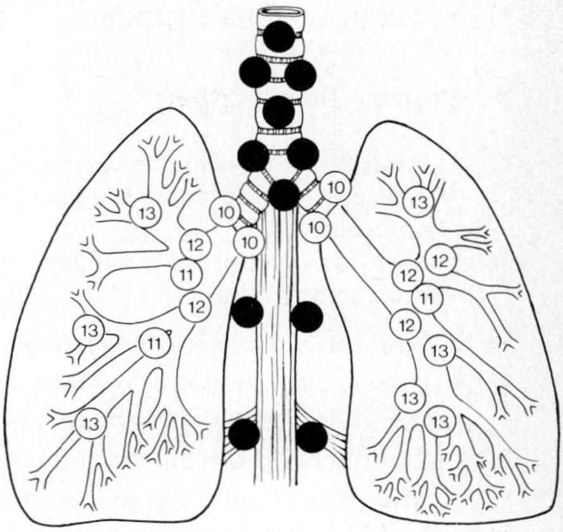

Fig. 187a

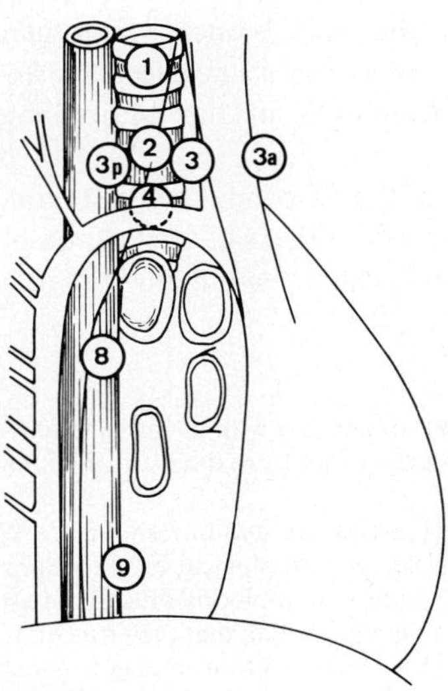

Fig. 187b

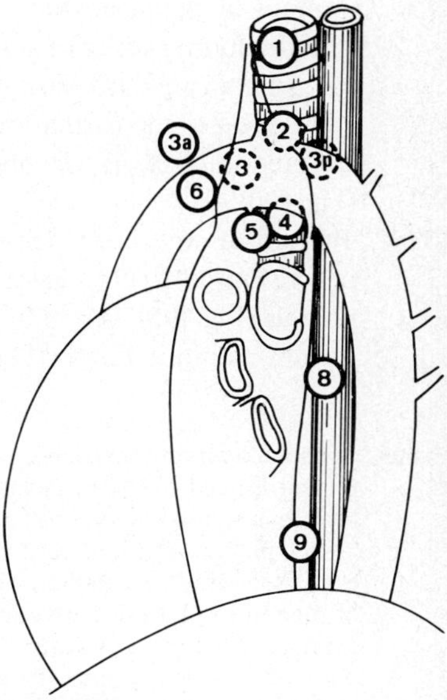

Fig. 187c

Fig. 187a–c. Lymph node map of Naruke. (Modified from Naruke T, Suemasu K, Ishikawa S (1978) Lymph node mapping and curability at various levels of metastasis in resected lung cancer. J Thorac Cardiavasc Surg 76: 832–839)

TNM Clinical Classification

T – Primary Tumour

TX Primary tumour cannot be assessed, *or* tumour proven by the presence of malignant cells in sputum or bronchial washings but not visualized by imaging or bronchoscopy

T0 No evidence of primary tumour

Tis Carcinoma in situ

T1 Tumour 3 cm or less in greatest dimension, surrounded by lung or visceral pleura, without bronchoscopic evidence of invasion more proximal than the lobar bronchus (i.e. not in the main bronchus)[1] (Fig. 188)

T2 Tumour with *any* of the following features of size or extent (Fig. 189):
More than 3 cm in greatest dimension
Involves main bronchus, 2 cm or more distal to the carina
Invades visceral pleura
Associated with atelectasis or obstructive pneumonitis which extends to the hilar region but does not involve the entire lung

T3 Tumour of any size which directly invades any of the following: chest wall (including superior sulcus tumours), diaphragm, mediastinal pleura, parietal pericardium; *or* tumour in the main bronchus less than 2 cm distal to the carina[1] but without involvement of the carina; *or* associated atelectasis or obstructive pneumonitis of the entire lung (Fig. 190)

T4 Tumour of any size which invades any of the following: mediastinum, heart (Figs. 191, 192), great vessels (Figs. 191, 193, 194), trachea, oesophagus (Fig. 195), vertebral body (Fig. 196), carina; *or* tumour with malignant pleural effusion[2] (Figs. 197, 198)

Notes: [1] The uncommon superficial spreading tumour of any size with its invasive component limited to the bronchial wall which may extend proximal to the main bronchus is also classified T1.

[2] Most pleural effusions associated with lung cancer are due to tumour. However, there are a few patients in whom multiple cytopathological examinations of pleural fluid are negative for tumour, the fluid is non-bloody and is not an exudate. Where these elements and clinical judgment dictate that the effusion is not related to the tumour, the effusion should be excluded as a staging element and the patient should be classified T1, T2 or T3.

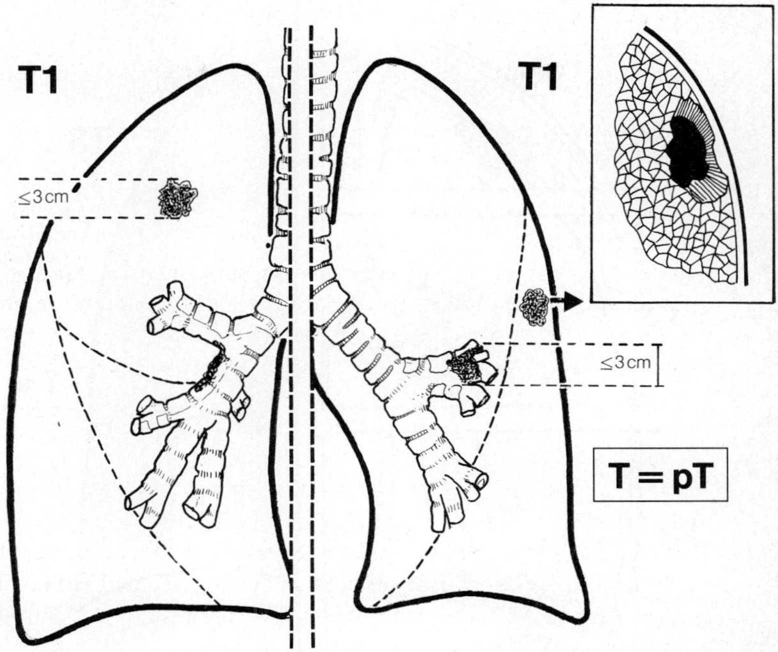

Fig. 188

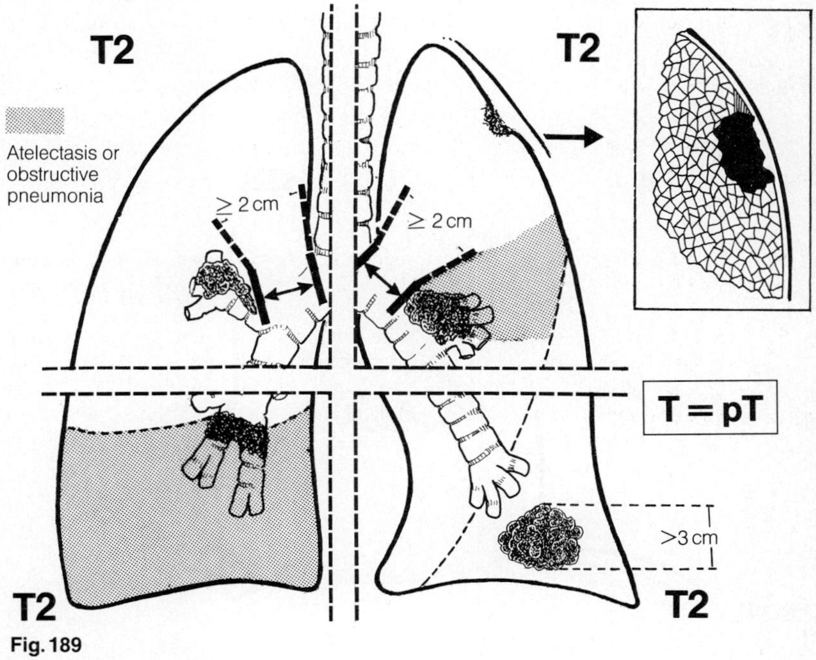

Fig. 189

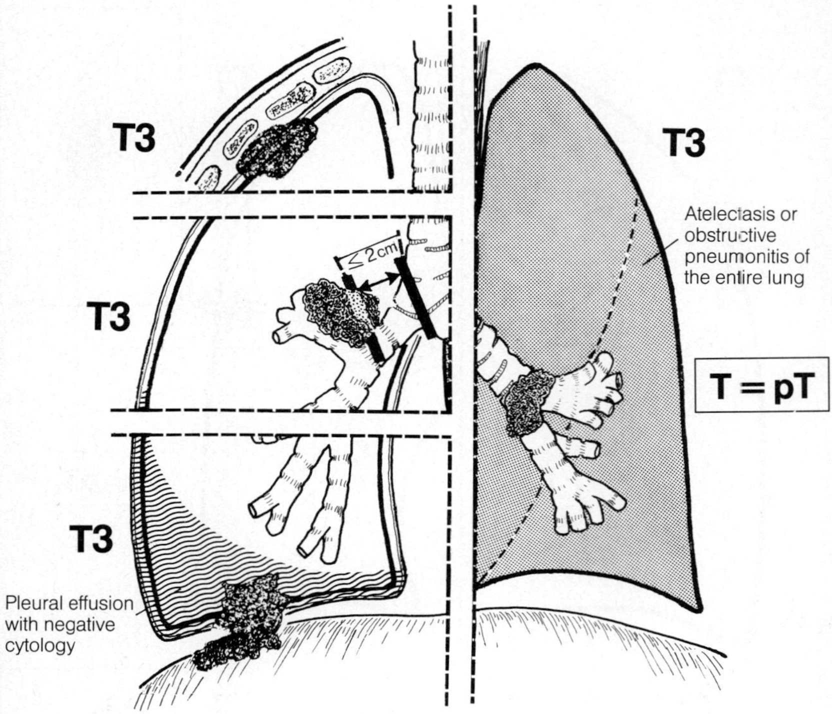

Fig. 190

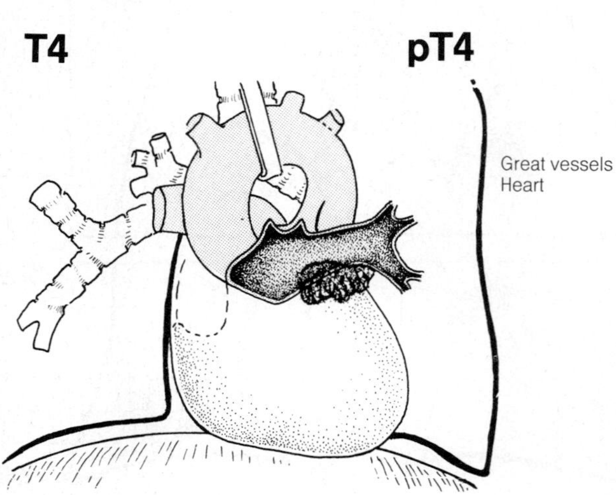

Fig. 191

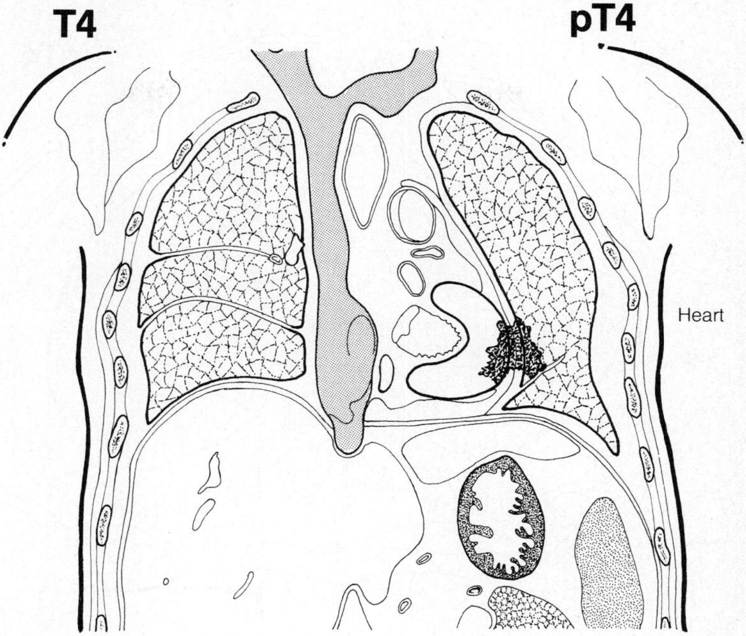

Fig. 192

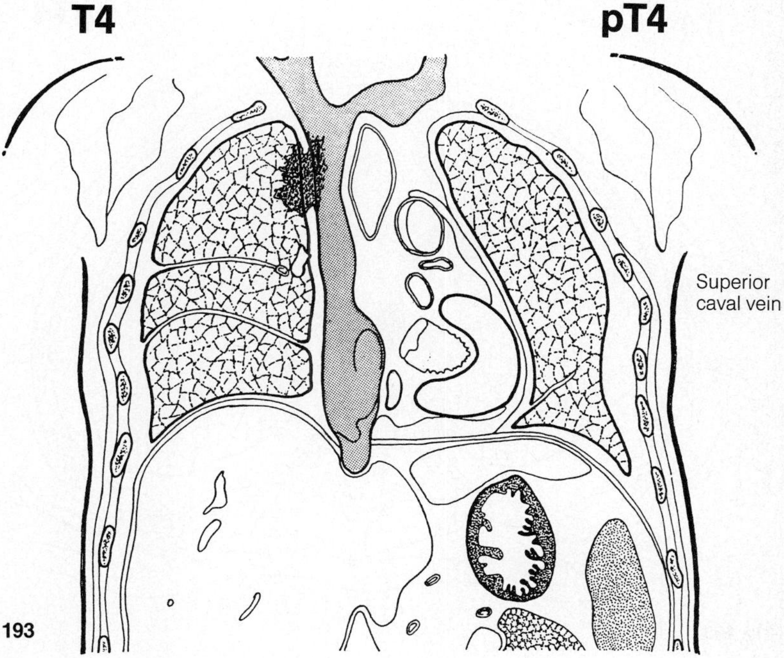

Fig. 193

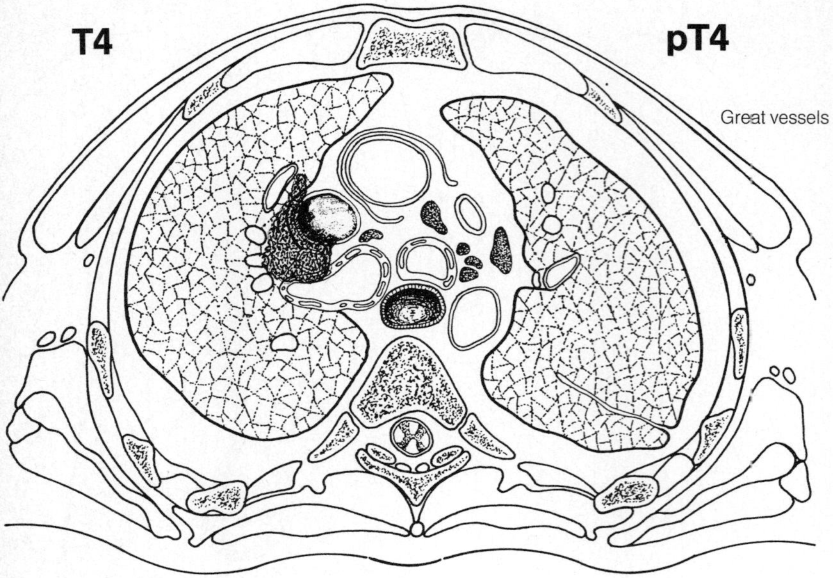

Fig. 194

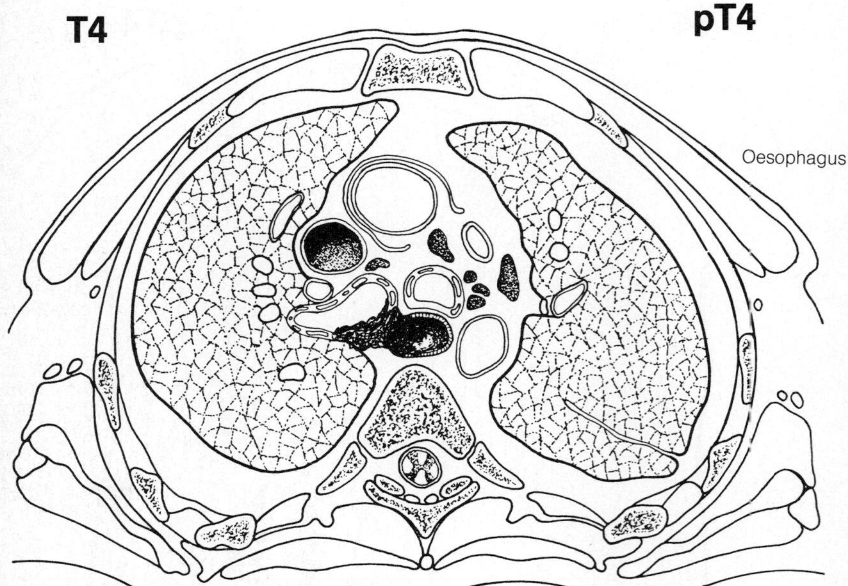

Fig. 195

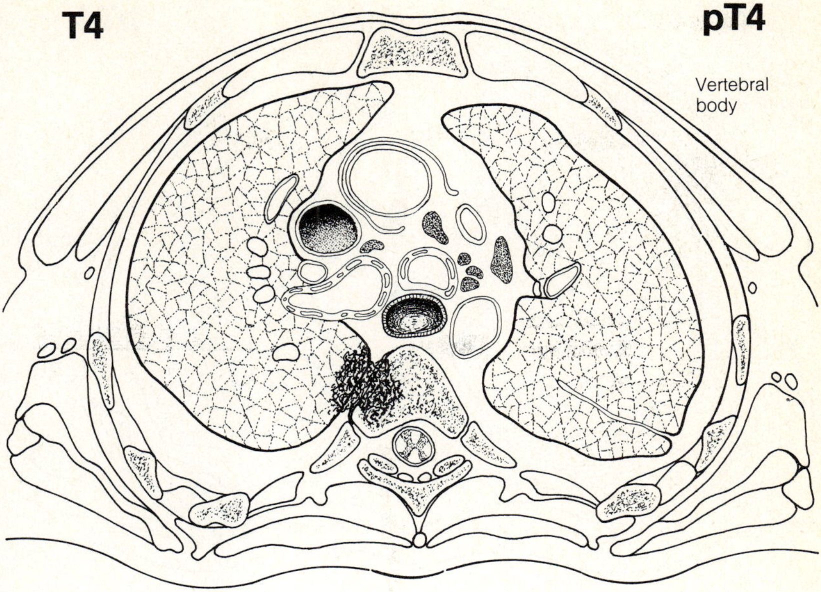

Fig. 196

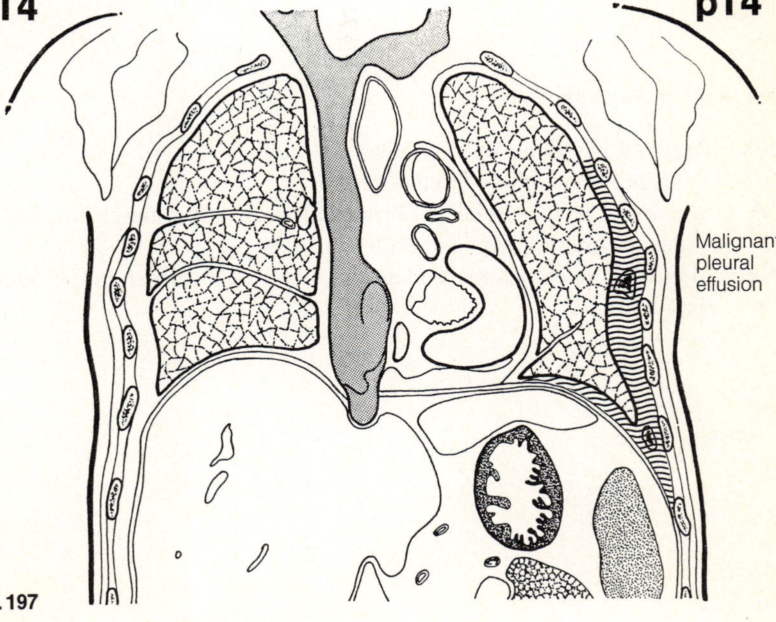

Fig. 197

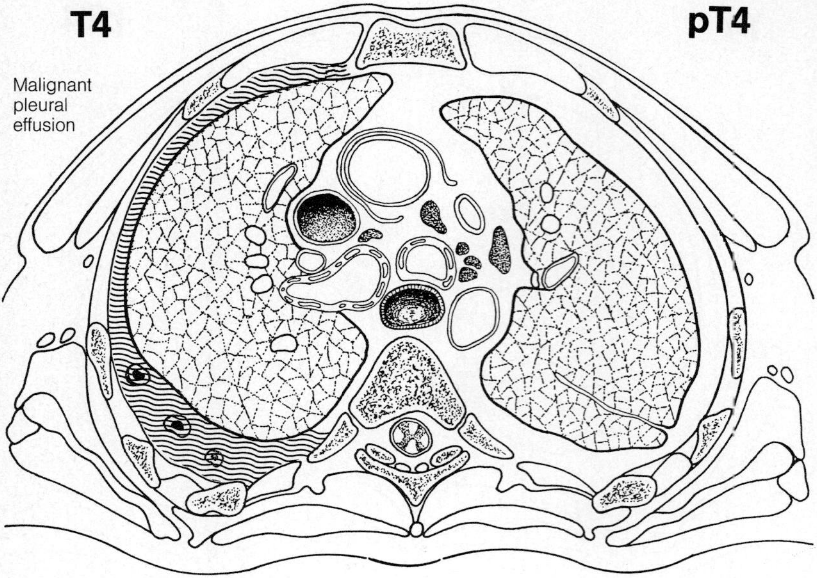

Fig. 198

N - Regional Lymph Nodes

NX Regional lymph nodes cannot be assessed

N0 No regional lymph node metastasis

N1 Metastasis in ipsilateral peribronchial and/or ipsilateral hilar lymph nodes, including direct extension (Fig. 199)

N2 Metastasis in ipsilateral mediastinal and/or subcarinal lymph node(s) (Fig. 200)

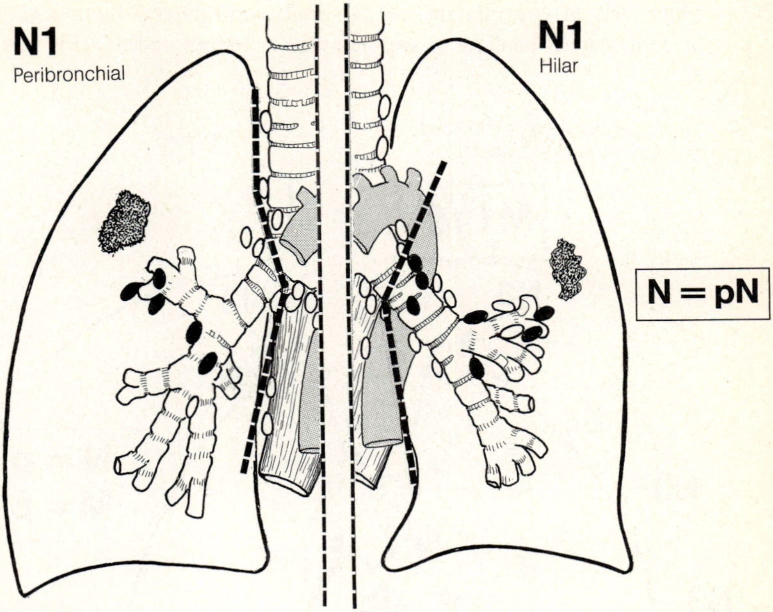

Fig. 199

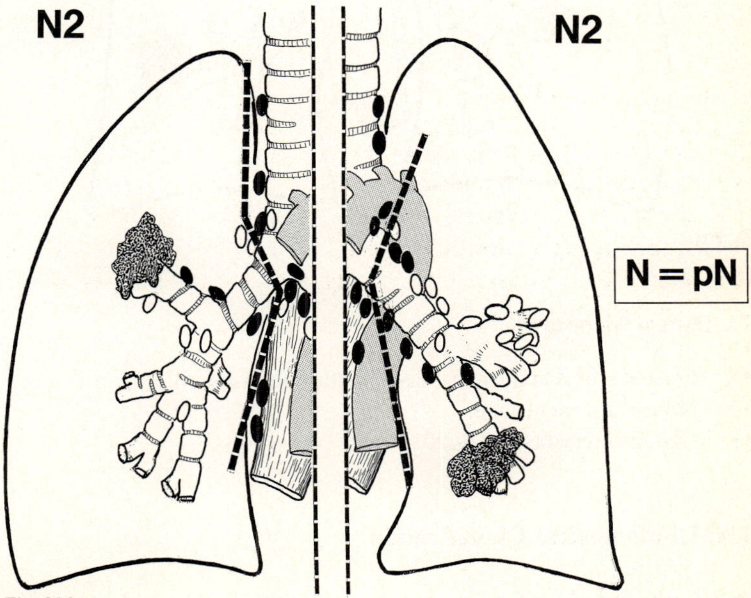

Fig. 200

N3 Metastasis in contralateral mediastinal, contralateral hilar, ipsilateral or contralateral scalene or supraclavicular lymph node(s) (Fig. 201)

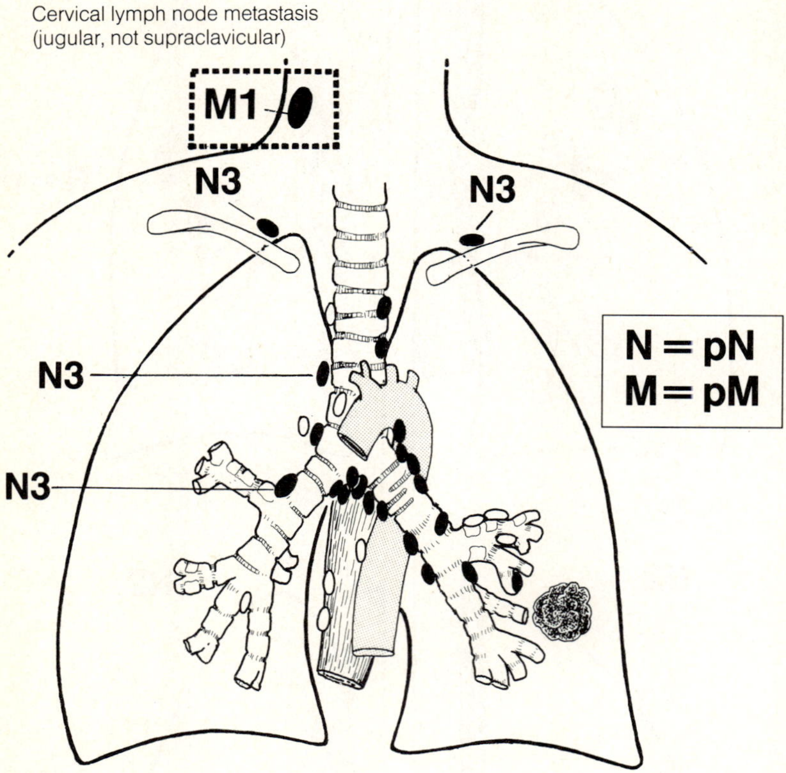

Fig. 201

M – Distant Metastasis

MX Presence of distant metastasis cannot be assessed
M0 No distant metastasis
M1 Distant metastasis (Fig. 201)

pTNM Pathological Classification

The pT, pN and pM categories correspond to the T, N and M categories.

TUMOURS OF BONE AND SOFT TISSUES

Introductory Notes

The following sites are included:

- Bone
- Soft tissues

Regional Lymph Nodes

The regional lymph nodes are those appropriate to the situation of the primary tumour (see Fig. 452, p. 343). The definitions of the N categories for all tumours of bone and soft tissues are:

N – Regional Lymph Nodes

NX Regional lymph nodes cannot be assessed
N0 No regional lymph node metastasis
N1 Regional lymph node metastasis

Bone (ICD-O 170)

Rules for Classification

The classification applies to all primary malignant bone tumours except multiple myeloma, juxtacortical osteosarcoma and juxtacortical chondrosarcoma. There should be histological confirmation of the disease to permit division of cases by histological type.

T Clinical Classification

T – Primary Tumour

TX Primary tumour cannot be assessed
T0 No evidence of primary tumour

T1 Tumour confined within the cortex (Fig. 202)
T2 Tumour invades beyond the cortex (Fig. 203)

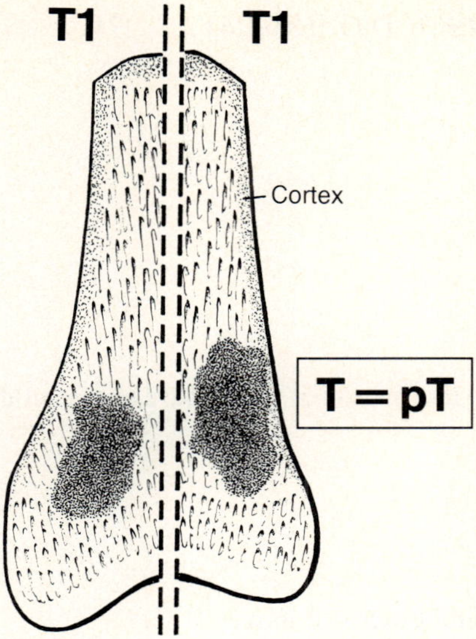

Fig. 202

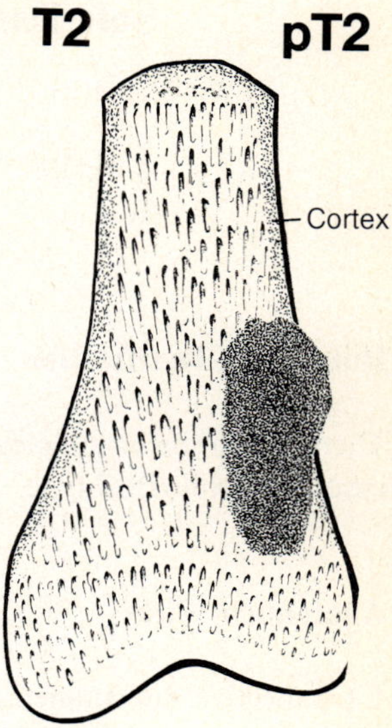

Fig. 203

pT Pathological Classification

The pT categories correspond to the T categories.

Soft Tissues (ICD-O 158.0, 164.2, 3, 171)

Rules for Classification

There should be histological confirmation of the disease to permit division of cases by histological type.

Anatomical Sites

1. Connective, subcutaneous and other soft tissues (171)
2. Retroperitoneum (158.0)
3. Mediastinum (164.2, 3)

Histological Types of Tumour

The following histological types of malignant tumours are included, the appropriate ICD-O morphology rubrics being indicated:

Alveolar soft-part sarcoma	9581/3
Angiosarcoma	9120/3
Epitheloid sarcoma	8804/3
Extraskeletal chondrosarcoma	9220/3
Extraskeletal osteosarcoma	9180/3
Fibrosarcoma	8810/3
Leiomyosarcoma	8890/3
Liposarcoma	8850/3
Malignant fibrous histiocytoma	8830/3
Malignant hemangiopericytoma	9150/3
Malignant mesenchymoma	8990/3
Malignant schwannoma	9560/3
Rhabdomyosarcoma	8900/3
Synovial sarcoma	9040/3
Sarcoma NOS (not otherwise specified)	8800/3

The following histological types of tumour are not included: Kaposi's sarcoma, dermatofibrosarcoma (protuberans), fibrosarcoma grade I (desmoid tumour) and sarcomata arising from the dura mater, brain, parenchymatous organs or hollow viscera.

T Clinical Classification

T - Primary Tumour

TX Primary tumour cannot be assessed
T0 No evidence of primary tumour
T1 Tumour 5 cm or less in greatest dimension (Figs. 204, 205)
T2 Tumour more than 5 cm in greatest dimension (Figs. 204, 206)

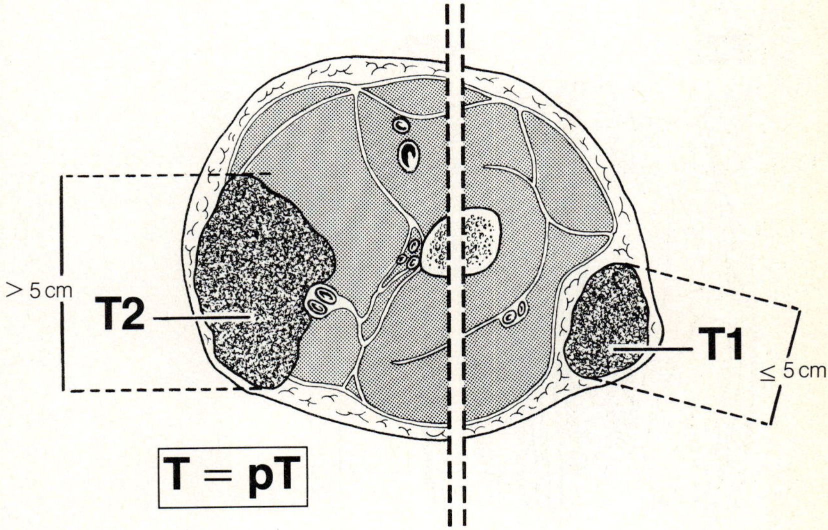

Fig. 204

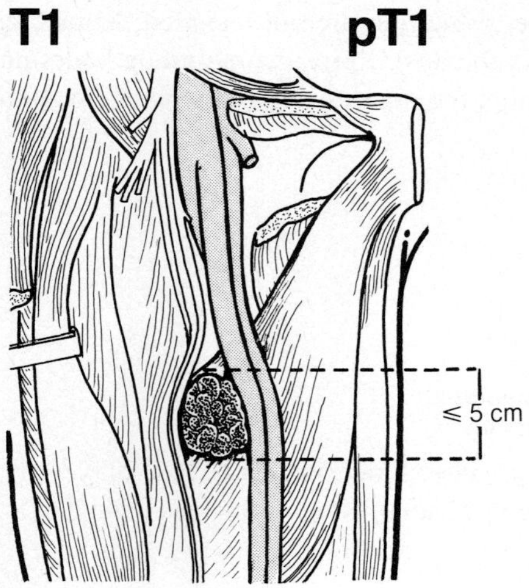

Fig. 205

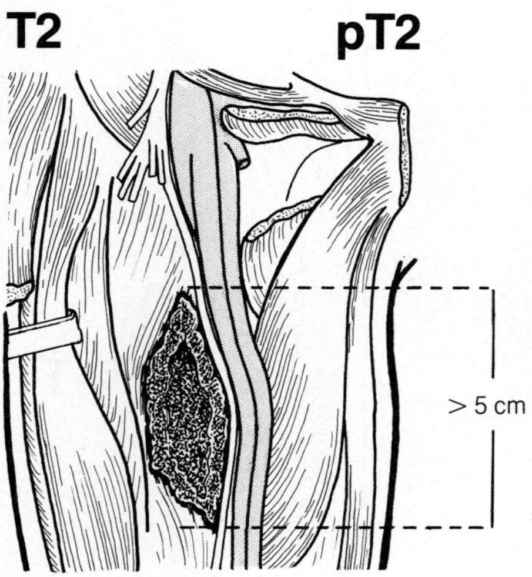

Fig. 206

pT Pathological Classification

The pT categories correspond to the T categories.

SKIN TUMOURS

Introductory Notes

The classification applies to carcinoma of the skin excluding eyelid (see p. 274), vulva (see p. 214), penis (see p. 237) and to melanoma of the skin.

Anatomical Sites

The following sites are identified by ICD-O topography rubrics:

1. Lip (excluding vermilion surface) (173.0)
2. Eyelid (173.1)
3. External ear (173.2)
4. Other parts of face (173.3)
5. Scalp and neck (173.4)
6. Trunk including anal margin and perianal skin (173.5)
7. Arm and shoulder (173.6)
8. Leg and hip (173.7)
9. Vulva (184.4)
10. Penis (187.4)
11. Scrotum (187.7)

Regional Lymph Nodes (Figs. 207, 208)

The regional lymph nodes are those appropriate to the site of the primary tumour.

Unilateral Tumours

Head, neck	Ipsilateral preauricular, submandibular, cervical and supraclavicular lymph nodes
Thorax	Ipsilateral axillary lymph nodes
Arm	Ipsilateral epitrochlear and axillary lymph nodes
Abdomen, loins and buttocks	Ipsilateral inguinal lymph nodes
Leg	Ipsilateral popliteal and inguinal lymph nodes
Anal margin and perianal skin	Ipsilateral inguinal lymph nodes

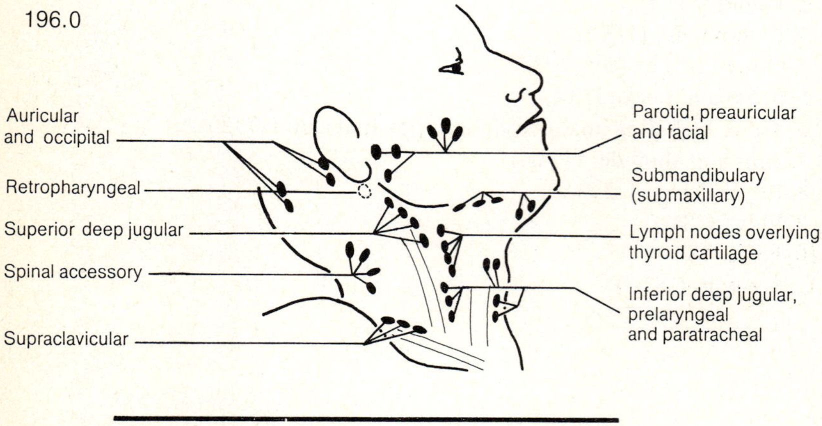

Fig. 207

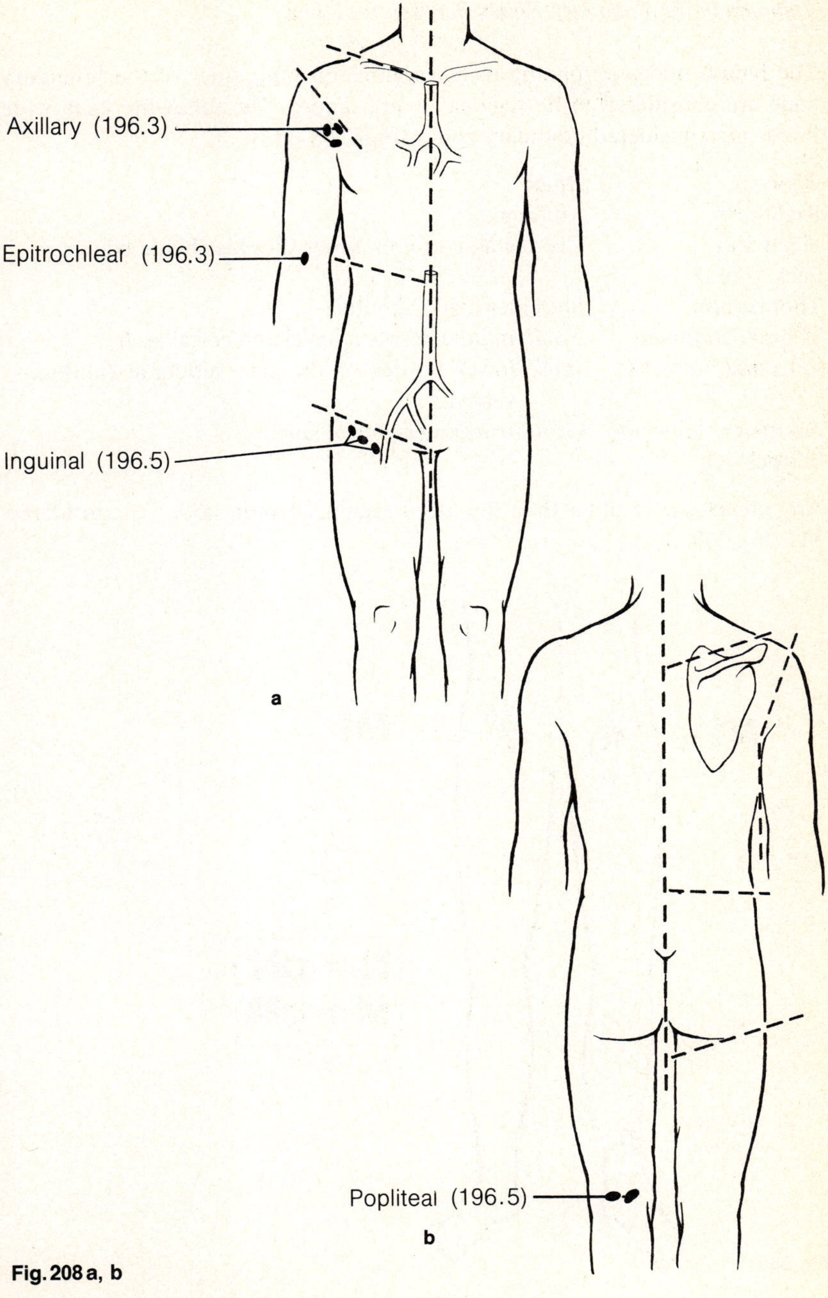
Axillary (196.3)
Epitrochlear (196.3)
Inguinal (196.5)
a
Popliteal (196.5)
b

Fig. 208 a, b

Tumours in the Boundary Zones Between the Above

The lymph nodes pertaining to the regions on both sides of the boundary zone are considered to be regional lymph nodes. The following 4-cm-wide bands are considered boundary zones (Figs. 208–213):

Between	*Along*
Right/left	Midline
Head and neck/thorax	Clavicula-acromion-upper shoulder blade edge
Thorax/arm	Shoulder-axilla-shoulder
Thorax/abdomen, loins and buttocks	*Front:* middle between navel and costal arch *Back:* lower border of thoracic vertebrae (midtransverse axis)
Abdomen, loins and buttock/leg	Groin-trochanter-gluteal sulcus

Any metastasis to other than the listed regional lymph nodes is considered M1 (Fig. 209–212).

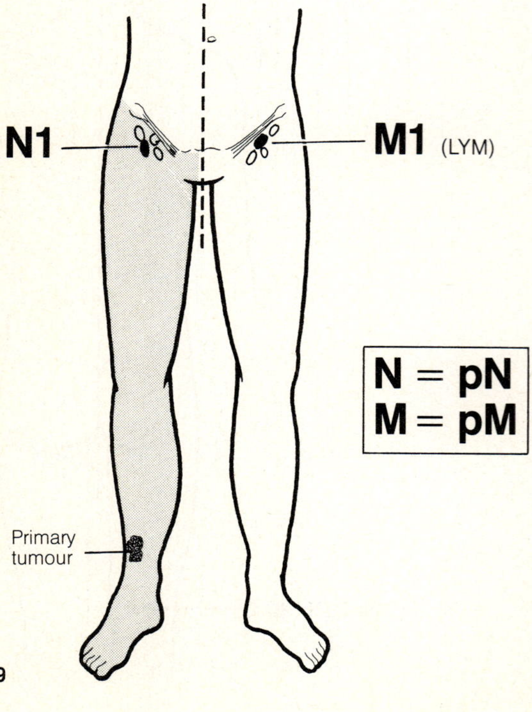

Fig. 209

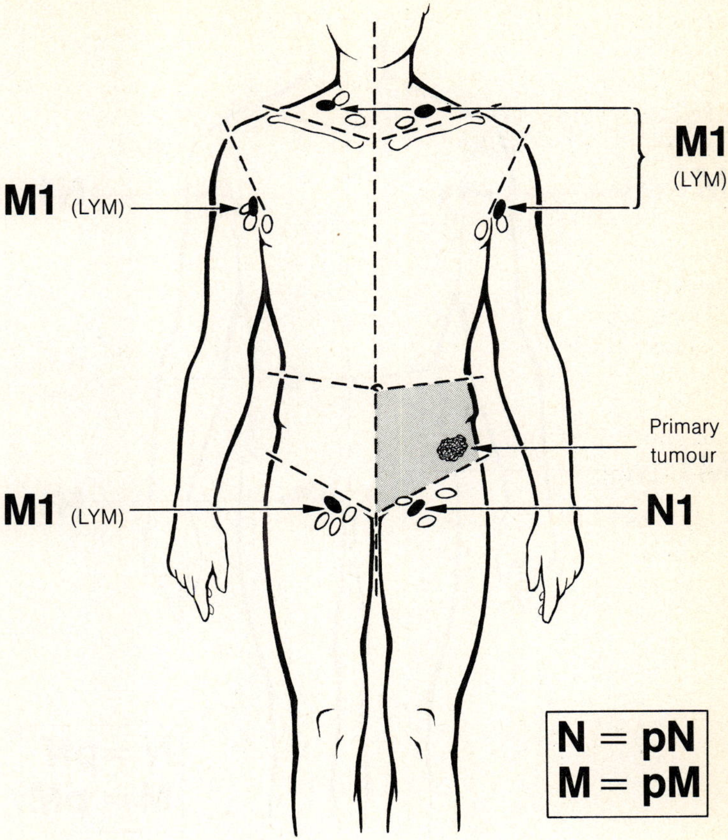

Fig. 210

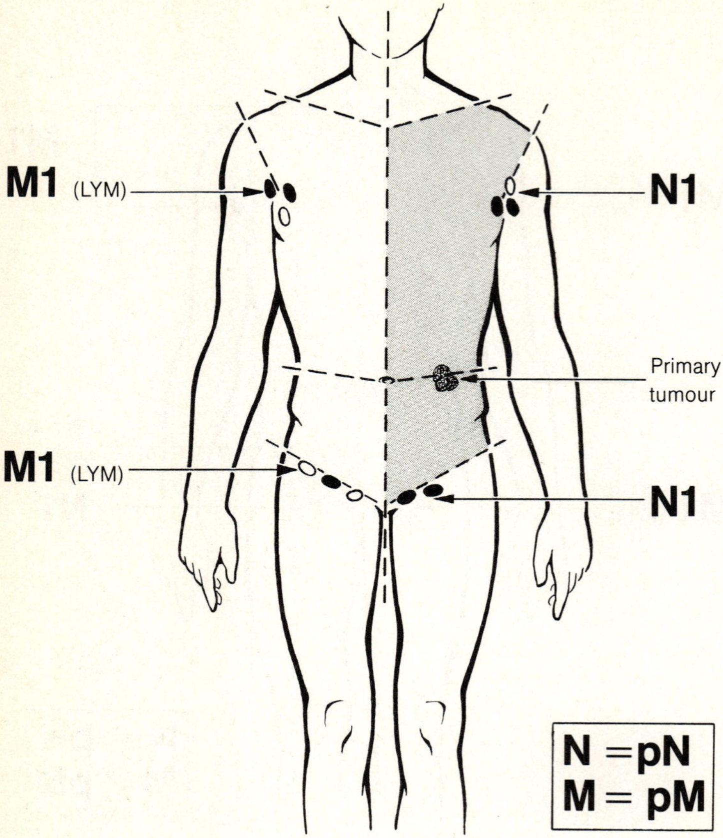

Fig. 211

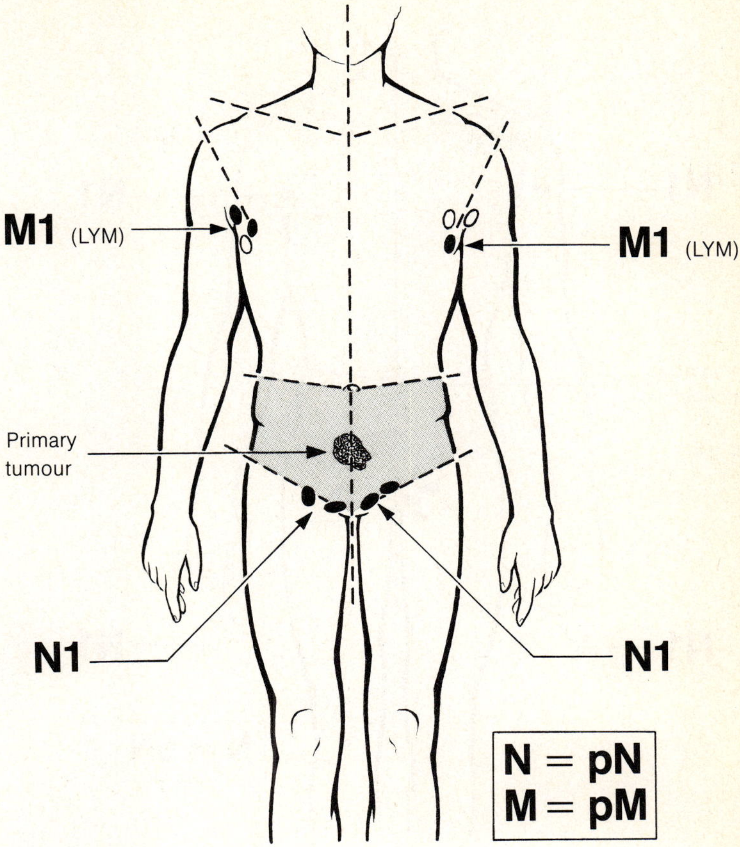

Fig. 212

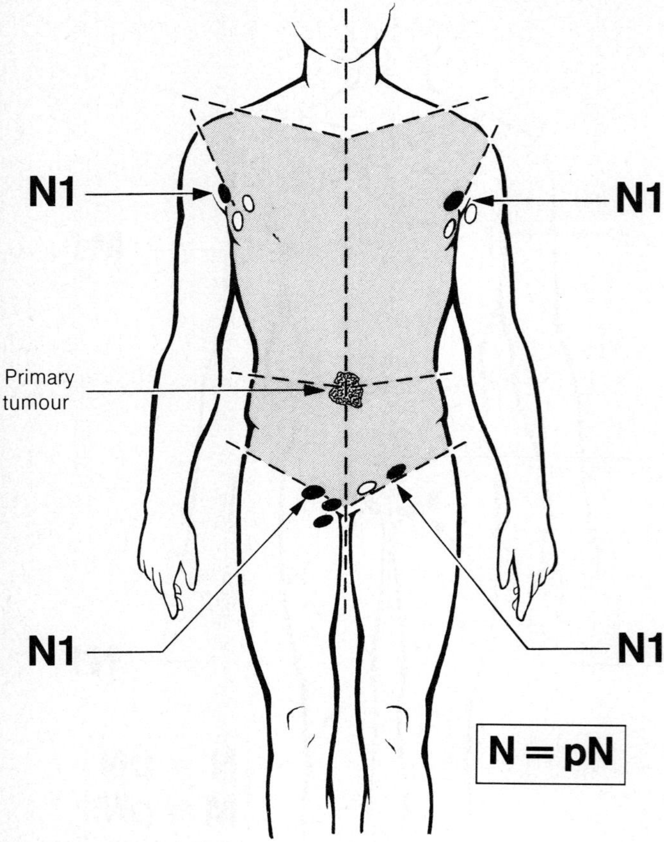

Fig. 213

Distant Metastasis

The definitions of the M categories for all skin tumours are:

M - Distant Metastasis

MX Presence of distant metastasis cannot be assessed
M0 No distant metastasis
M1 Distant metastasis (Figs. 209-212)

Carcinoma of Skin (excluding eyelid, vulva and penis)

(ICD-O 173.0,2–9, 187.7)

Rules for Classification

The classification applies only to carcinoma. There should be histological confirmation of the disease to permit division of cases by histological type.

Regional Lymph Nodes

See p. 152

TNM Clinical Classification

T – Primary Tumour

TX Primary tumour cannot be assessed
T0 No evidence of primary tumour
Tis Carcinoma in situ (Fig. 214)

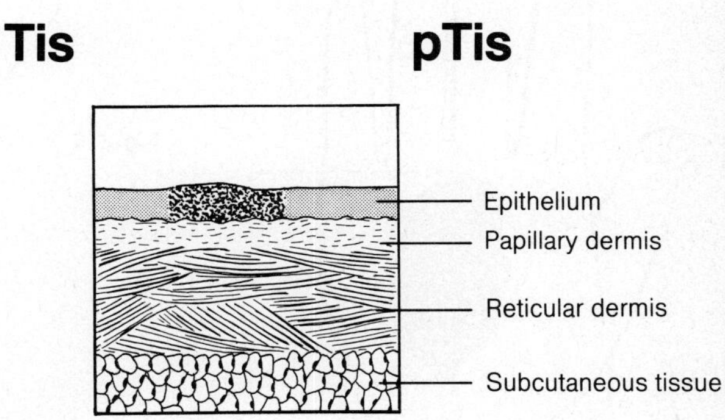

Fig. 214

T1 Tumour 2 cm or less in greatest dimension (Fig. 215)

T2 Tumour more than 2 cm but not more than 5 cm in greatest dimension (Fig. 216)

T3 Tumour more than 5 cm in greatest dimension (Fig. 217)

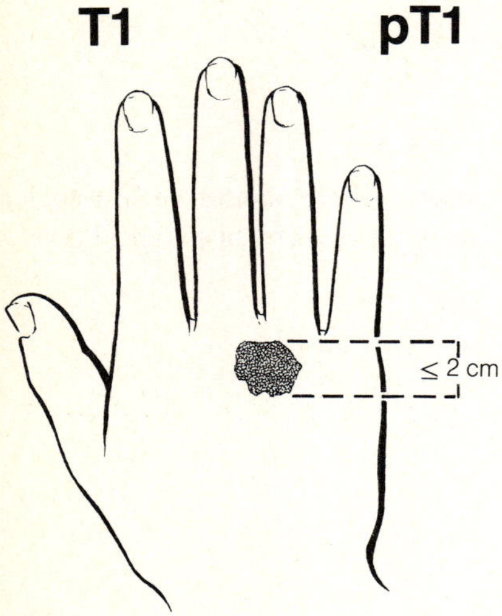

Fig. 215

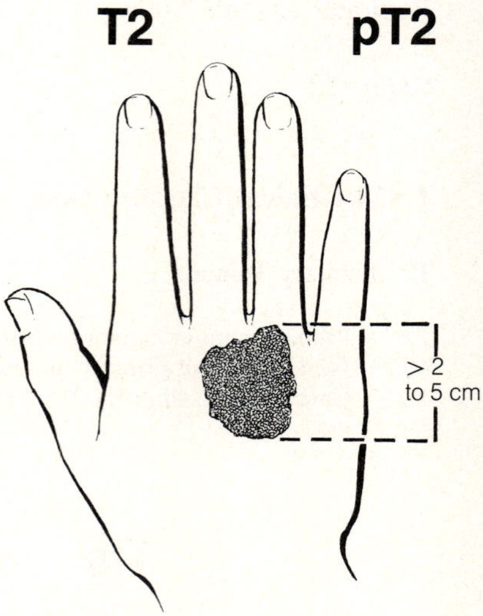

Fig. 216

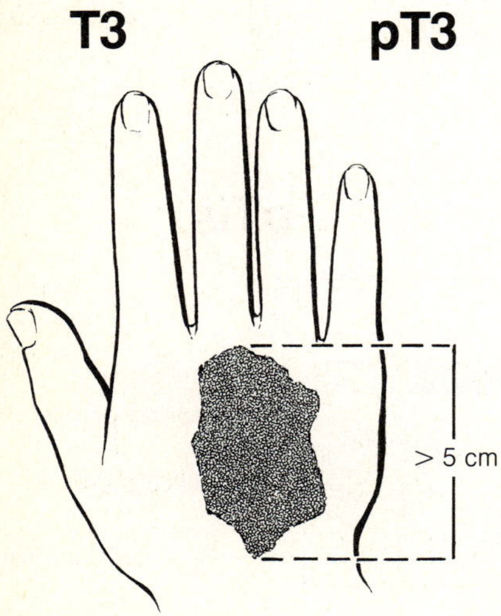

Fig. 217

T4 Tumour invades deep extradermal structures, i.e. cartilage, skeletal muscle or bone (Fig. 218)

Note: In the case of multiple simultaneous tumours, the tumour with the highest T category will be classified, and the number of separate tumours will be indicated in parenthesis, e.g. T2 (5) (Fig. 219).

T4 **pT4**

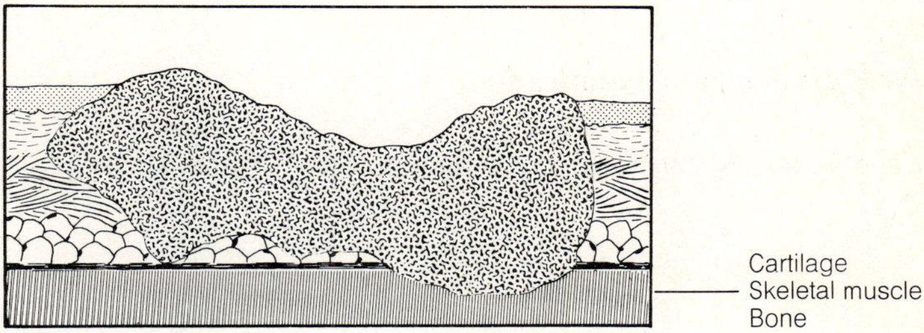

Fig. 218

T2(5) **pT2**(5)

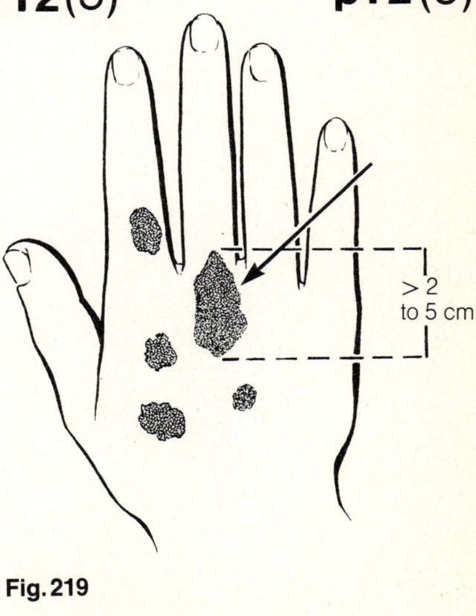

Fig. 219

N - Regional Lymph Nodes

NX Regional lymph nodes cannot be assessed
N0 No regional lymph node metastasis
N1 Regional lymph node metastasis (see Figs. 209-213, pp. 154-158)

M - Distant Metastasis

See p. 158

pTNM Pathological Classification

The pT, pN and pM categories correspond to the T, N and M categories.

Melanoma of Skin (ICD-O 173, 184.4, 187.4, 187.7)

Rules for Classification

There should be histological confirmation of the disease.

Regional Lymph Nodes

See p. 152

TNM Clinical Classification

T – Primary Tumour

The extent of tumour is classified after excision, see pT, p. 170.

N – Regional Lymph Nodes (See also Figs. 209–213, pp. 154–158)

NX Regional lymph nodes cannot be assessed
N0 No regional lymph node metastasis
N1 Metastasis 3 cm or less in greatest dimension in any regional node(s) (Figs. 220, 221)
N2 Metastasis more than 3 cm in greatest dimension in any regional lymph node(s) and/or in-transit metastasis
  N2a Metastasis more than 3 cm in greatest dimension in any regional lymph node(s) (Fig. 222)
  N2b In-transit metastasis (Figs. 223, 224)
  N2c Both (Fig. 225)

Note: In-transit metastasis involves skin or subcutaneous tissue more than 2 cm from the primary tumour but not beyond the regional lymph nodes (see also Fig. 229, p. 169).

N1 **pN1**

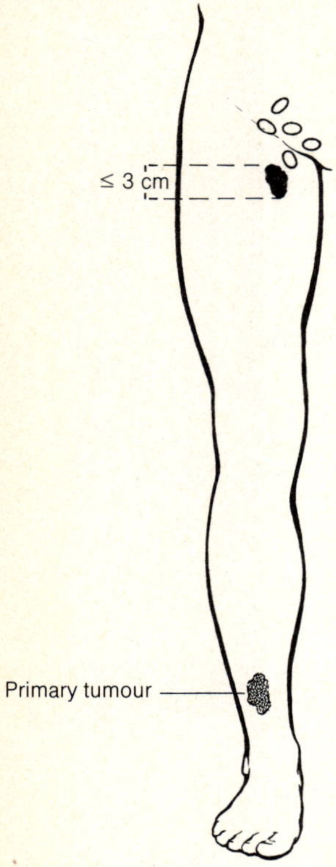

Fig. 220

N1 **pN1**

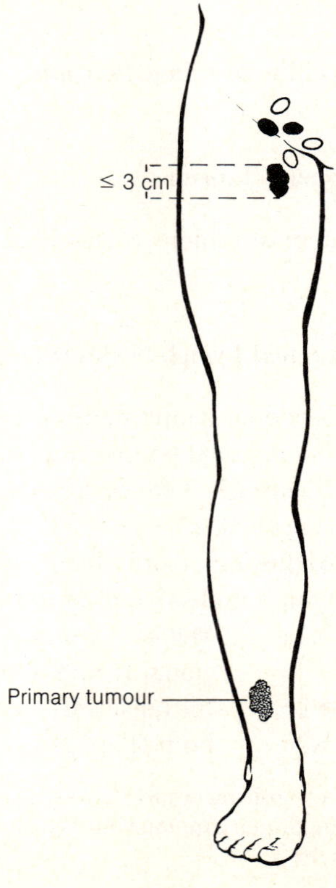

Fig. 221

N2a **pN2a**

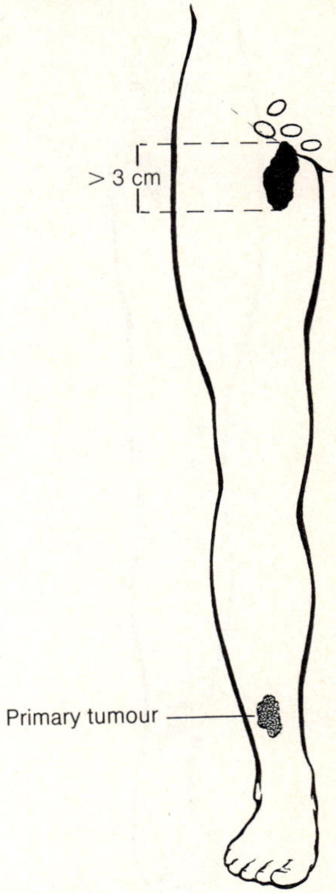

Fig. 222

N2b **pN2b**

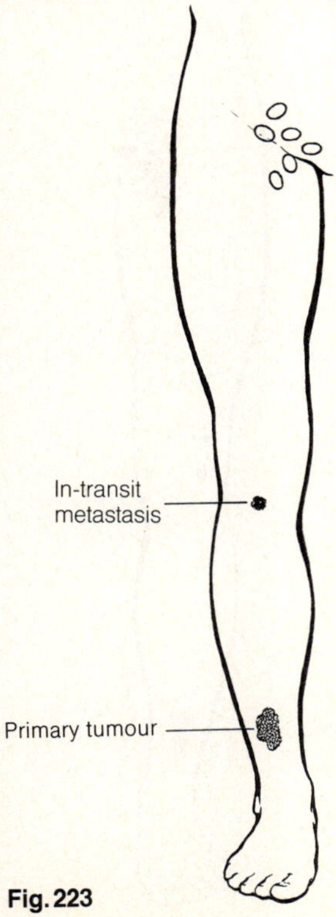

Fig. 223

N2b **pN2b**

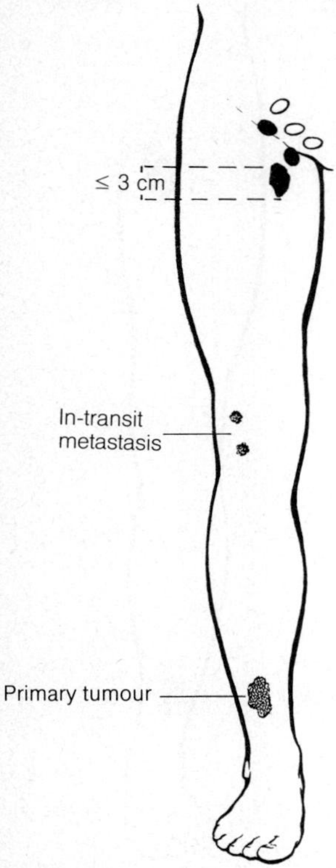

Fig. 224

N2c **pN2c**

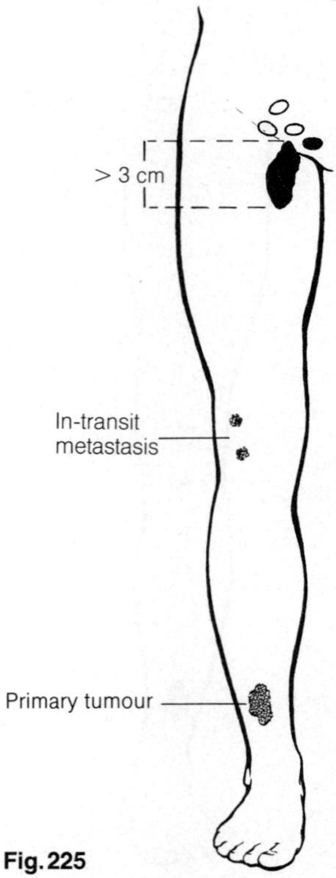

Fig. 225

M– Distant Metastasis

MX Presence of distant metastasis cannot be assessed
M0 No distant metastasis
M1 Distant metastasis
- M1a Metastasis in skin or subcutaneous tissue or lymph node(s) beyond the regional lymph nodes (see Figs. 209–212, pp. 154–157)
- M1b Visceral metastasis

pTNM Pathological Classification

Introductory Note

The pT classification of malignant melanoma considers three histological criteria:

1. Tumour thickness (Breslow) according to the largest vertical diameter of the tumour in millimetres (Fig. 226) (melanoma cells within the epithelium of structures such as hair and sebaceous glands of the skin are not taken into consideration)
2. Clark's "levels" (Fig. 227)
3. Absence or presence of satellites within 2 cm of the primary tumour (Figs. 228, 229)

The definitive pT category is based on these three criteria (Fig. 230).
In case of discrepancy between tumour thickness and level, the pT category is based on the *less favourable finding*.

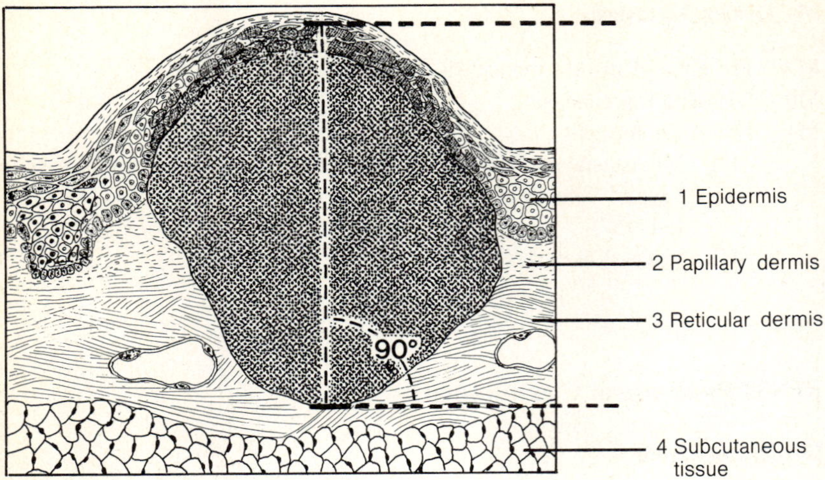
90°
1 Epidermis
2 Papillary dermis
3 Reticular dermis
4 Subcutaneous tissue

a

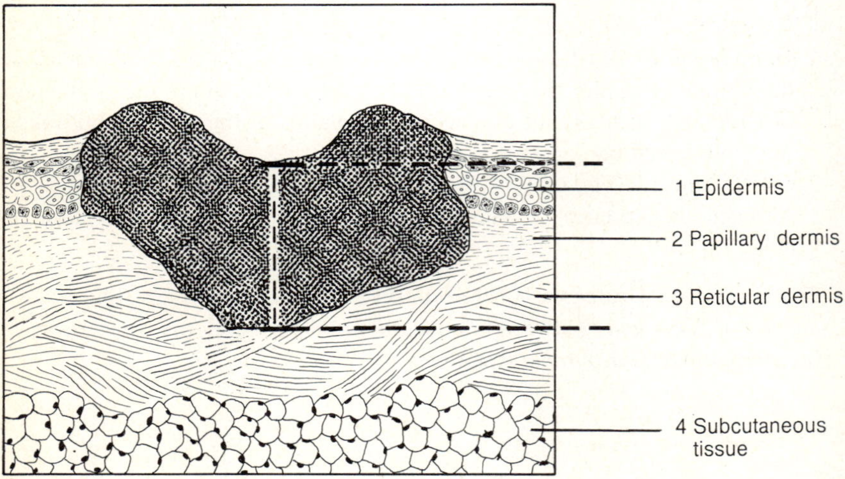
1 Epidermis
2 Papillary dermis
3 Reticular dermis
4 Subcutaneous tissue

b

Fig. 226 a, b

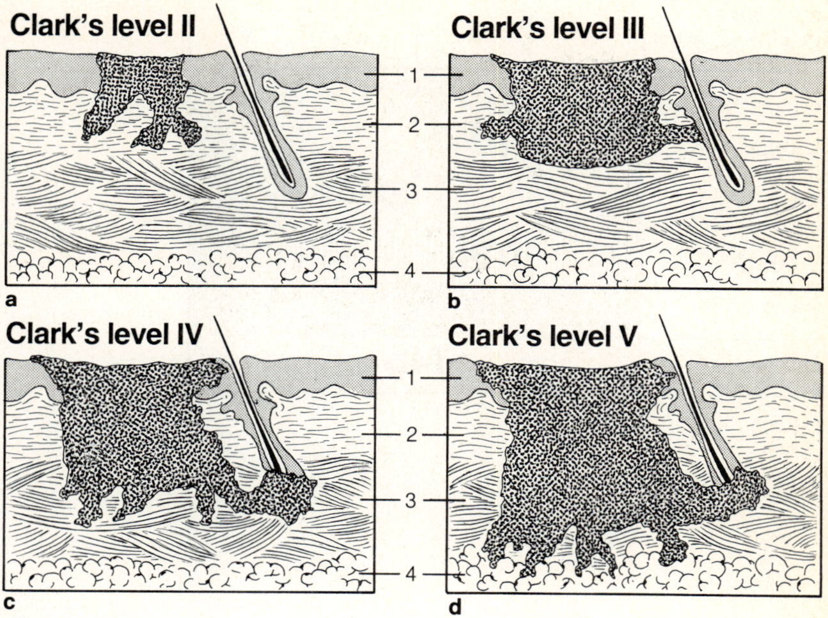

Fig. 227 a-d

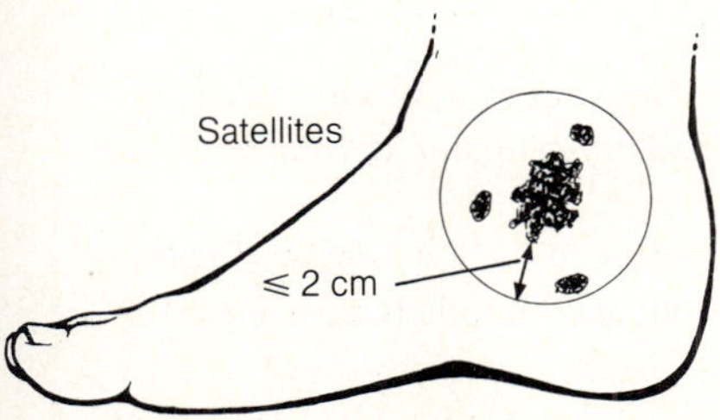

Fig. 228

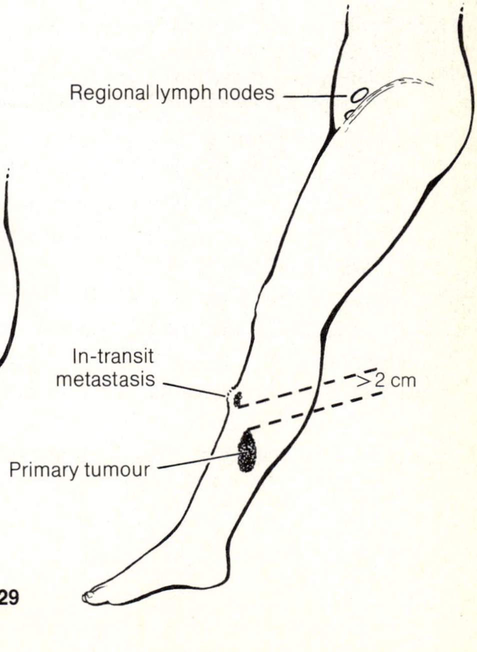

Fig. 229

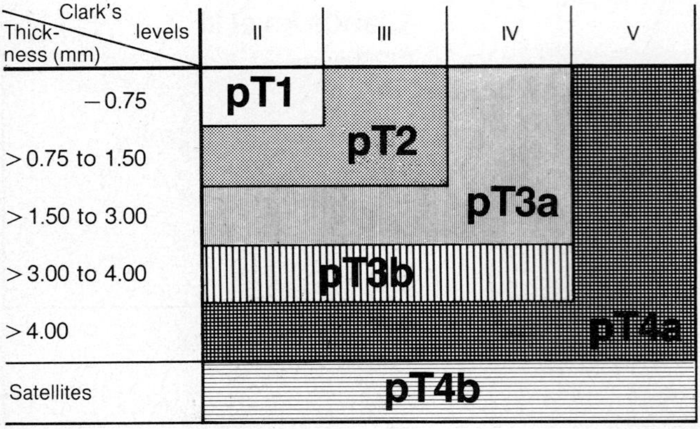

Fig. 230

pT – Primary Tumour

pTX Primary tumour cannot be assessed
pT0 No evidence of primary tumour
pTis Melanoma in situ (Clark's level I) (atypical melanocytic hyperplasia, severe melanocytic dysplasia, not an invasive malignant lesion)

pT1 Tumour 0.75 mm or less in thickness (Fig. 231) and invading the papillary dermis (Clark's level II) (Fig. 227a)

pT2 Tumour more than 0.75 mm but not more than 1.5 mm in thickness (Fig. 232) and/or invading to the papillary-reticular dermal interface (Clark's level III) (Fig. 227b)

pT3 Tumour more than 1.5 mm but not more than 4.0 mm in thickness (Figs. 233, 234) and/or invading the reticular dermis (Clark's level IV) (Fig. 227c)

pT3a Tumour more than 1.5 mm but not more than 3.0 mm in thickness (Fig. 233)

pT3b Tumour more than 3.0 mm but not more than 4.0 mm in thickness (Fig. 234)

pT1

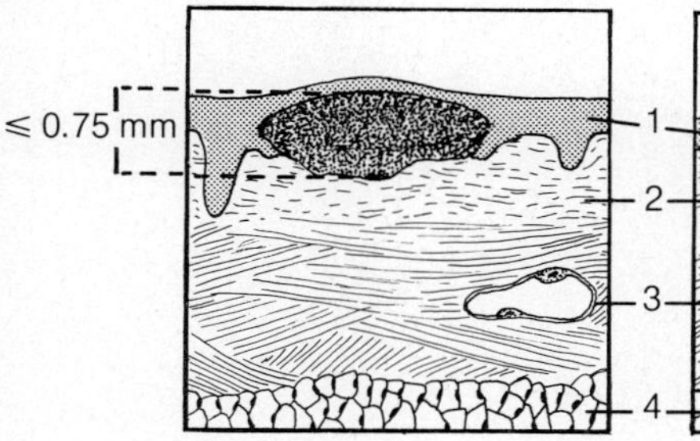

Fig. 231

pT2

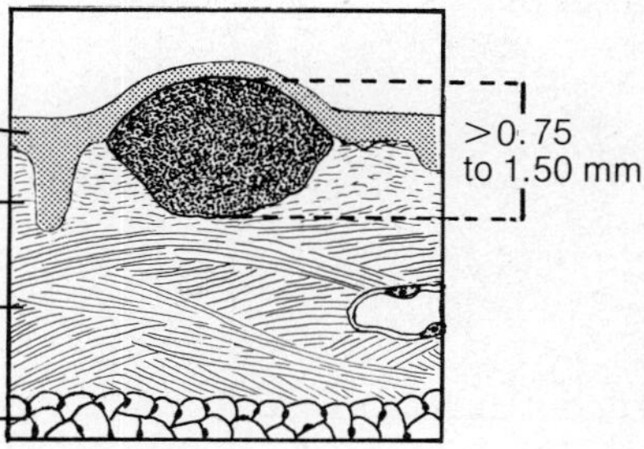

Fig. 232

pT3a

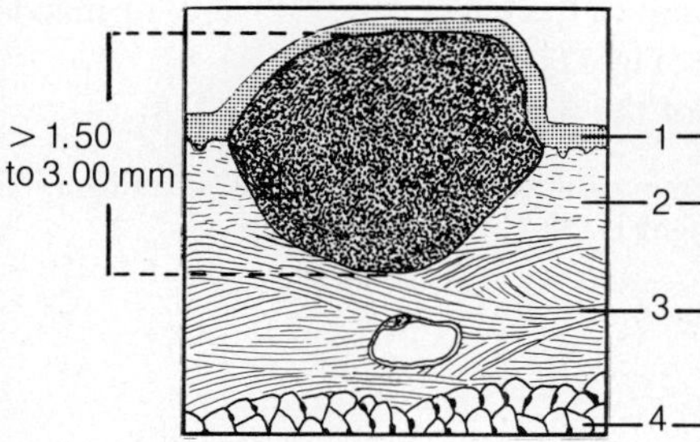

Fig. 233

pT3b

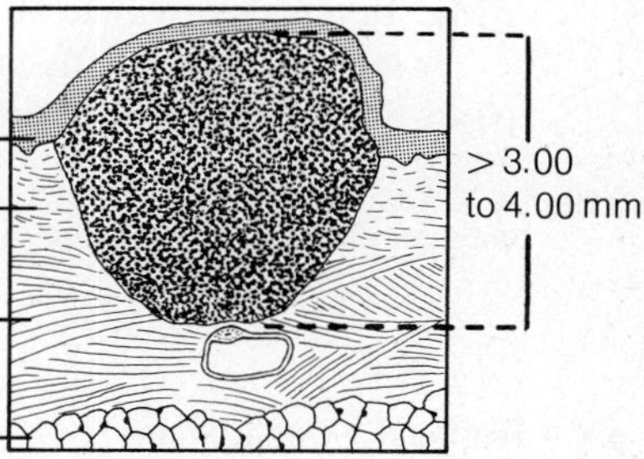

Fig. 234

pT4

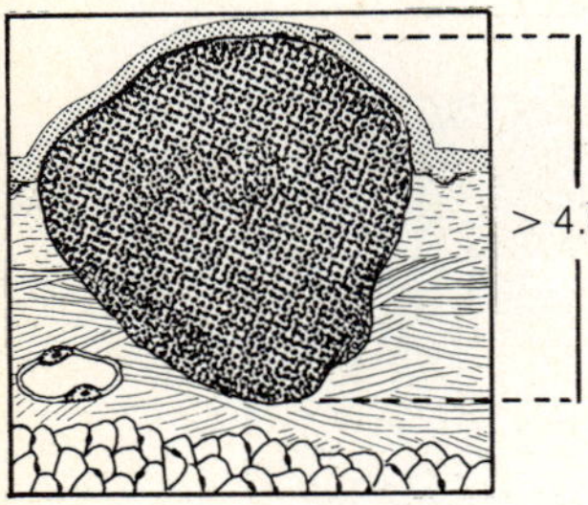

Fig. 235

pT4 Tumour more than 4.0 mm in thickness (Fig. 235) and/or invading subcutaneous tissue (Clark's level V) (Fig. 227 d) and/or satellite(s) within 2 cm of the primary tumour (Fig. 228)

- pT4a Tumour more than 4.0 mm in thickness (Fig. 235) and/or invading subcutaneous tissue (Fig. 227 d)
- pT4b Satellite(s) within 2 cm of the primary tumour (Fig. 228)

Note: In case of discrepancy between tumour thickness and level, the pT category is based on the less favourable finding (Fig. 230).

pN - Regional Lymph Nodes

The pN categories correspond to the N categories.

pM - Distant Metastasis

The pM categories correspond to the M categories.

BREAST TUMOURS (ICD-O 174, 175)

Rules for Classification

The classification applies only to carcinoma. There should be histological confirmation of the disease. The anatomical subsite of origin should be recorded but is not considered in classification.
In the case of multiple simultaneous tumours in one breast, the tumour with the highest T category should be used for classification. Simultaneous bilateral breast cancers should be classified independently.

Anatomical Sites and Subsites (Fig. 236)

Female breast (174):

1. Nipple (174.0)
2. Central portion (174.1)
3. Upper inner quadrant (174.2)
4. Lower inner quadrant (174.3)
5. Upper outer quadrant (174.4)
6. Lower outer quadrant (174.5)
7. Axillary tail (174.6)

Male breast (175)

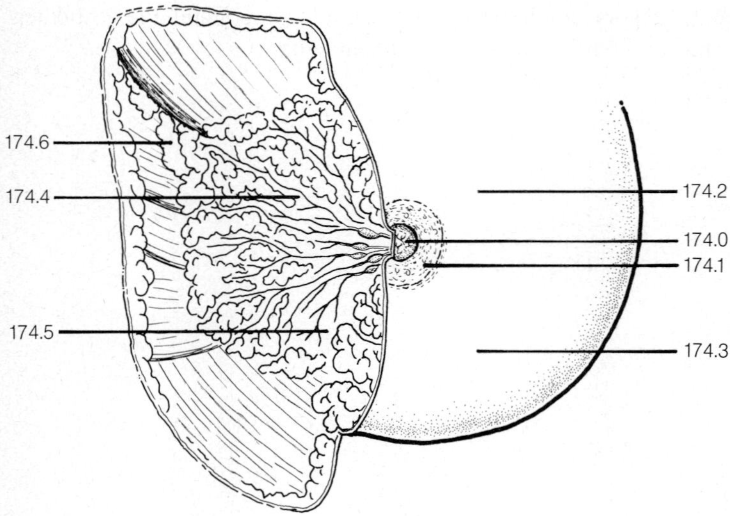

Fig. 236

Regional Lymph Nodes (Fig. 237)

The regional lymph nodes are:

1. *Axillary* (ipsilateral): interpectoral (Rotter's) nodes and lymph nodes along the axillary vein and its tributaries which may be divided into the following levels:
   i) *Level I* (low axilla): lymph nodes lateral to the lateral border of pectoralis minor muscle
   ii) *Level II* (mid-axilla): lymph nodes between the medial and lateral borders of the pectoralis minor muscle and the interpectoral (Rotter's) lymph nodes
   iii) *Level III* (apical axilla): lymph nodes medial to the medial margin of the pectoralis minor muscle including those designated as subclavicular, infraclavicular or apical

   Note: Intramammary lymph nodes are coded as axillary lymph nodes.

2. *Internal mammary* (ipsilateral): lymph nodes in the intercostal spaces along the edge of the sternum in the endothoracic fascia.

Any other lymph node metastasis is coded as a distant metastasis (M1), including supraclavicular, cervical, or contralateral internal mammary lymph nodes (see Fig. 248, p. 181).

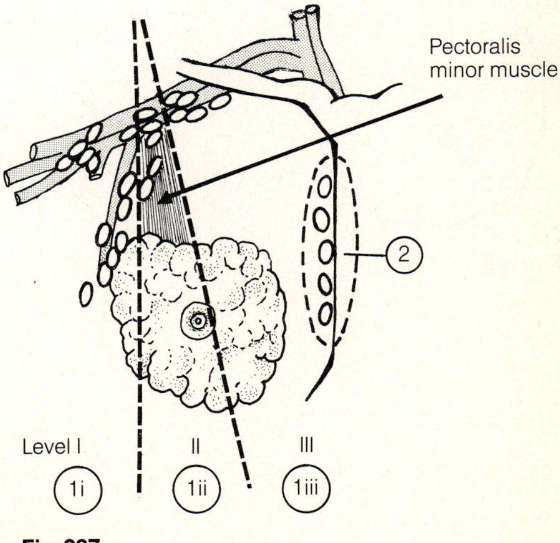

Fig. 237

TN Clinical Classification

T - Primary Tumour

TX Primary tumour cannot be assessed
T0 No evidence of primary tumour
Tis Carcinoma in situ: intraductal carcinoma, *or* lobular carcinoma in situ, *or* Paget's disease of the nipple with no tumour (Fig. 238)

Note: Paget's disease associated with a tumour is classified according to the size of the tumour.

T1 Tumour 2 cm or less in greatest dimension (Fig. 239)
- T1a 0.5 cm or less in greatest dimension
- T1b More than 0.5 cm but not more than 1 cm in greatest dimension
- T1c More than 1 cm but not more than 2 cm in greatest dimension

T2 Tumour more than 2 cm but not more than 5 cm in greatest dimension (Fig. 240)
T3 Tumour more than 5 cm in greatest dimension (Fig. 240)
T4 Tumour of any size with direct extension to chest wall or skin

Note: Chest wall includes ribs, intercostal muscles and serratus anterior muscle but not pectoral muscle.

Tis **pTis**

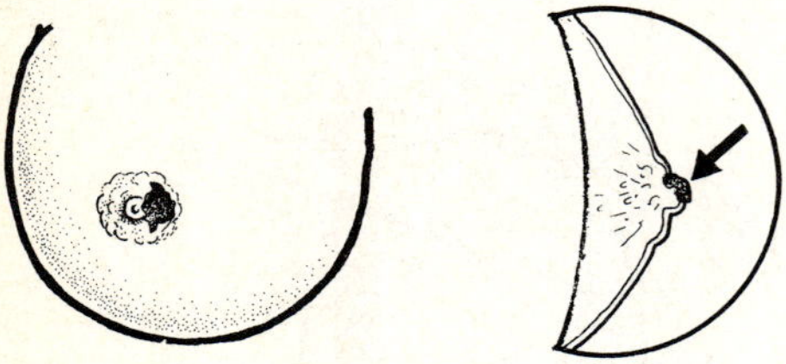

Fig. 238

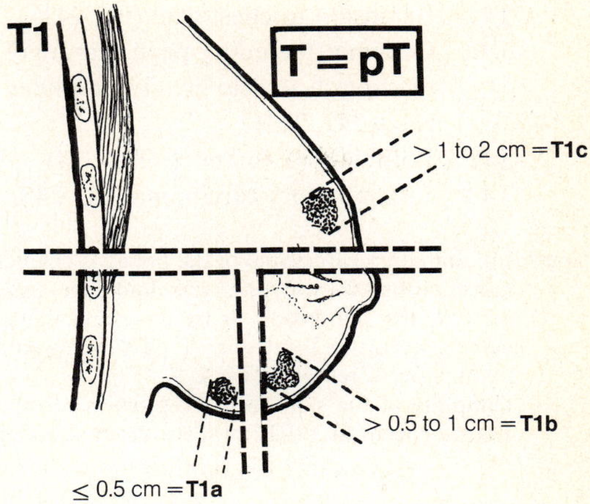

Fig. 239

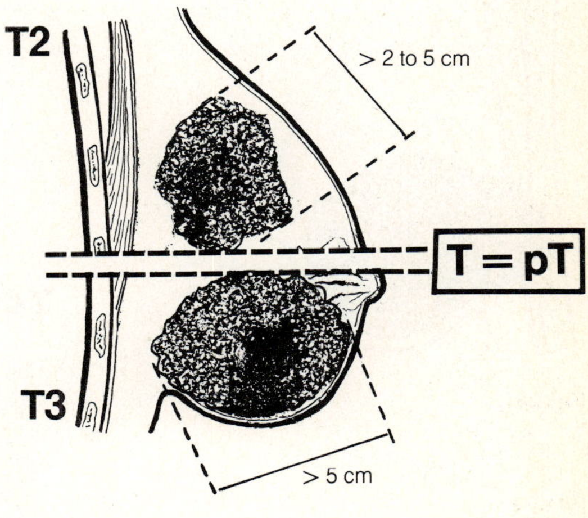

Fig. 240

T4a Extension to chest wall (Fig. 241)

T4b Oedema (including peau d'orange), *or* ulceration of the skin of the breast, *or* satellite skin nodules confined to the same breast (Figs. 242, 243)

T4c Both 4a and 4b above (Fig. 244)

T4d Inflammatory carcinoma (Fig. 245)

Notes: Inflammatory carcinoma of the breast is characterized by diffuse, brawny, induration of the skin with an erysipeloid edge, usually with no underlying palpable mass. If the skin biopsy is negative and there is no localized measurable primary cancer, the T category is pTX when pathologically staging a clinical inflammatory carcinoma (T4d).

Dimpling of the skin, nipple retraction or other skin changes, except those in T4, may occur in T1, T2 or T3 without affecting the classification.

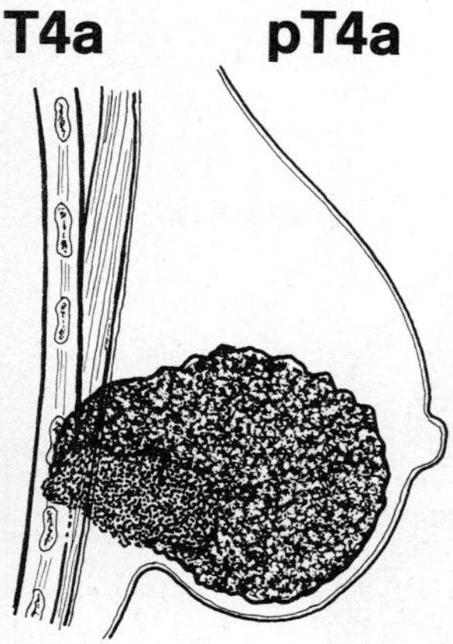

Fig. 241

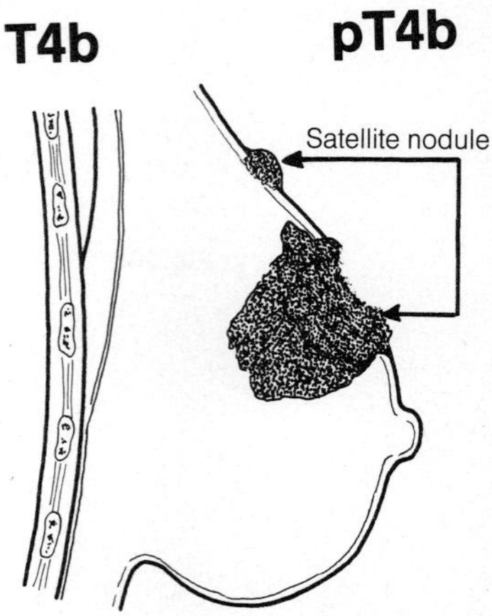

Fig. 242

T4b pT4b

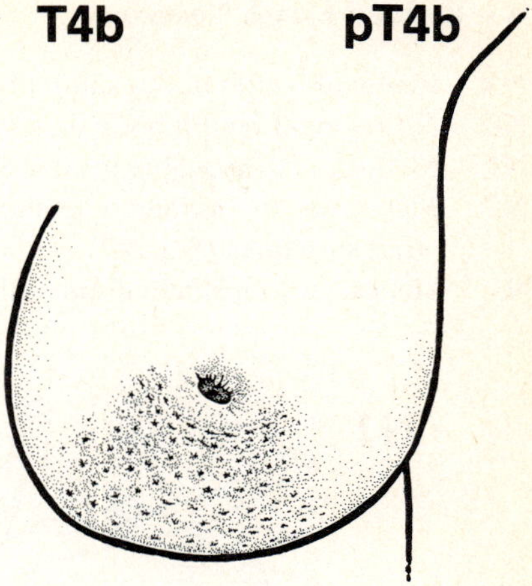

Fig. 243

T4c pT4c

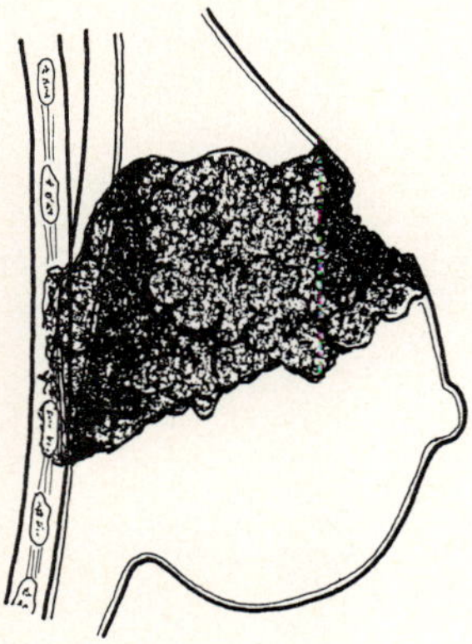

Fig. 244

T4d pT4d

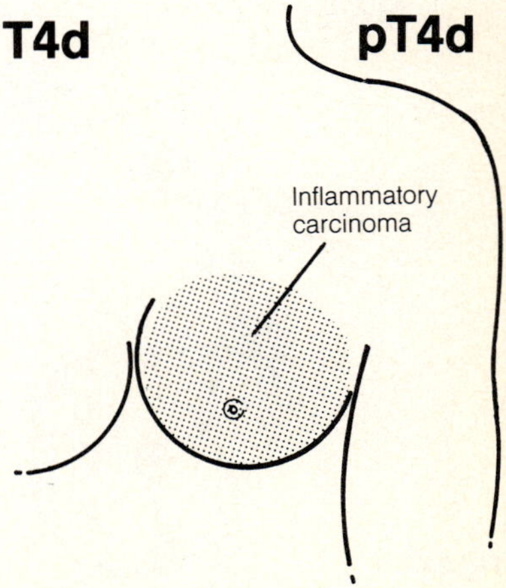

Fig. 245

N – Regional Lymph Nodes

NX Regional lymph nodes cannot be assessed (e.g. previously removed)
N0 No regional lymph node metastasis
N1 Metastasis to movable ipsilateral axillary node(s) (Fig. 246)
N2 Metastasis to ipsilateral axillary node(s) fixed to one another or to other structures (Fig. 247)
N3 Metastasis to ipsilateral internal mammary lymph node(s) (Fig. 248)

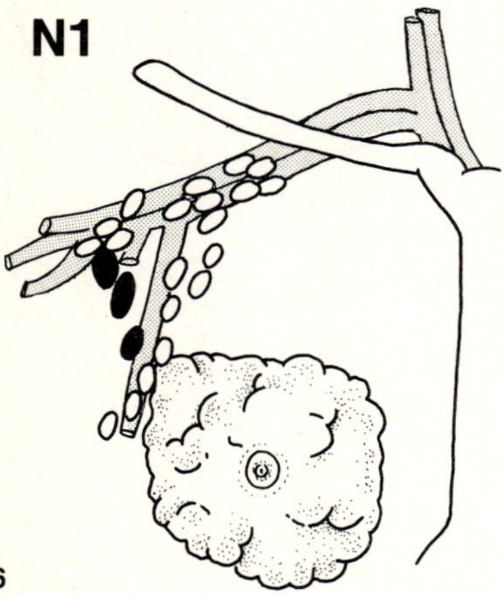

Fig. 246

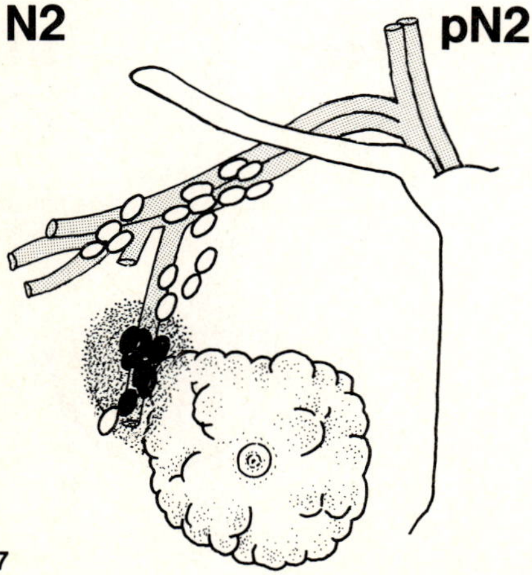

Fig. 247

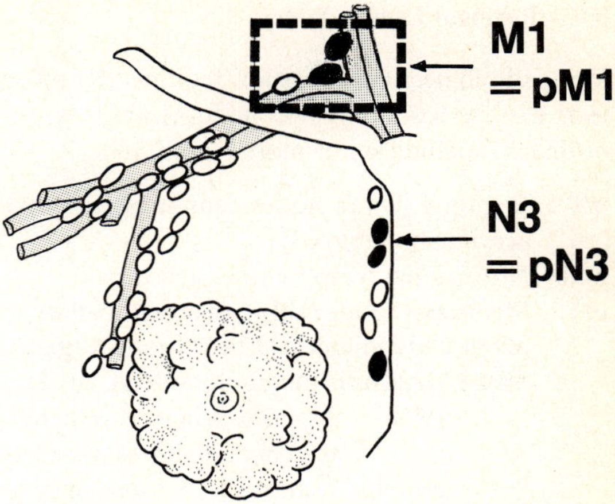

Fig. 248

pTN Pathological Classification

pT – Primary Tumour

The pathological classification requires the examination of the primary carcinoma with no gross tumour at the margins of resection. A case can be classified pT if there is only microscopic tumour in a margin.

The pT categories correspond to the T categories.

When classifying pT the tumour size is a measurement of the *invasive* component. If there is a large in situ component (e.g. 4 cm) and a small invasive component (e.g. 0.5 cm), the tumour is coded pT1a.

pN - Regional Lymph Nodes

The pathological classification requires the resection and examination of at least the low axillary lymph nodes (level I) (see p. 175). Such a resection will ordinarily include six or more lymph nodes.

pNX Regional lymph nodes cannot be assessed (not removed for study or previously removed)

pN0 No regional lymph node metastasis

pN1 Metastasis to movable ipsilateral axillary node(s)

- pN1a Only micrometastasis (none larger than 0.2 cm) (Fig. 249)
- pN1b Metastasis to lymph node(s), any larger than 0.2 cm (Fig. 250)
  - pN1bi Metastasis in one to three lymph nodes, any more than 0.2 cm and all less than 2.0 cm in greatest dimension
  - pN1bii Metastasis to four or more lymph nodes, any more than 0.2 cm and all less than 2.0 cm in greatest dimension
  - pN1biii Extension of tumour beyond the capsule of a lymph node, metastasis less than 2.0 cm in greatest dimension
  - pN1biv Metastasis to a lymph node 2.0 cm or more in greatest dimension

pN2 Metastasis to ipsilateral axillary lymph nodes that are fixed to one another or to other structures (Fig. 247, see p. 180)

pN3 Metastasis to ipsilateral internal mammary lymph node(s) (Fig. 248, see p. 181)

pN1a

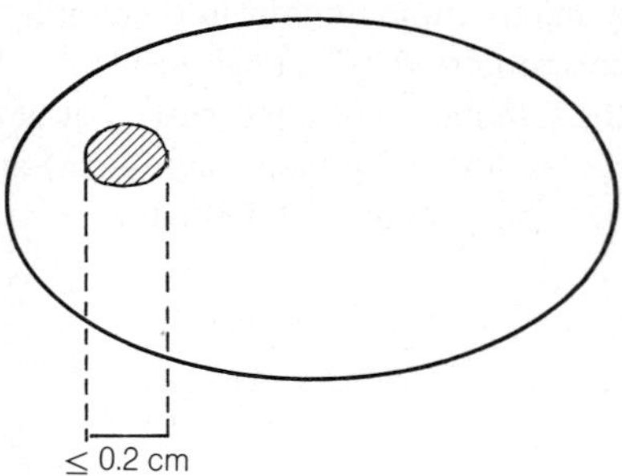

Fig. 249

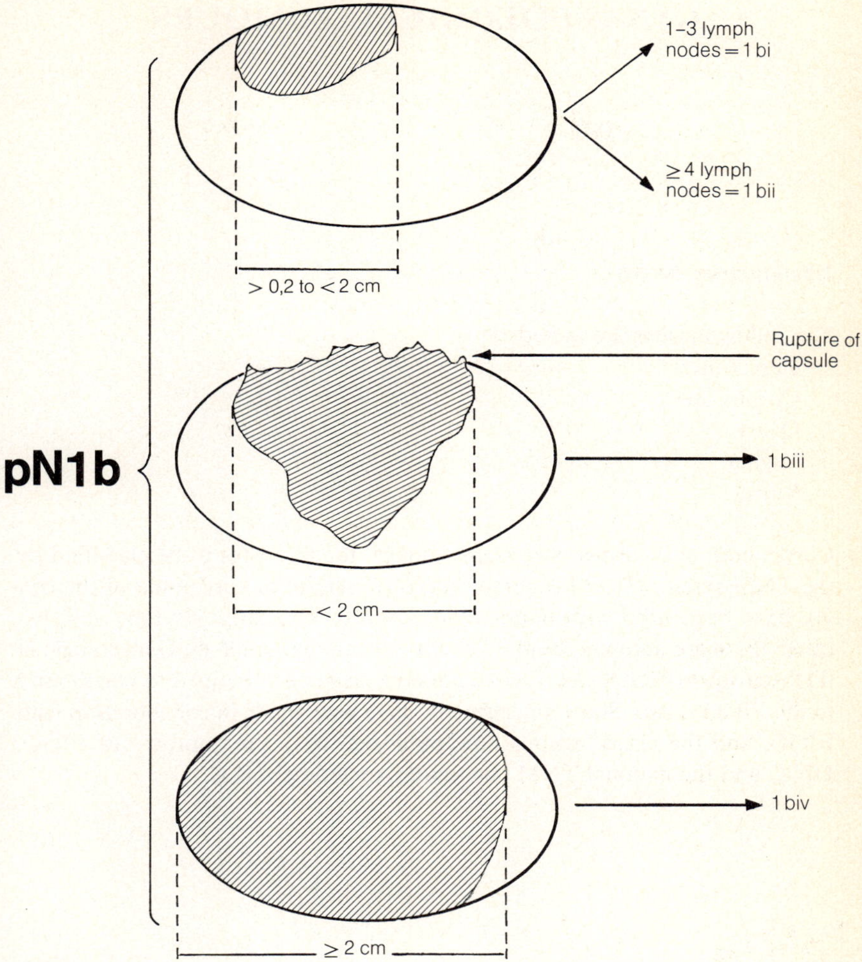
1–3 lymph nodes = 1 bi
≥ 4 lymph nodes = 1 bii
> 0,2 to < 2 cm
Rupture of capsule
1 biii
< 2 cm
1 biv
≥ 2 cm
pN1b

Fig. 250

GYNAECOLOGICAL TUMOURS

Introductory Notes

The following sites are included:

Cervix uteri
Corpus uteri
Ovary
Vagina
Vulva

Cervix uteri and corpus uteri were amongst the first sites to be classified by the TNM system. The "League of Nations" stages for carcinoma of the cervix have been used with minor modifications for nearly 50 years, and, because these are accepted by the Fédération Internationale de Gynécologie et d'Obstétrique (FIGO), the TNM categories have been defined to correspond to the FIGO stages. Some amendments have been made in collaboration with FIGO, and the classifications now published have the approval of FIGO, UICC and the national TNM committees including AJCC.

Cervix Uteri (ICD-O 180)

The definitions of the T categories correspond to the several stages accepted by FIGO. Both systems are included for comparison.

Rules for Classification

The classification applies only to carcinoma. There should be histological confirmation of the disease.

Anatomical Subsites (See Fig. 251)

1. Endocervix (180.0)
2. Exocervix (180.1)

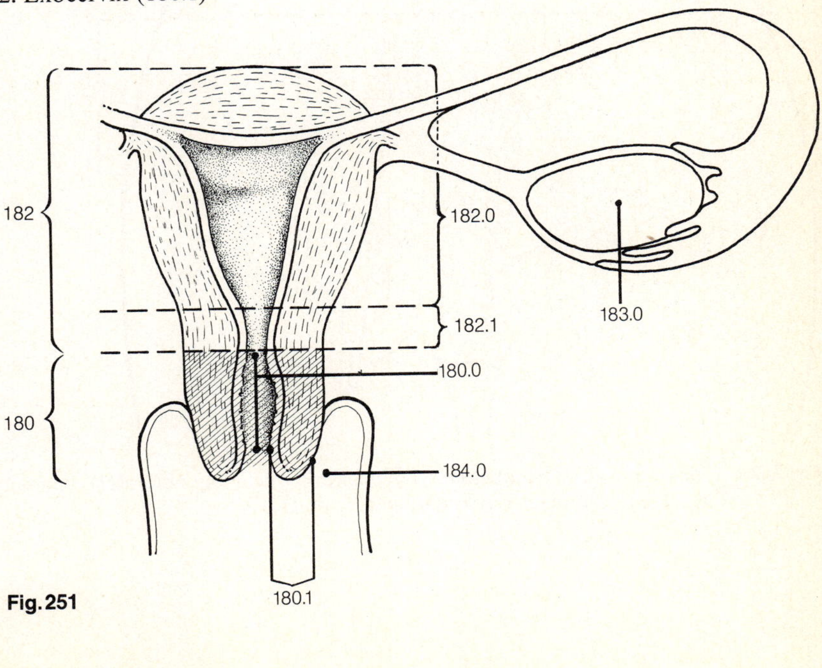

Fig. 251

Regional Lymph Nodes (Fig. 252)

The regional lymph nodes are
(1) paracervical nodes
(2) parametrial nodes
(3) hypogastric (obturator), internal iliac nodes
(4) external iliac nodes
(5) common iliac nodes
(6) presacral nodes
(not shown in Fig. 252) lateral sacral nodes

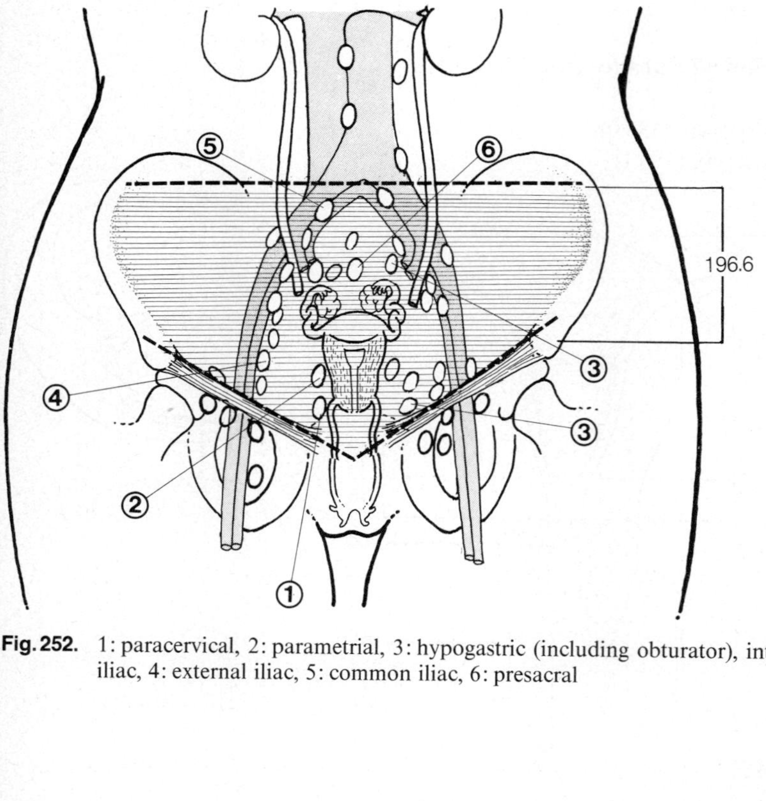

Fig. 252. 1: paracervical, 2: parametrial, 3: hypogastric (including obturator), internal iliac, 4: external iliac, 5: common iliac, 6: presacral

TN Clinical Classification

T - Primary Tumour

TNM categories	FIGO stages	
TX		Primary tumour cannot be assessed
T0		No evidence of primary tumour
Tis	0	Carcinoma in situ
T1	I	Cervical carcinoma confined to uterus (extension to corpus should be disregarded)
T1a	IA	Preclinical invasive carcinoma, diagnosed by microscopy only
T1a1	IA1	Minimal microscopic stromal invasion (Fig. 253)
T1a2	IA2	Tumour with invasive component 5 mm or less in depth, taken from the base of the epithelium, *and* 7 mm or less in horizontal spread (Fig. 254)
T1b	IB	Tumour larger than T1a2 (Fig. 255)
T2	II	Cervical carcinoma invades beyond uterus but not to pelvic wall or to lower third of the vagina (Fig. 256)
T2a	IIA	Without parametrial invasion
T2b	IIB	With parametrial invasion
T3	III	Cervical carcinoma extends to pelvic wall and/or involves the lower third of the vagina and/or causes hydronephrosis or non-functioning kidney (Fig. 257)
T3a	IIIA	Tumour involves lower third of the vagina, no extension to pelvic wall
T3b	IIIB	Tumour extends to pelvic wall and/or causes hydronephrosis or non-functioning kidney
T4	IVA	Tumour invades *mucosa* of bladder or rectum and/or extends beyond true pelvis (Fig. 258)
		Note: The presence of bullous oedema is not sufficient evidence to classify a tumour T4.
M1	IVB	Distant metastasis

TNM: **T1a1** **pT1a1**
FIGO: IA1

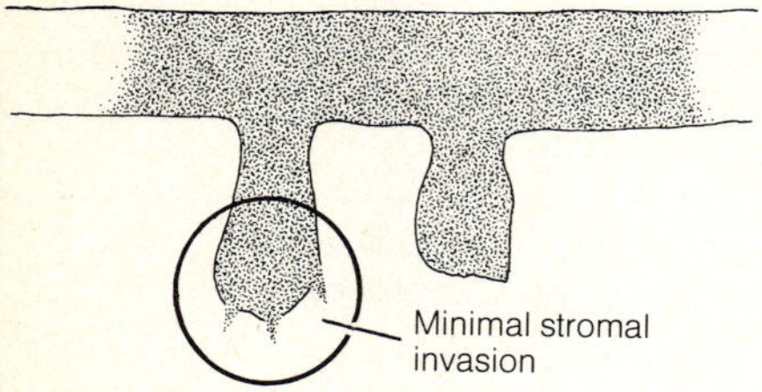

Fig. 253

TNM: **T1a2** **pT1a2**
FIGO: IA2

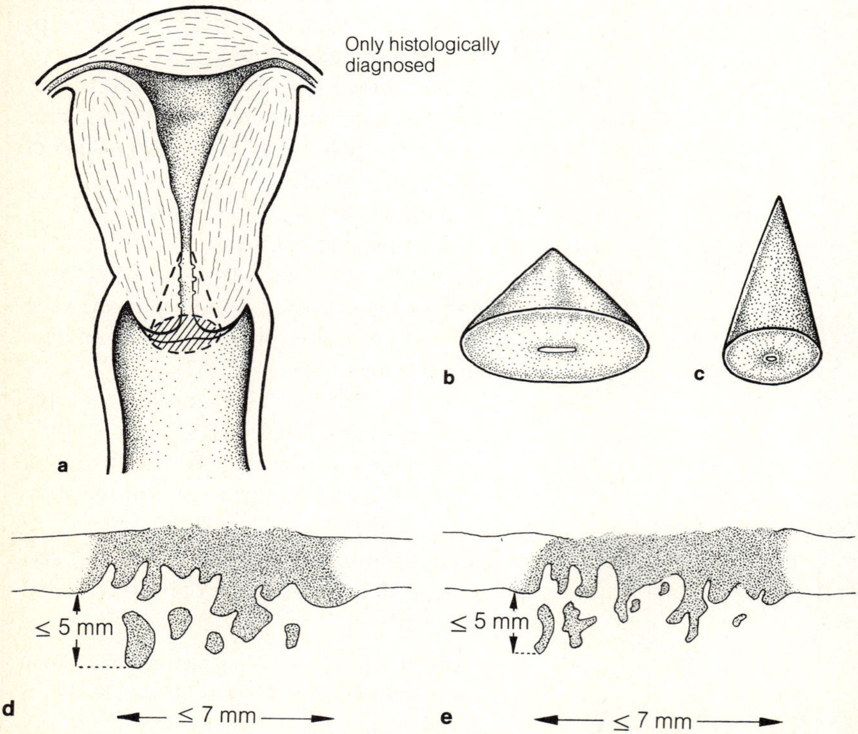

Fig. 254 a-e

TNM: **T1b** **pT1b**

FIGO: IB

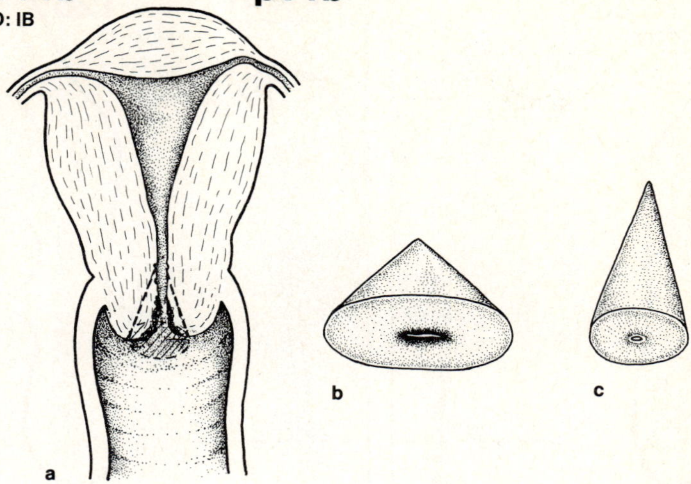

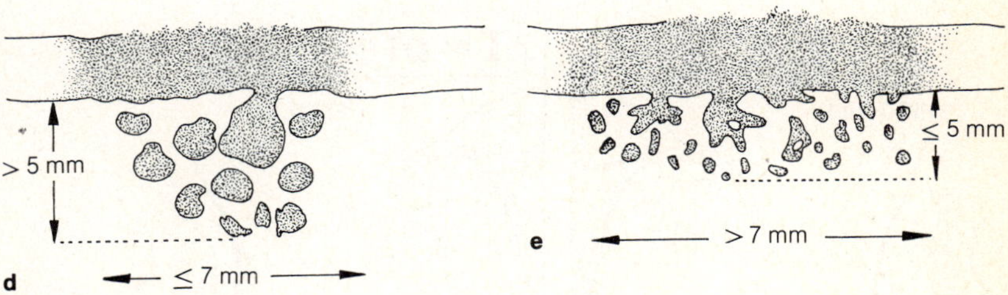

Fig. 255 a-e

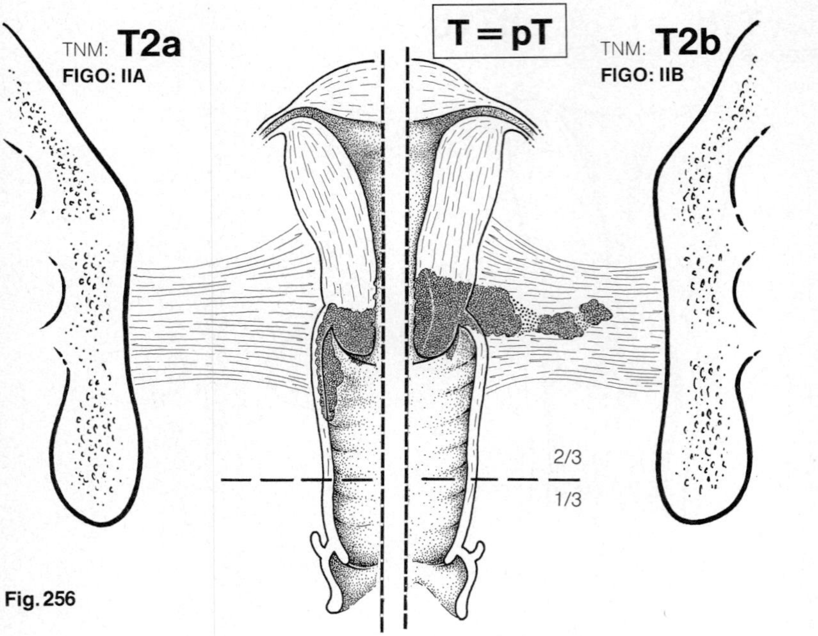

Fig. 256

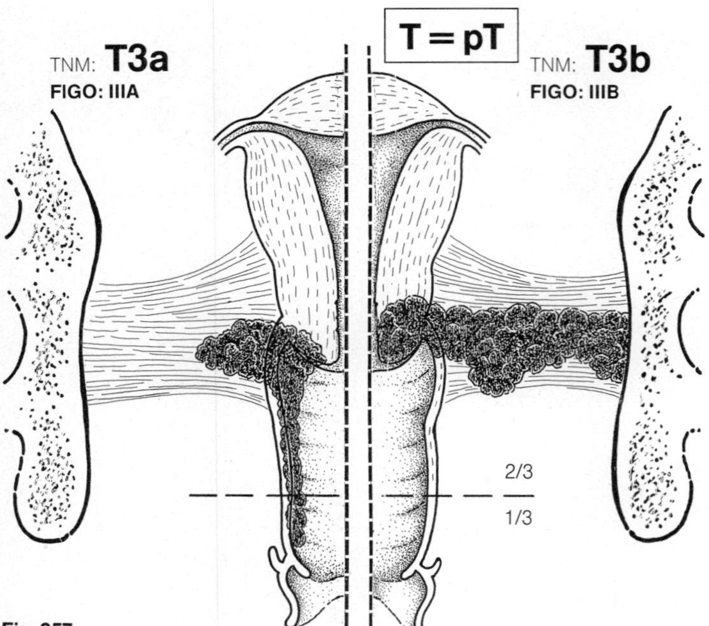

Fig. 257

TNM: **T4**
FIGO: IVA

pT4

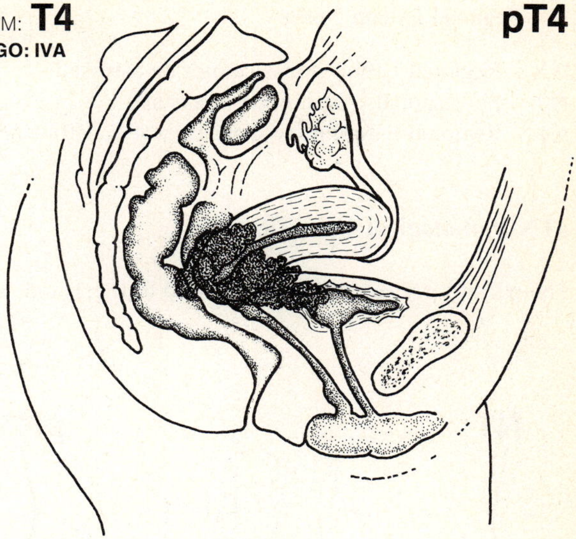

Fig. 258

N – Regional Lymph Nodes

NX Regional lymph nodes cannot be assessed
N0 No regional lymph node metastasis
N1 Regional lymph node metastasis (Fig. 259)

pTN Pathological Classification

The pT and pN categories correspond to the T and N categories.

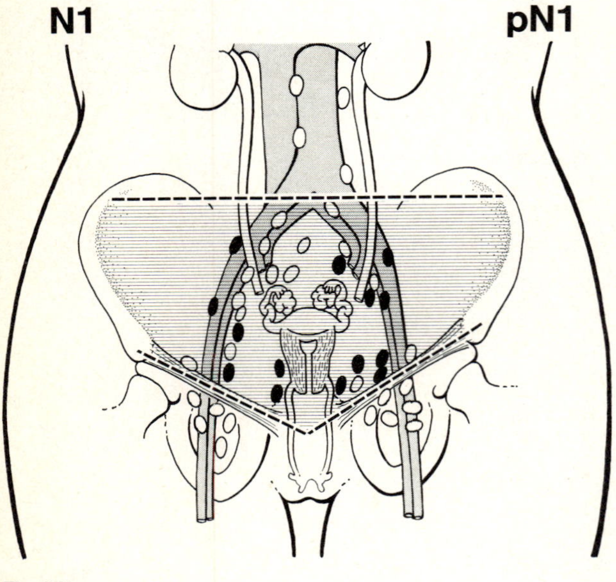

Fig. 259

Corpus Uteri (ICD-O 182)

The definitions of the T categories correspond to the several stages accepted by FIGO. Both systems are included for comparison.

Rules for Classification

The classification applies only to carcinoma. There should be histological verification and grading of the tumour. The diagnosis should be based on examination of specimens taken by endometrial biopsy.

Anatomical Subsites (See Fig. 251, p. 185)

1. Corpus uteri (182.0)
2. Isthmus uteri (182.1)

Regional Lymph Nodes (See Fig. 265, p. 199)

The regional lymph nodes are:
1. The pelvic nodes
- hypogastric (obturator, internal iliac) nodes *(1)*
- common iliac nodes *(2)*
- external iliac nodes *(3)*
- parametrial nodes *(not shown)*
- sacral nodes *(4)*

and
2. The para-aortic nodes *(5)*

TN Clinical Classification

T - Primary Tumour

TNM categories	FIGO stages	
TX		Primary tumour cannot be assessed
T0		No evidence of primary tumour
Tis	0	Carcinoma in situ
T1	I	Tumour confined to corpus (Fig. 260)
T1a	IA	Tumour limited to endometrium
T1b	IB	Invasion ≤1/2 myometrium
T1c	IC	Invasion >1/2 myometrium
T2	II	Tumour invades cervix but does not extend beyond uterus (Fig. 261)
T2a	IIA	Endocervical glandular involvement only
T2b	IIB	Cervical stromal invasion
T3 and/or N1	III	Local and/or regional spread as specified in T3a, b, N1 and FIGO IIIA, B, C below
T3a	IIIA	Tumour involves serosa and/or adnexa (direct extension or metastasis) and/or positive peritoneal cytology (Fig. 262)
T3b	IIIB	Vaginal involvement (Fig. 262) (direct extension or metastasis)
N1	IIIC	Metastasis to pelvic and/or para-aortic lymph nodes (Fig. 264)
T4	IVA	Tumour invades bladder mucosa and/or bowel mucosa (Fig. 263)
M1	IVB	Distant metastasis (excluding metastasis to vagina, pelvic serosa or adnexa, including metastasis to intra-abdominal lymph nodes other than para-aortic and/or inguinal lymph nodes)

Note: For histological grading see the following publications: FIGO (1989) Annual report on the results of treatment of gynecological cancer. Int J Gynecol Obstet 28: 189-193; FIGO (1990) Changes in gynecologic staging by the International Federation of Gynecology and Obstetrics. Am J Obstet Gynecol 162: 610-611.

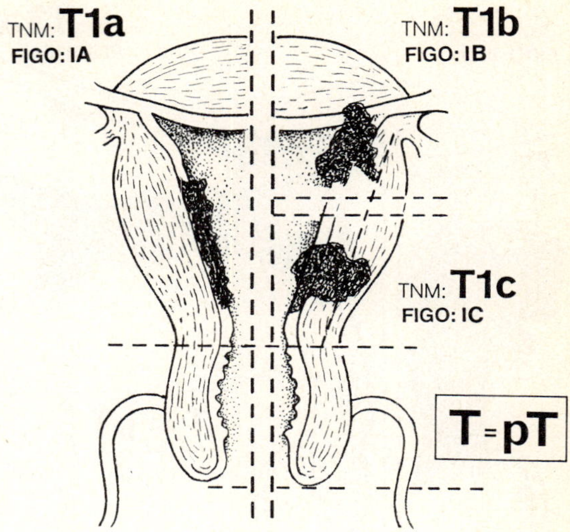

Fig. 260

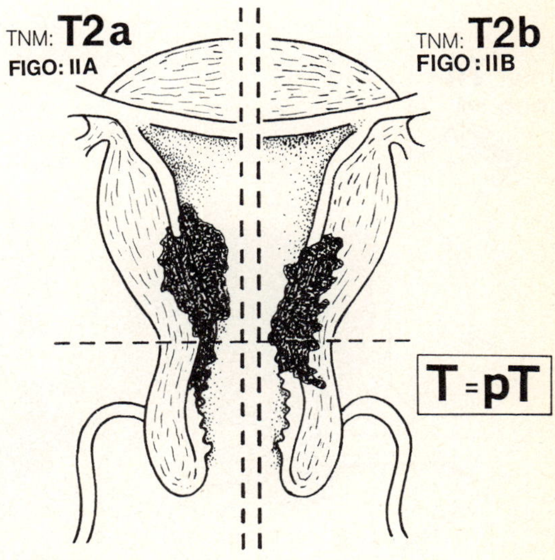

Fig. 261

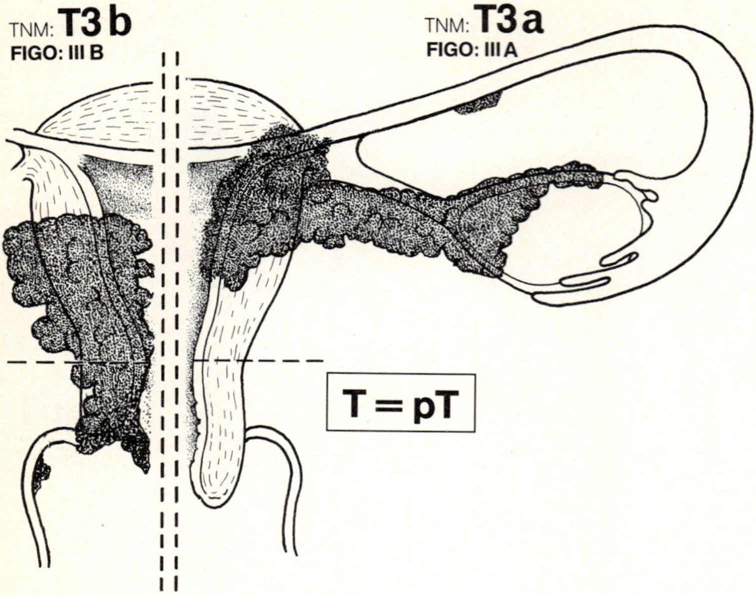

Fig. 262

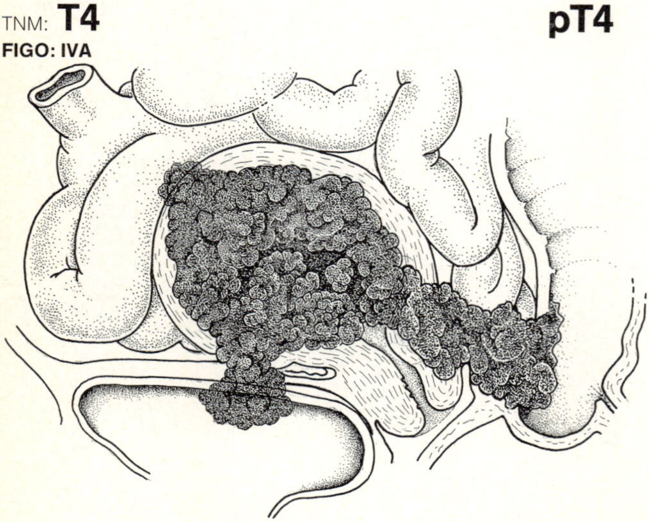

Fig. 263

N - Regional Lymph Nodes

NX Regional lymph nodes cannot be assessed
N0 No regional lymph node metastasis
N1 Regional lymph node metastasis (Fig. 264)

pTN Pathological Classification

The pT and pN categories correspond to the T and N categories.

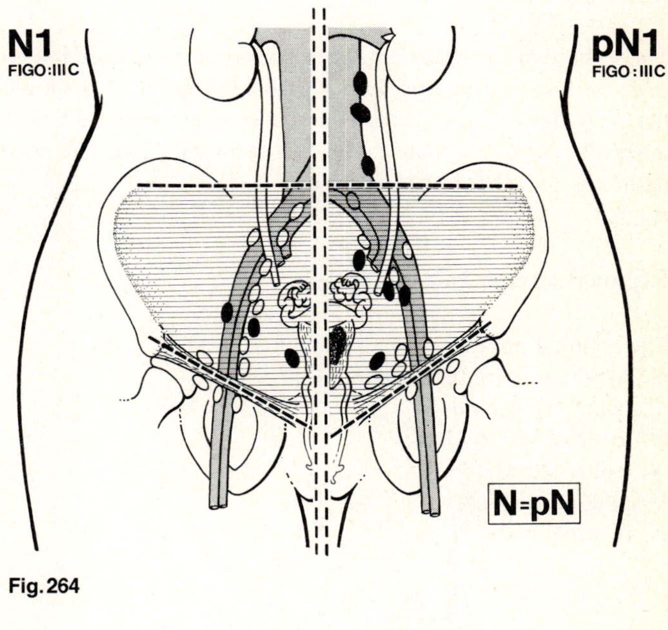

Fig. 264

Ovary (ICD-O 183.0) (See Fig. 251, p. 185)

The definitions of the T categories correspond to the several stages accepted by FIGO. Both systems are included for comparison.

Rules for Classification

There should be histological confirmation of the disease to permit division of cases by histological type. In accordance with FIGO, a simplified version of the WHO histological typing (International Histological Classification of Tumours No. 9, WHO, Geneva 1973) is recommended. The degree of differentiation (grade) should be recorded.

Regional Lymph Nodes (Fig. 265)

The regional nodes are
(1) hypogastric (obturator) nodes
(2) common iliac nodes
(3) external iliac nodes
(4) lateral sacral nodes
(5) para-aortic nodes
(6) inguinal nodes

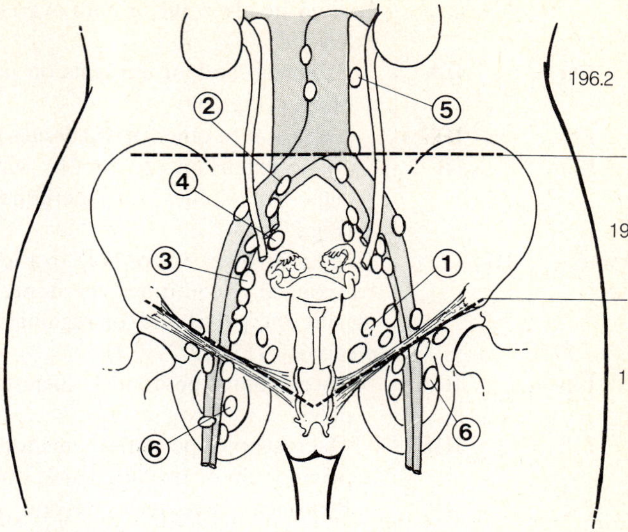

Fig. 265. *1* hypogastric; *2* common iliac; *3* external iliac; *4* lateral sacral; *5* para-aortic; *6* inguinal

TNM Clinical Classification

T – Primary Tumour

TNM categories	FIGO stages	
TX		Primary tumour cannot be assessed
T0		No evidence of primary tumour
T1	I	Tumour limited to ovaries
T1a	IA	Tumour limited to one ovary; capsule intact, no tumour on ovarian surface (Fig. 266)
T1b	IB	Tumour limited to both ovaries; capsules intact, no tumour on ovarian surface (Fig. 267)
T1c	IC	Tumour limited to one or both ovaries with any of the following: capsule ruptured, tumour on ovarian surface, malignant cells in ascites or peritoneal washing (Fig. 268)

T2	II	Tumour involves one or both ovaries with pelvic extension
T2a	IIA	Extension and/or implants on uterus and/or tube(s) (Fig. 269)
T2b	IIB	Extension to other pelvic tissues (Fig. 270)
T2c	IIC	Pelvic extension (2a or 2b) with malignant cells in ascites or peritoneal washing (Fig. 271)
T3 and/ or N1	III	Tumour involves one or both ovaries with microscopically confirmed peritoneal metastasis outside the pelvis and/or regional lymph node metastasis (Figs. 272–274)
T3a	IIIA	Microscopic peritoneal metastasis beyond pelvis
T3b	IIIB	Macroscopic peritoneal metastasis beyond pelvis, 2 cm or less in greatest dimension
T3c and/ or N1	IIIC	Peritoneal metastasis beyond pelvis more than 2 cm in greatest dimension and/or regional lymph node metastasis
M1	IV	Distant metastasis (excludes peritoneal metastasis) (Fig. 273)

Note: Liver capsule metastasis is T3/stage III, liver parenchymal metastasis M1/stage IV. Pleural effusion must have positive cytology for M1/stage IV (Fig. 273).

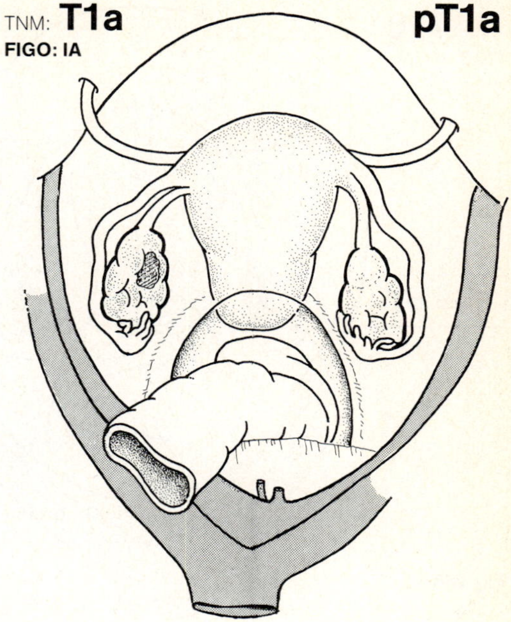

Fig. 266

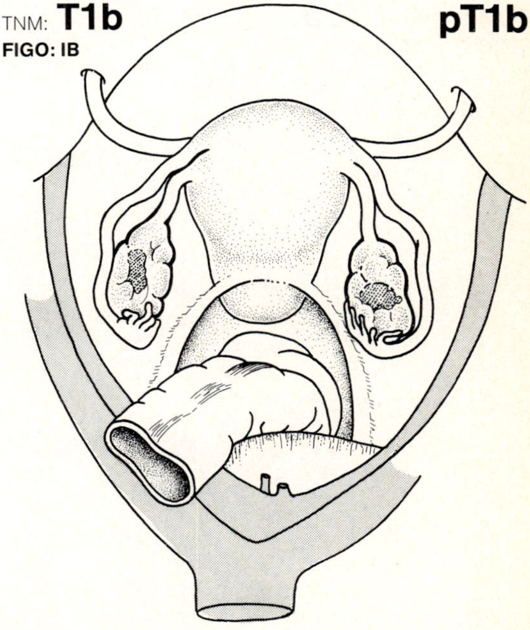

Fig. 267

TNM: **T1c**
FIGO: IC

TNM: **T1c**
FIGO: IC

T = pT

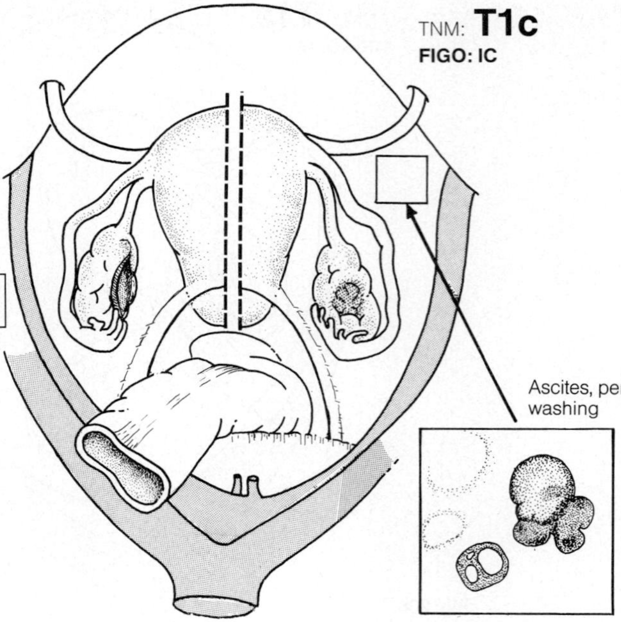

Fig. 268

TNM: **T2a**
FIGO: IIA

pT2a

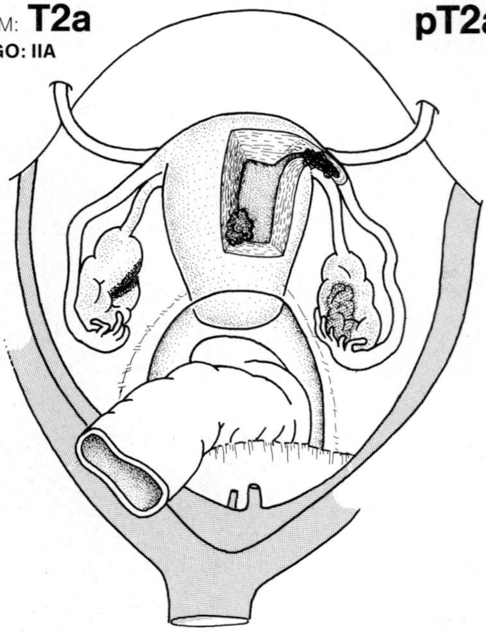

Fig. 269

TNM: **T2b** **pT2b**

FIGO: IIB

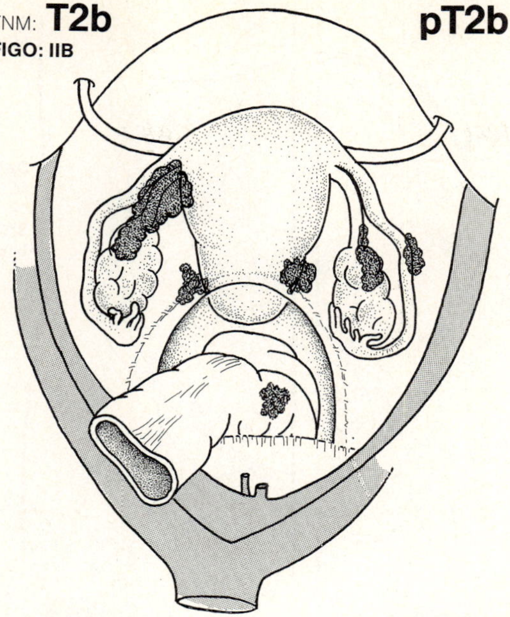

Fig. 270

TNM: **T2c** **pT2c**

FIGO: IIC

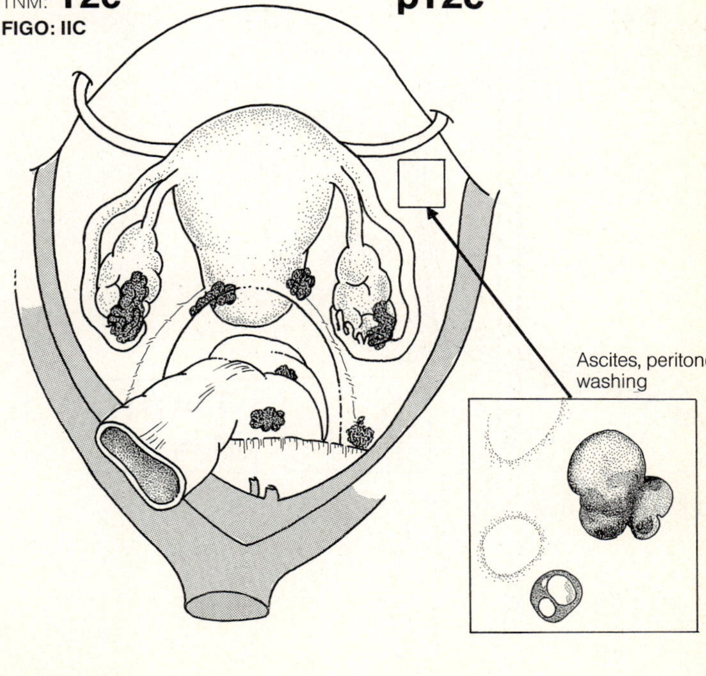

Fig. 271

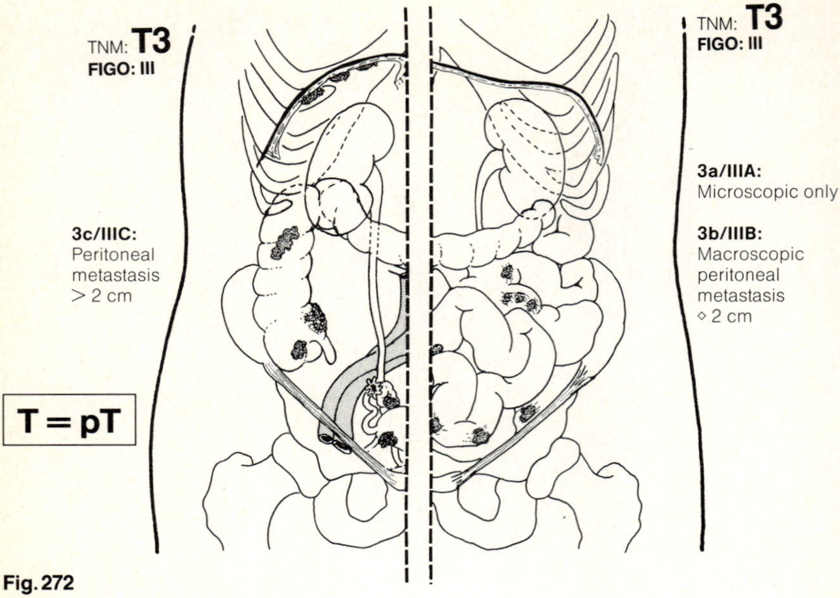

Fig. 272

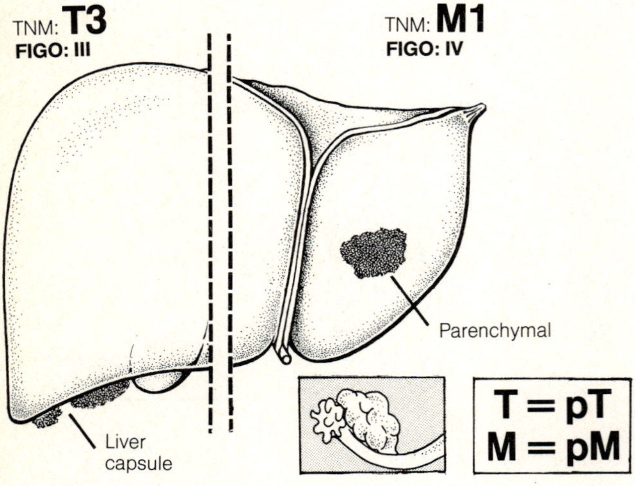

Fig. 273

N – Regional Lymph Nodes

NX Regional lymph nodes cannot be assessed
N0 No regional lymph node metastasis
N1 Regional lymph node metastasis (Fig. 274)

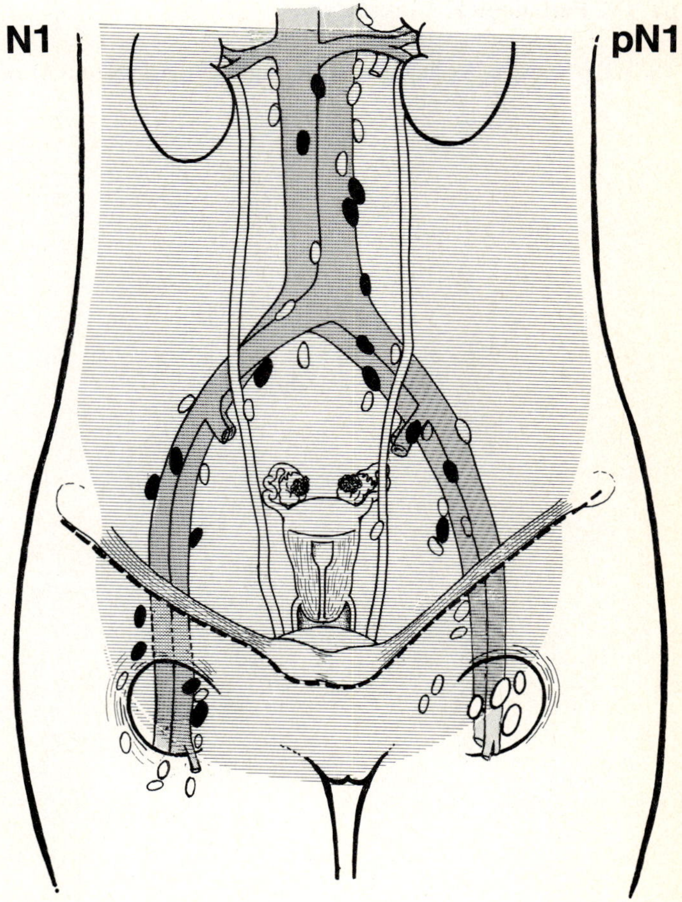

Fig. 274

M – Distant Metastasis

MX Presence of distant metastasis cannot be assessed
M0 No distant metastasis
M1 Distant metastasis (Fig. 273)

pTNM Pathological Classification

The pT, pN and pM categories correspond to the T, N and M categories.

Vagina (ICD-O 184.0) (Fig. 275)

The definitions of the T categories correspond to the several stages accepted by FIGO. Both systems are included for comparison.

Rules for Classification

The classification applies to primary carcinoma only.
Tumours present in the vagina as secondary growths from either genital or extragenital sites should be excluded.
A tumour that has extended to the portio and reached the external os should be classified as carcinoma of the cervix.
A tumour involving the vulva should be classified as carcinoma of the vulva.
There should be histological confirmation of the disease.

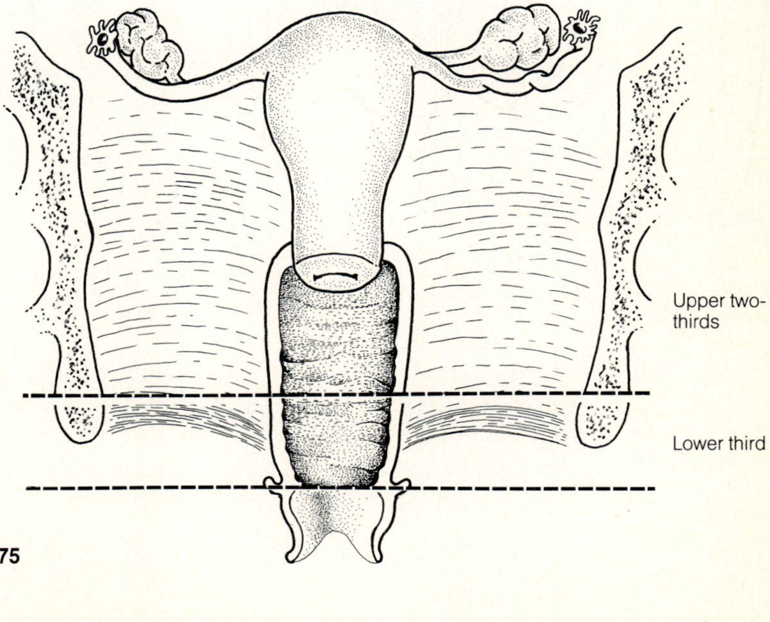

Fig. 275

Regional Lymph Nodes

Upper Two-Thirds of Vagina
The pelvic nodes (Fig. 276)

Lower Third of Vagina
The inguinal nodes (Fig. 277)

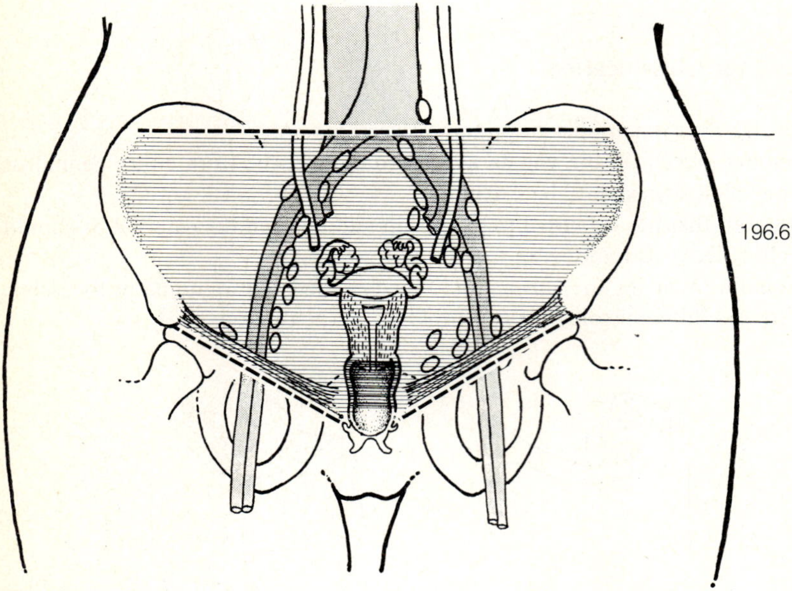

Fig. 276

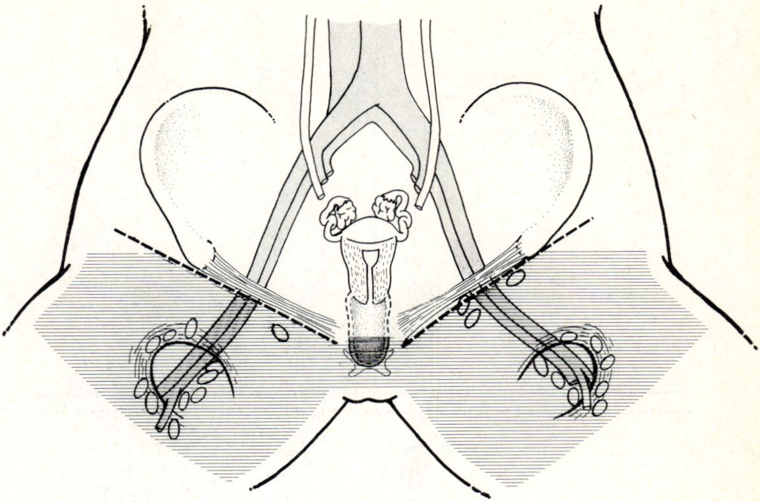

Fig. 277

TN Clinical Classification

T - Primary Tumour

TNM categories	FIGO stages	
TX		Primary tumour cannot be assessed
T0		No evidence of primary tumour
Tis	0	Carcinoma in situ
T1	I	Tumour confined to vagina (Fig. 278)
T2	II	Tumour invades paravaginal tissues but does not extend to pelvic wall (Fig. 279)
T3	III	Tumour extends to pelvic wall (Fig. 280)
T4	IVA	Tumour invades mucosa of bladder or rectum and/or extends beyond the true pelvis (Fig. 281) **Note:** The presence of bullous oedema is not sufficient evidence to classify a tumour T4.
M1	IVB	Distant metastasis

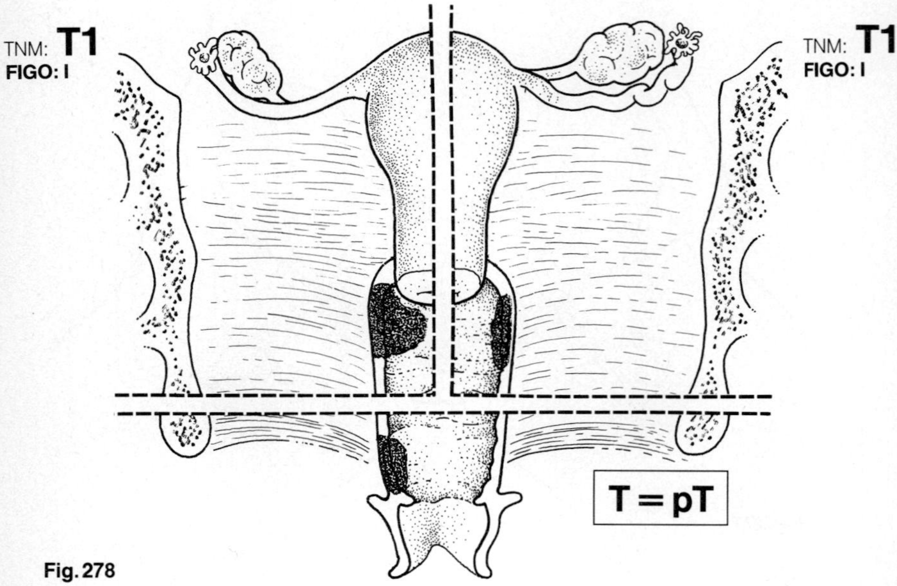

Fig. 278

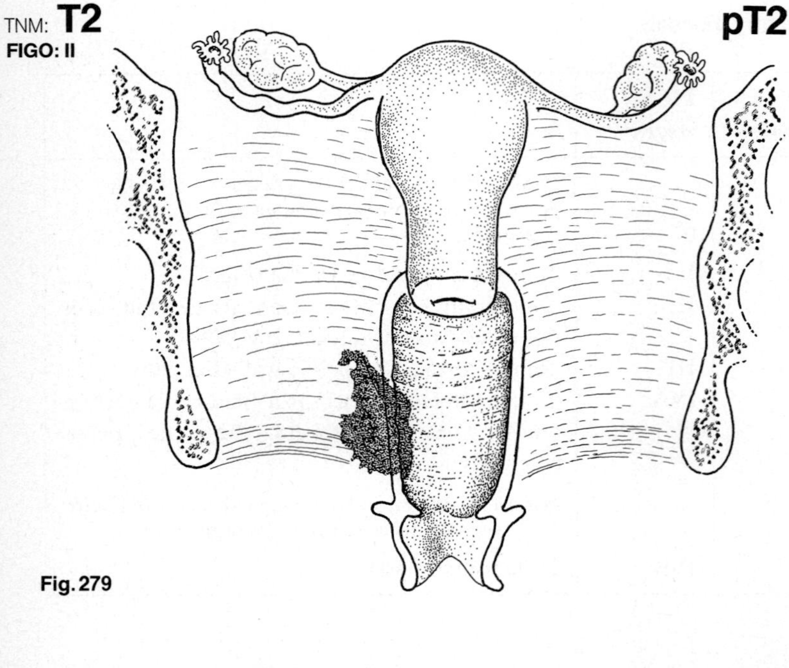

Fig. 279

TNM: **T3**
FIGO: III

pT3

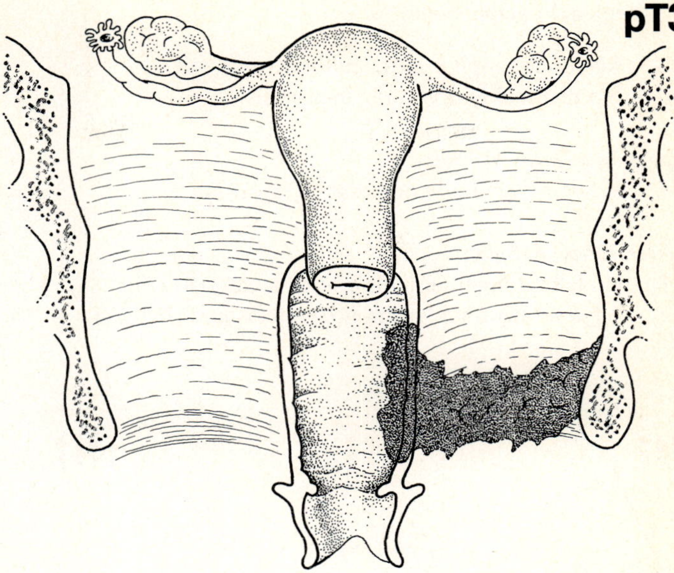

Fig. 280

TNM: **T4**
FIGO: IVA

pT4

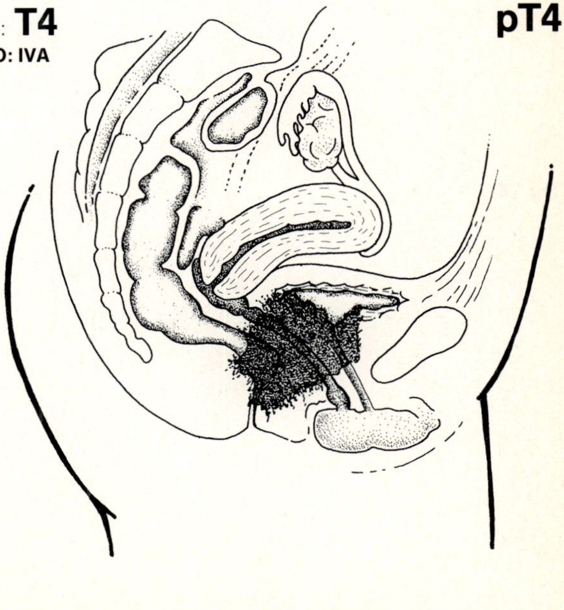

Fig. 281

N – Regional Lymph Nodes

NX Regional lymph nodes cannot be assessed
N0 No regional lymph node metastasis

Upper Two-Thirds of Vagina
N1 Pelvic lymph node metastasis (Fig. 282)

Lower Third of Vagina
N1 Unilateral inguinal lymph node metastasis (Fig. 283)
N2 Bilateral inguinal lymph node metastasis (Fig. 284)

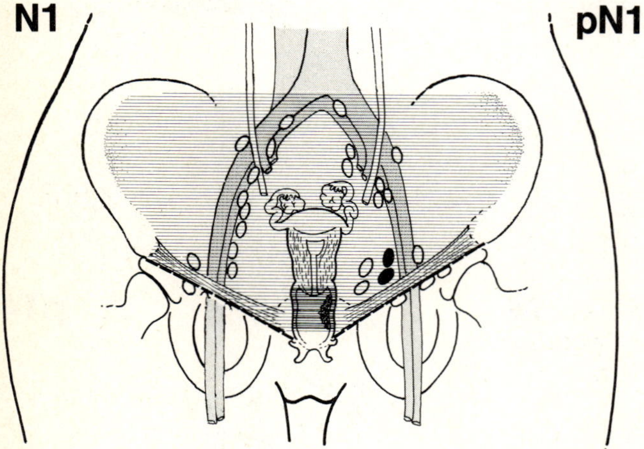

Fig. 282

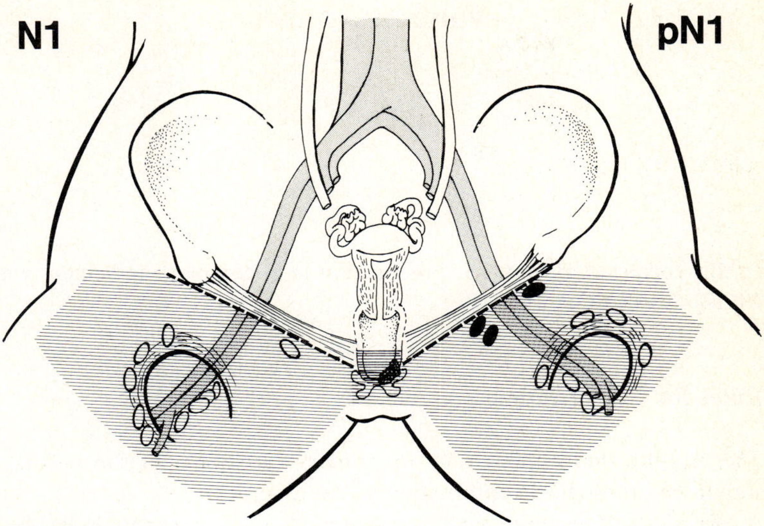

Fig. 283

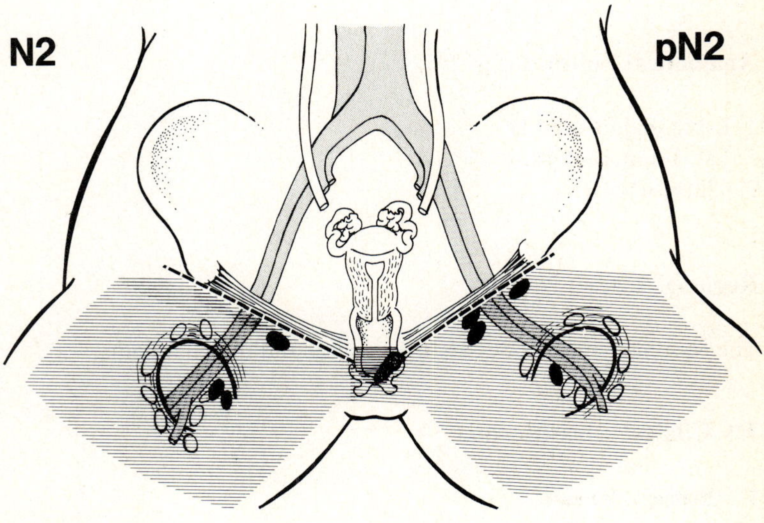

Fig. 284

pTN Pathological Classification

The pT and pN categories correspond to the T and N categories.

Vulva (ICD-O 184.1-4)

In this corrected reprint the classification is in complete agreement with the FIGO classification 1989/90.

Rules for Classification

The classification applies only to primary carcinoma of the vulva. There should be histological confirmation of the disease.
A carcinoma of the vulva that has extended to the vagina should be classified as carcinoma of the vulva.

Anatomical Subsites (Fig. 285)

1. Labia majora (184.1)
2. Labia minora (184.2)
3. Clitoris (184.3)

Regional Lymph Nodes

The regional lymph nodes are the femoral and inguinal nodes.

TN Clinical Classification

T - Primary Tumour

TX	Primary tumour cannot be assessed
T0	No evidence of primary tumour
Tis	Carcinoma in situ (preinvasive carcinoma)

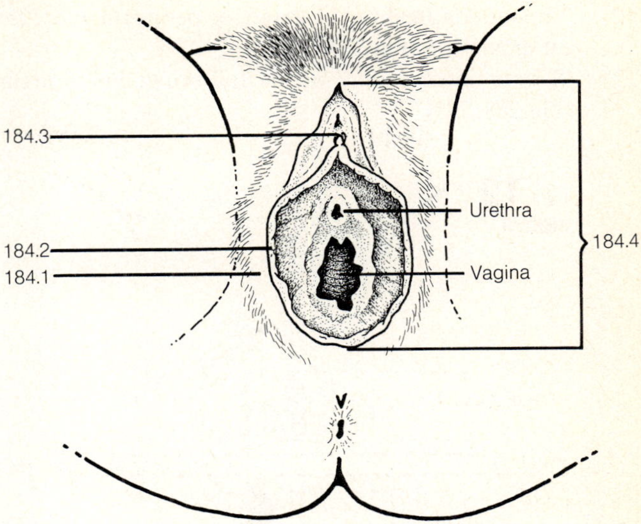

Fig. 285

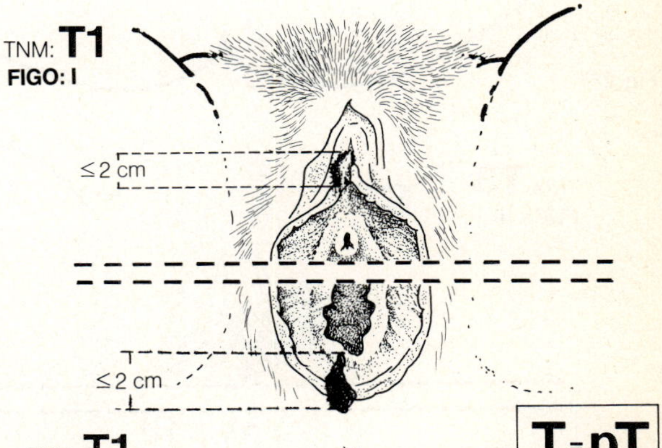

Fig. 286

T1 Tumour confined to vulva and/or perineum, 2 cm or less in greatest dimension (Fig. 286)

T2 Tumour confined to vulva and/or perineum, more than 2 cm in greatest dimension (Fig. 287)

T3 Tumour involves any of the following: lower urethra, vagina, anus (Fig. 288, 289)

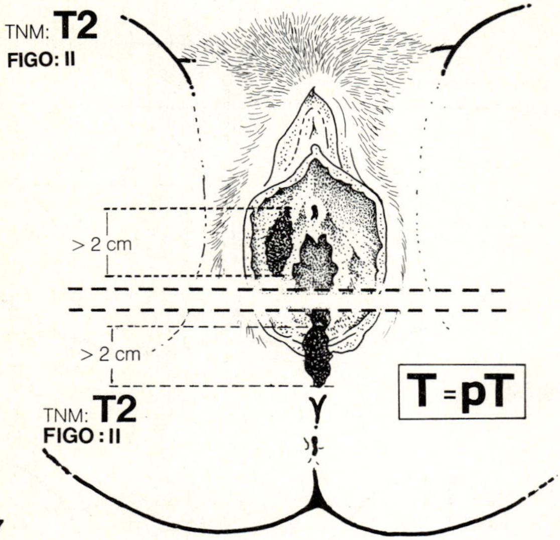

Fig. 287

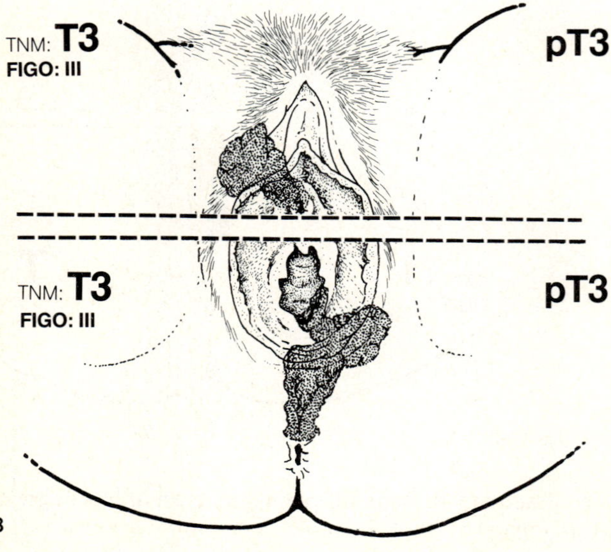

Fig. 288

T4 Tumour involves any of the following: bladder mucosa, rectal mucosa, upper urethra, pelvic bone (Fig. 290)

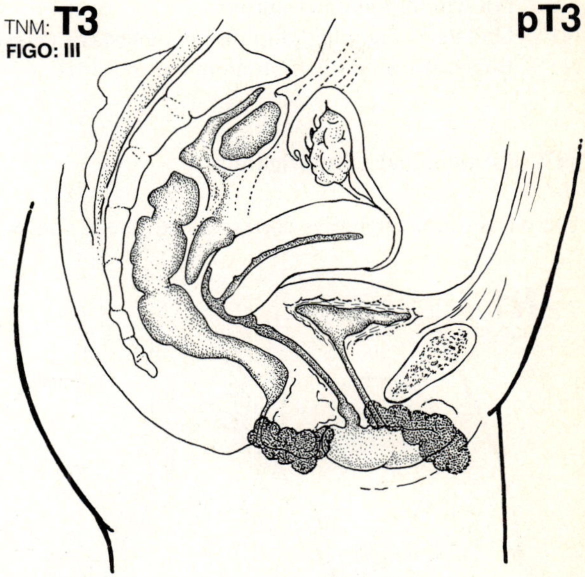

Fig. 289

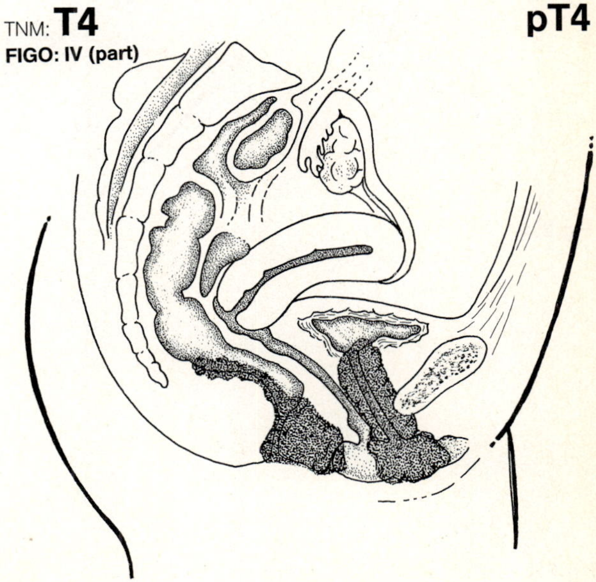

Fig. 290

N – Regional Lymph Nodes

NX Regional lymph nodes cannot be assessed
N0 No lymph node metastasis
N1 Unilateral regional lymph node metastasis (Fig. 291)
N2 Bilateral regional lymph node metastasis (Fig. 292)

pTN Pathological Classification

The pT and pN categories correspond to the T and N categories.

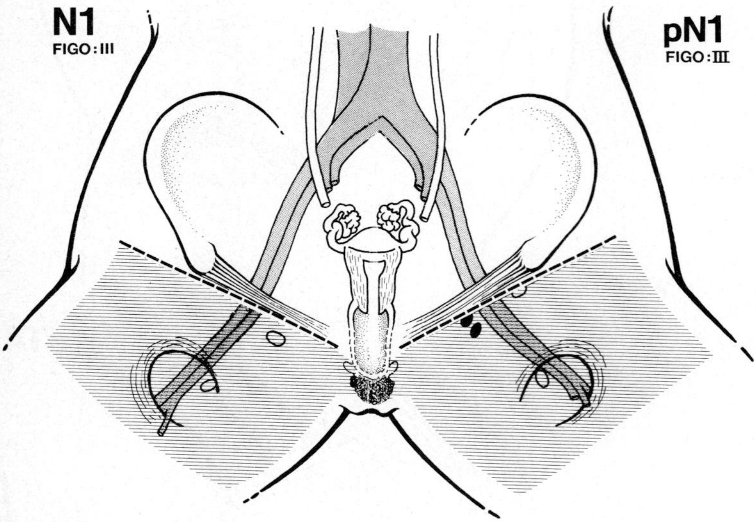

Fig. 291

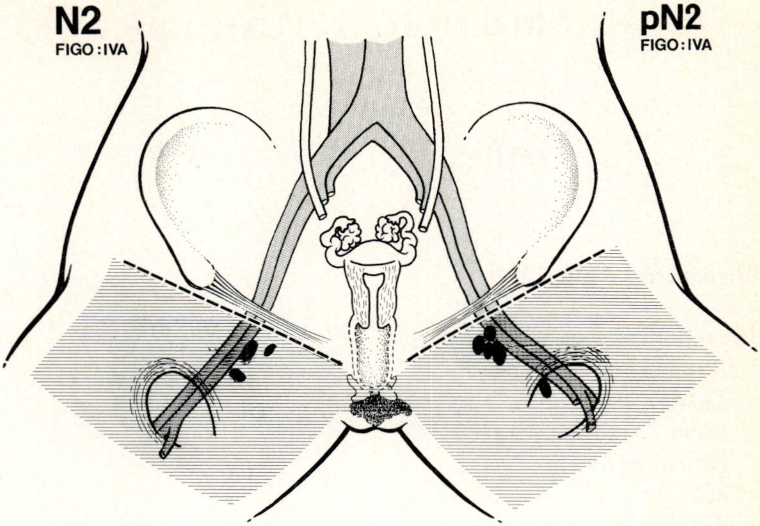

Fig. 292

UROLOGICAL TUMOURS

Introductory Notes

The following sites are included:

- Prostate
- Testis
- Penis
- Urinary bladder
- Kidney
- Renal pelvis and ureter
- Urethra

Prostate (ICD-O 185) (Figs. 293, 333 [see p. 245])

Rules for Classification

The classification applies only to carcinoma. There should be histological confirmation of the disease.

Regional Lymph Nodes (Fig. 294)

The regional lymph nodes are the nodes of the true pelvis which essentially are the pelvic nodes below the bifurcation of the common iliac arteries. Laterality does not affect the N classification.

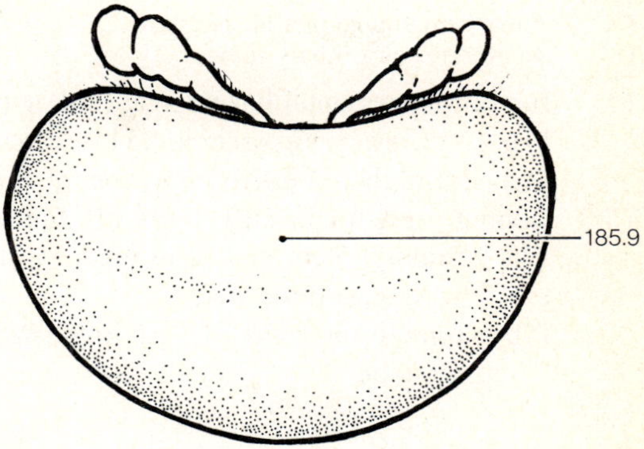

Fig. 293

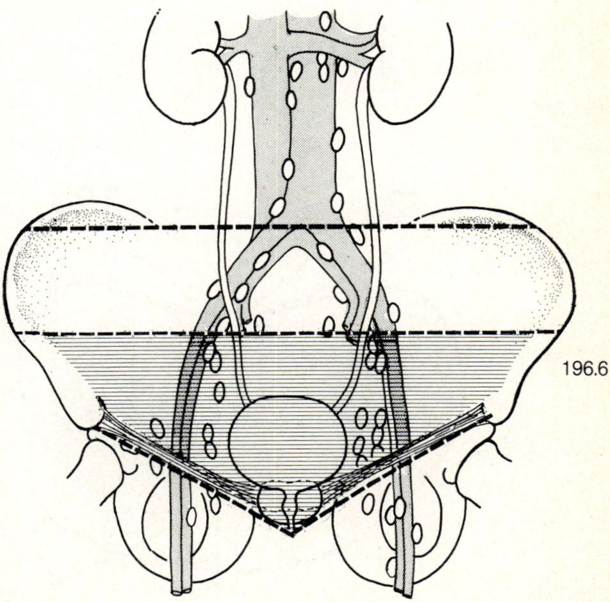

Fig. 294

TN Clinical Classification

T – Primary Tumour

TX Primary tumour cannot be assessed

T0 No evidence of primary tumour

T1 Tumour is incidental histological finding (Fig. 295)

- T1a 3 or fewer microscopic foci of carcinoma
- T1b More than 3 microscopic foci of carcinoma

T2 Tumour present clinically or grossly, limited to the gland (Fig. 296)

- T2a Tumor 1.5 cm or less in greatest dimension with normal tissue on at least three sides
- T2b Tumour more than 1.5 cm in greatest dimension *or* in more than one lobe

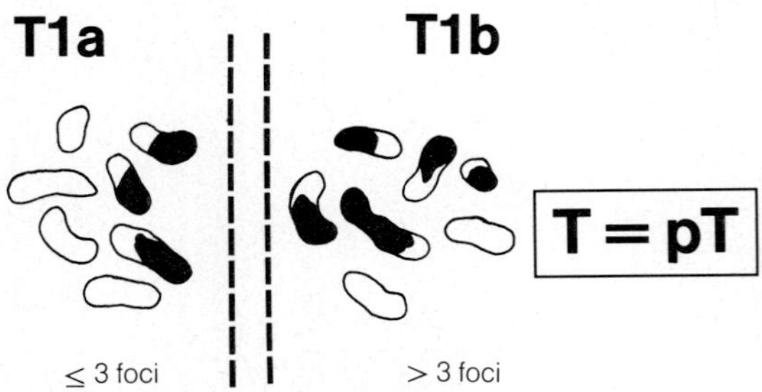

Fig. 295

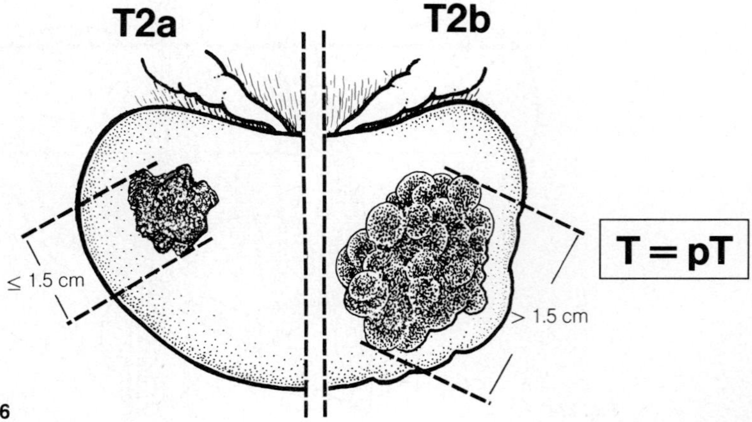

Fig. 296

T3 Tumour invades into the prostatic apex or into or beyond the prostatic capsule or bladder neck or seminal vesicle, but is not fixed (Fig. 297)

T4 Tumour is fixed *or* invades adjacent structures other than those listed in T3 (Fig. 298)

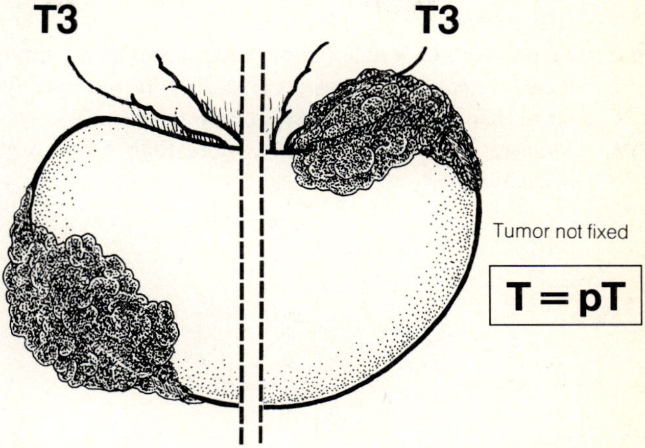

Fig. 297

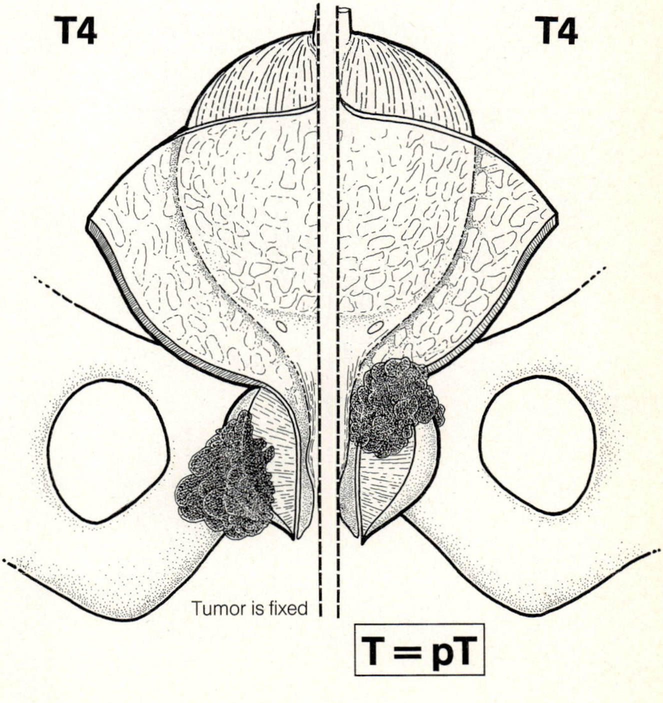

Fig. 298

N - Regional Lymph Nodes

NX Regional lymph nodes cannot be assessed
N0 No regional lymph node metastasis
N1 Metastasis in a single lymph node, 2 cm or less in greatest dimension (Fig. 299)
N2 Metastasis in a single lymph node, more than 2 cm but not more than 5 cm in greatest dimension (Fig. 300), *or* multiple lymph nodes, none more than 5 cm in greatest dimension (Fig. 301)
N3 Metastasis in a lymph node, more than 5 cm in greatest dimension (Figs. 302, 303)

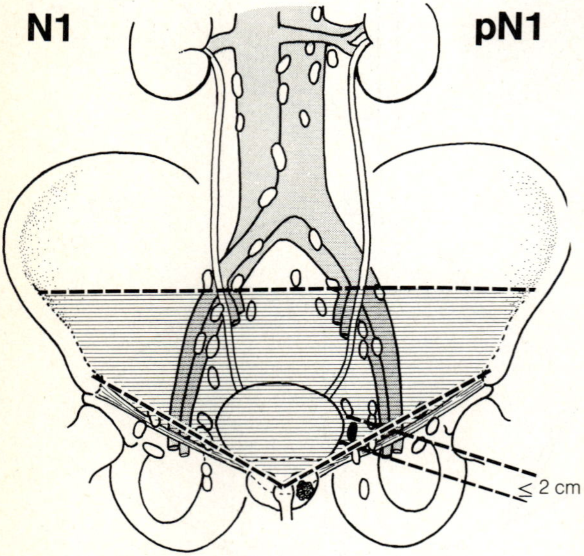

Fig. 299

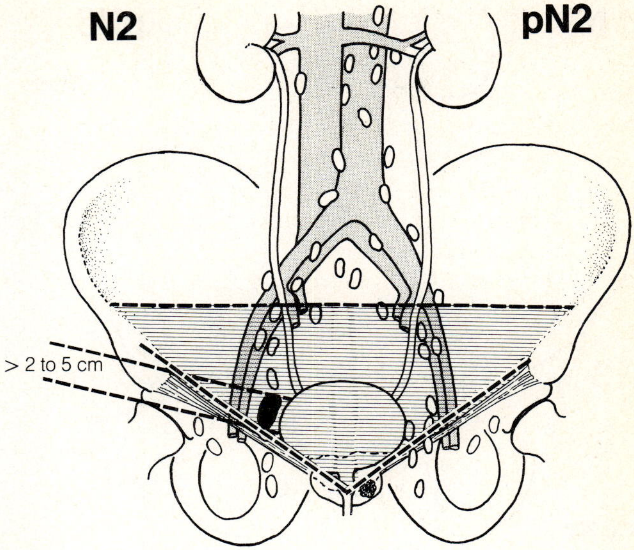

Fig. 300

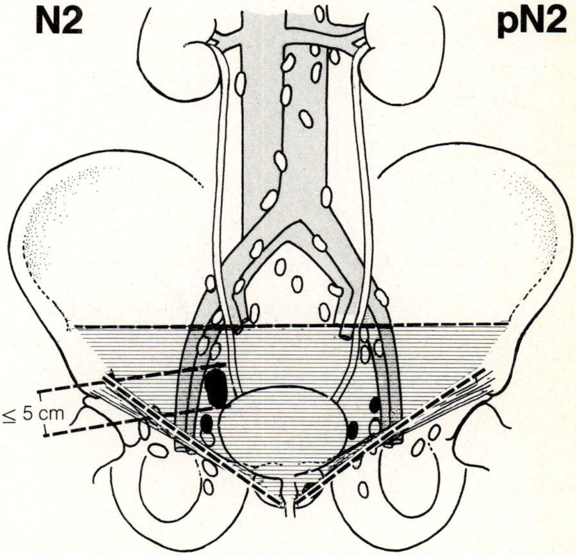

Fig. 301

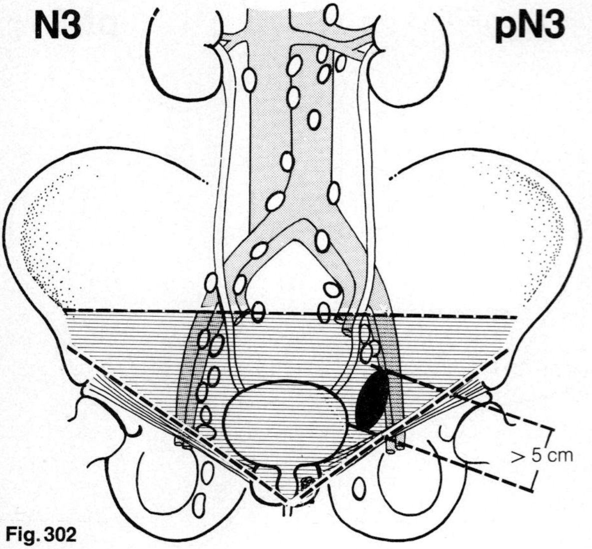

Fig. 302

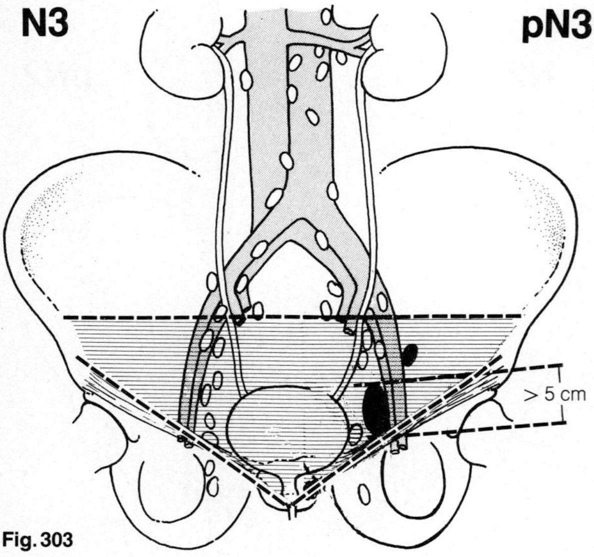

Fig. 303

pTN Pathological Classification

The pT and pN categories correspond to the T and N categories.

Testis (ICD-O 186) Fig. 304)

Rules for Classification

Testis refers to the body of the testis and excludes the epididymis. There should be histological confirmation of the disease to permit division of cases by histological type. Malignant lymphoma is excluded.

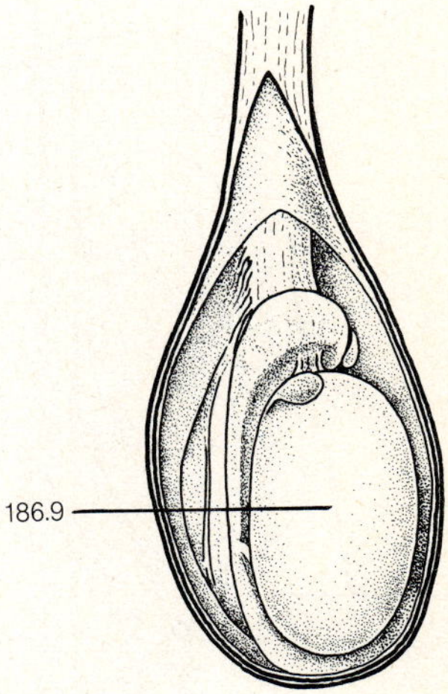

Fig. 304

Regional Lymph Nodes (Fig. 305)

The regional lymph nodes are the abdominal para-aortic and paracaval nodes, the intrapelvic nodes and the inguinal nodes after scrotal or inguinal surgery. Laterality does not affect the N classification.

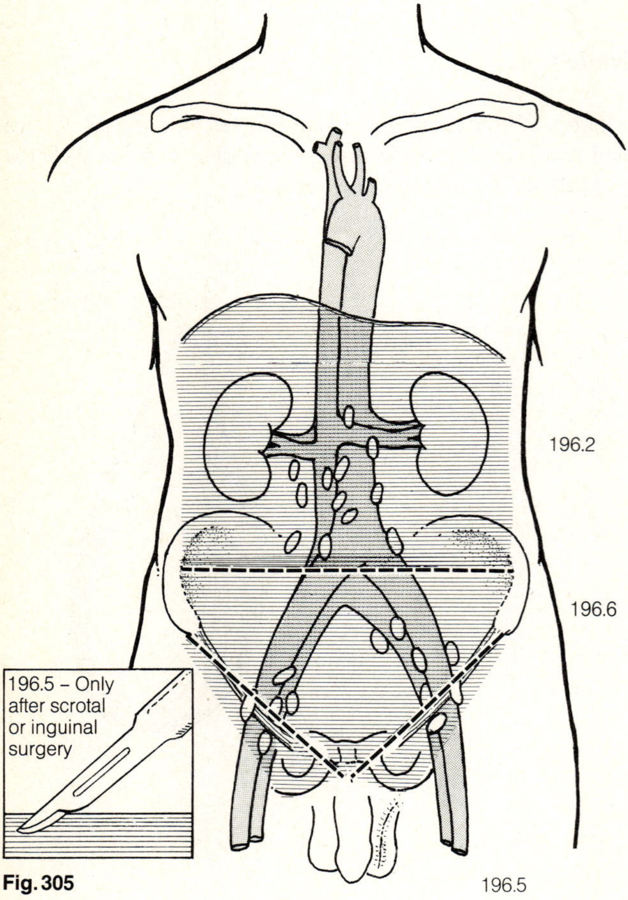

Fig. 305

TN Clinical Classification

T – Primary Tumour

The extent of primary tumour is classified after radical orchiectomy, see pT. In the absence of radical orchiectomy TX is used.

N – Regional Lymph Nodes

NX Regional lymph nodes cannot be assessed
N0 No regional lymph node metastasis
N1 Metastasis in a single lymph node, 2 cm or less in greatest dimension (Figs. 306, 307)
N2 Metastasis in a single lymph node, more than 2 cm but not more than 5 cm in greatest dimension (Fig. 308), *or* multiple lymph nodes, none more than 5 cm in greatest dimension (Figs. 309–311)
N3 Metastasis in a lymph node, more than 5 cm in greatest dimension (Figs. 312–315)

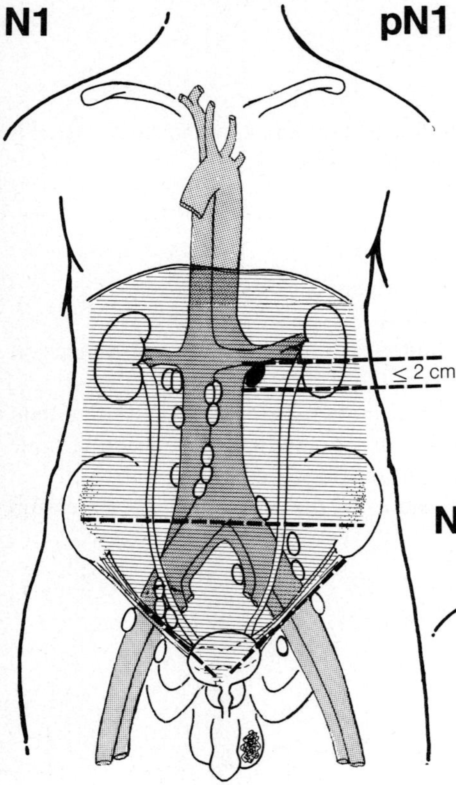

Fig. 306

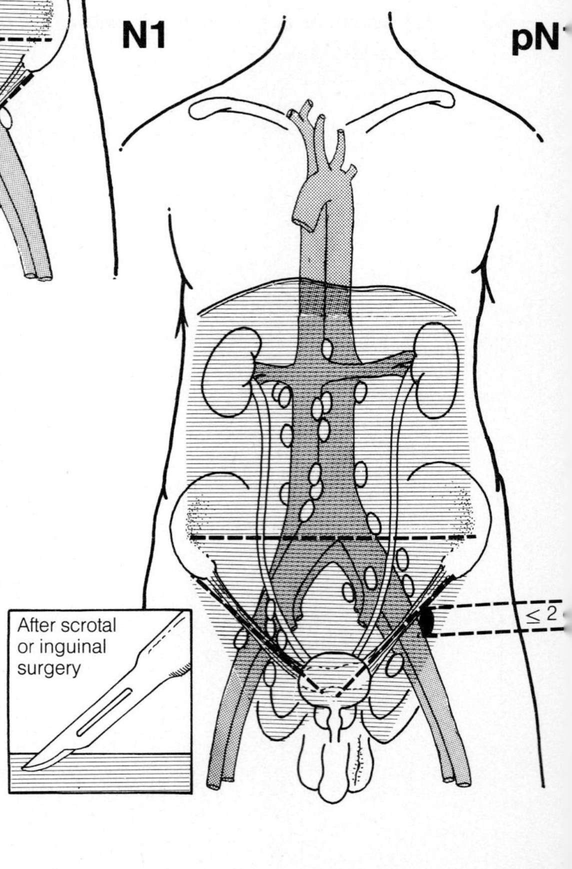

Fig. 307

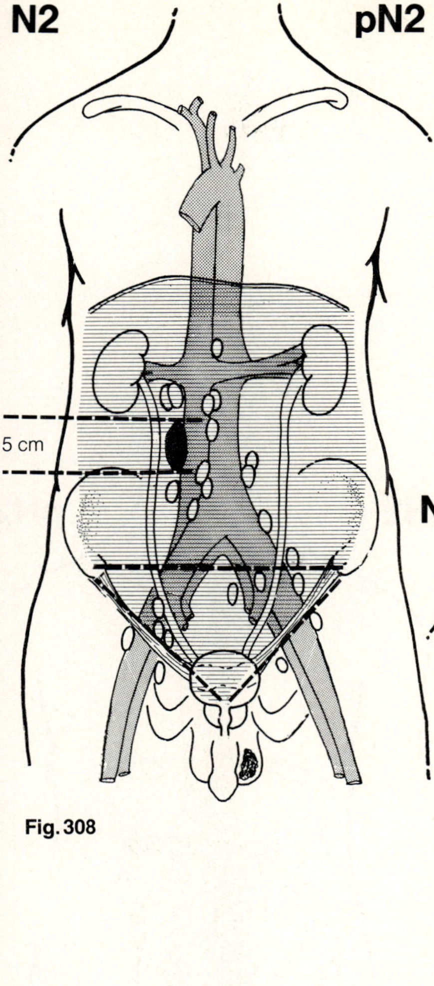

Fig. 308

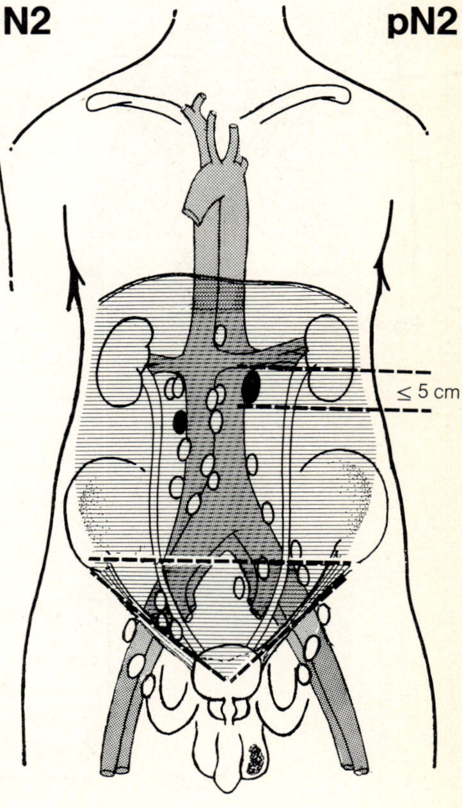

Fig. 309

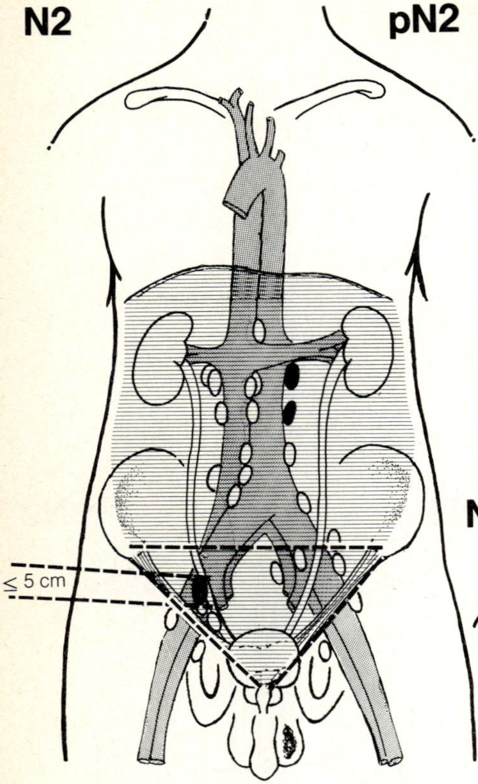

Fig. 310

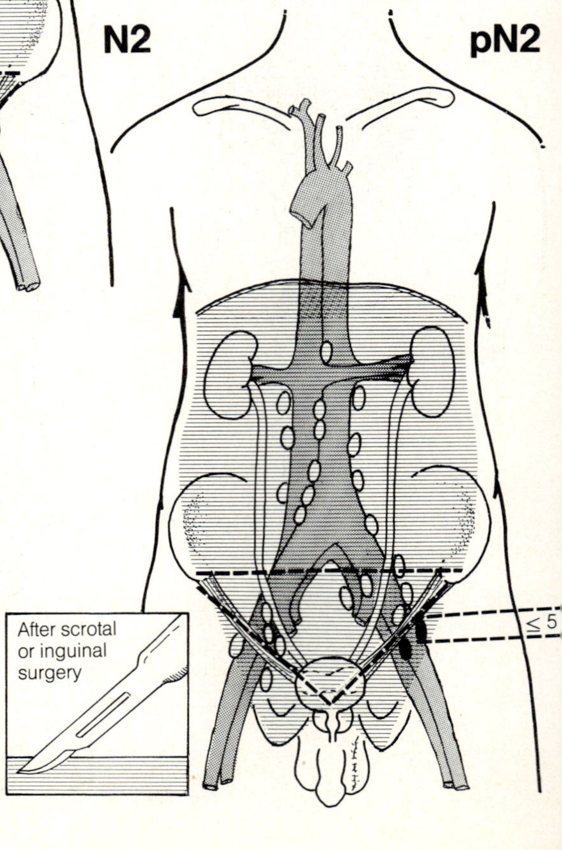

Fig. 311

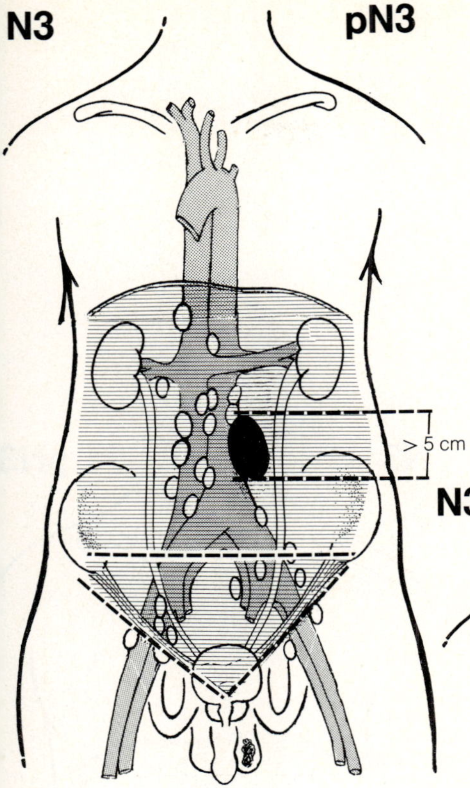

Fig. 312

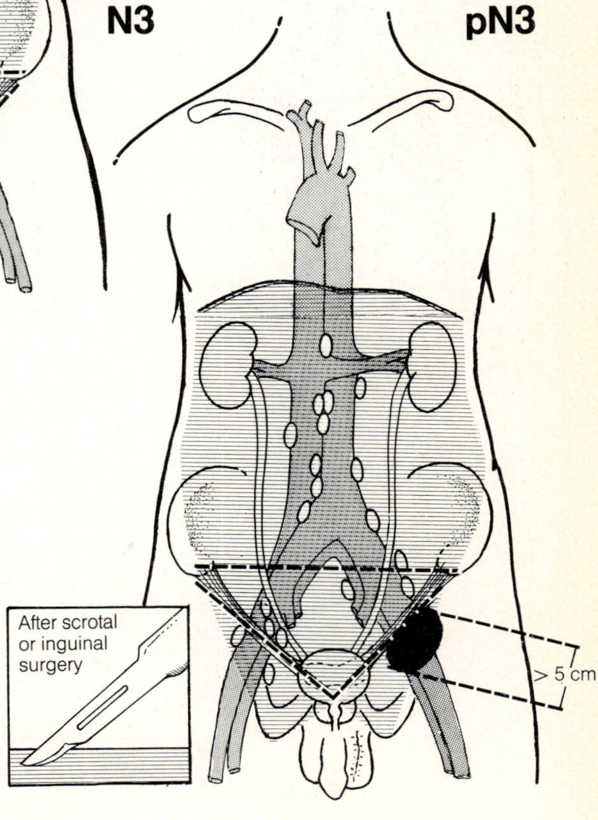

Fig. 313

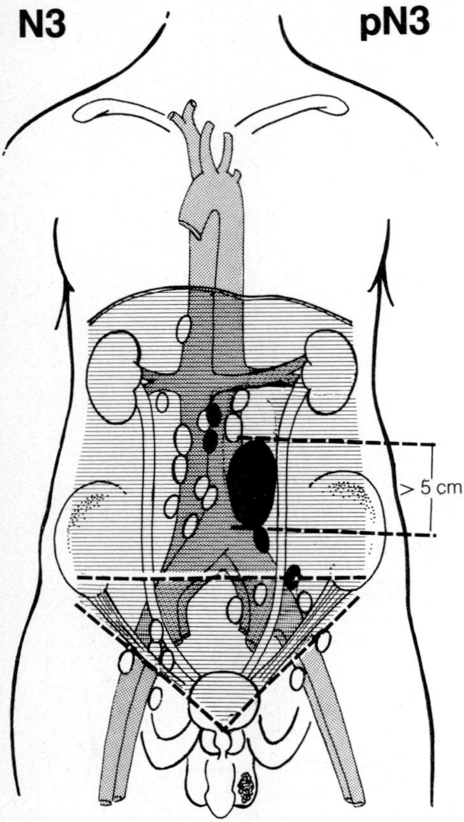

Fig. 314

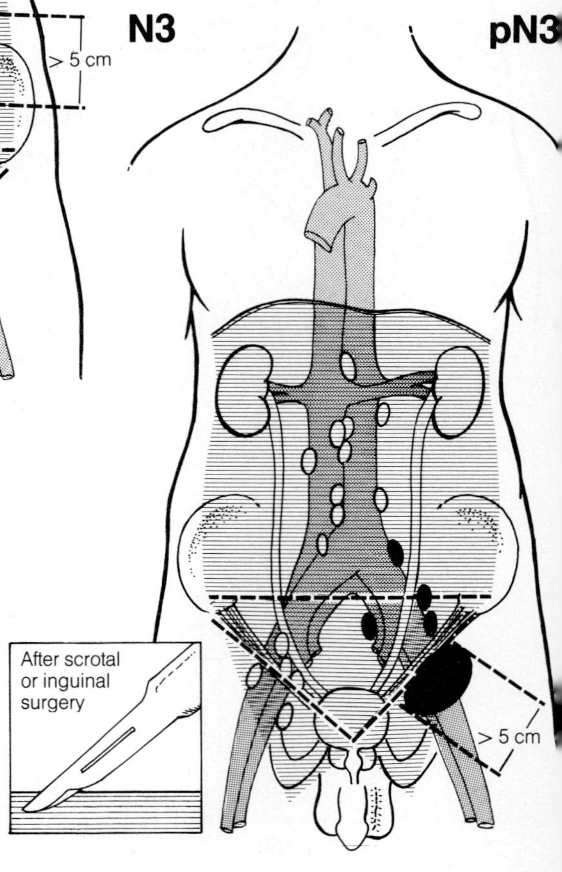

Fig. 315

pTN Pathological Classification

pT - Primary Tumour

pTX Primary tumour cannot be assessed (in the absence of radical orchiectomy TX is used)
pT0 Histological scar or no evidence of primary tumour
pTis Intratubular tumour: preinvasive cancer
pT1 Tumour limited to testis, including rete testis (Fig. 316)
pT2 Tumour invades beyond tunica albuginea or into epididymis (Fig. 316)

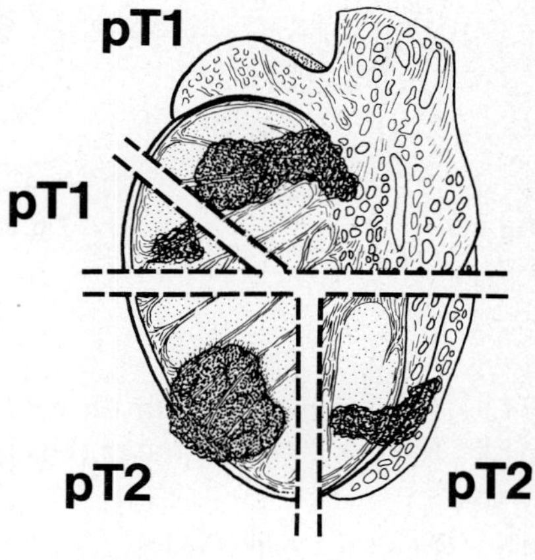

Fig. 316

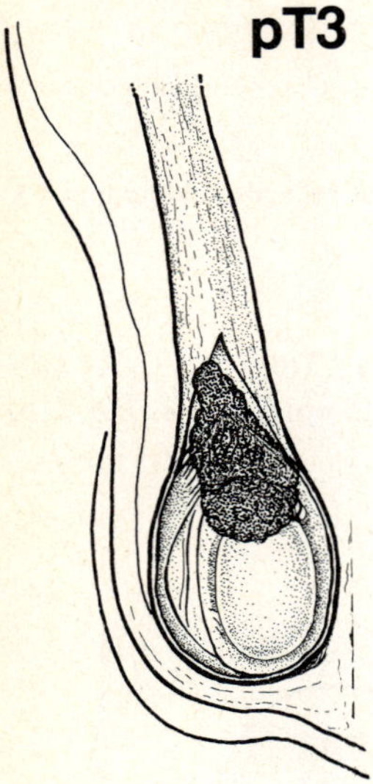

Fig. 317

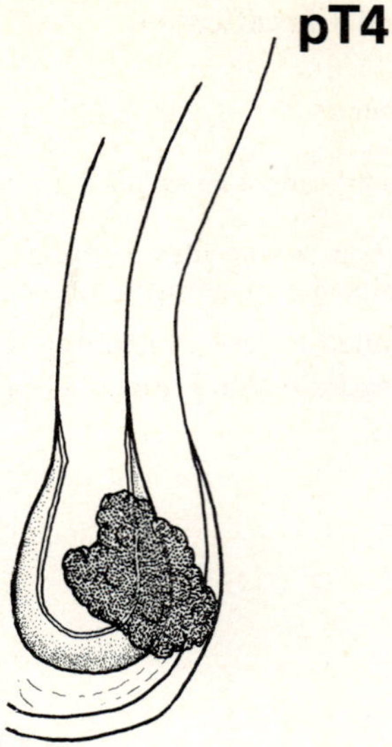

Fig. 318

pT3 Tumour invades spermatic cord (Fig. 317)
pT4 Tumour invades scrotum (Fig. 318)

pN - Regional Lymph Nodes

The pN categories correspond to the N categories.

Penis (ICD-O 187.1–4)

Rules for Classification

The classification applies only to carcinoma. There should be histological confirmation of the disease.

Anatomical Subsites (Fig. 319)

1. Preputium or prepuce (187.1)
2. Glans penis (187.2)
3. Shaft of penis (187.3)

Regional Lymph Nodes

The regional lymph nodes are the superficial and deep inguinal and the pelvic nodes.

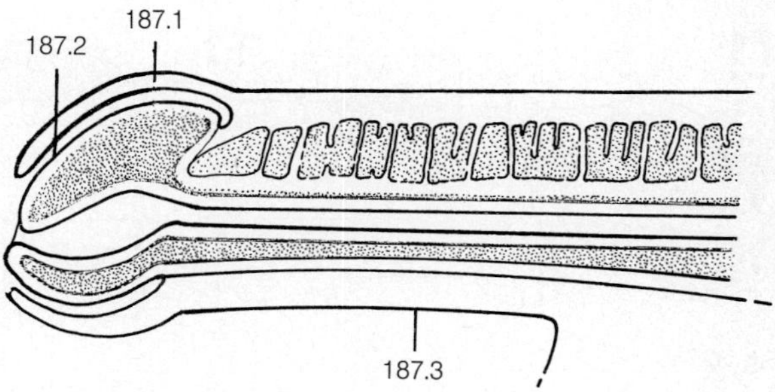

Fig. 319

TN Clinical Classification

T – Primary Tumour

TX Primary tumour cannot be assessed
T0 No evidence of primary tumour
Tis Carcinoma in situ
  Ta Non-invasive verrucous carcinoma (Fig. 320)

T1 Tumour invades subepithelial connective tissue (Fig. 321)
T2 Tumour invades corpus spongiosum or cavernosum (Fig. 322)
T3 Tumour invades urethra (Fig. 323) or prostate (Fig. 324)
T4 Tumour invades other adjacent structures (Figs. 325, 326)

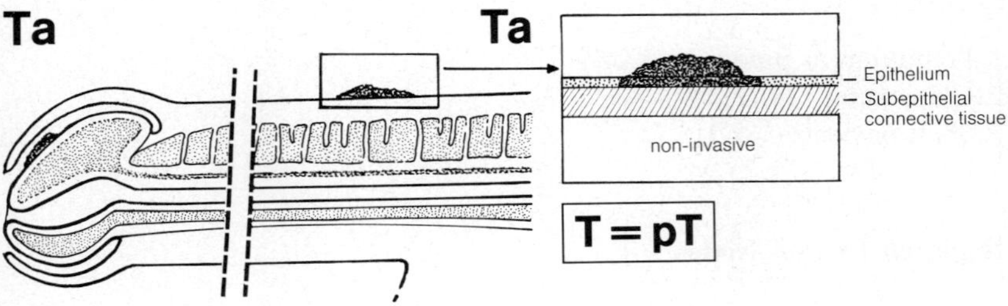

Fig. 320

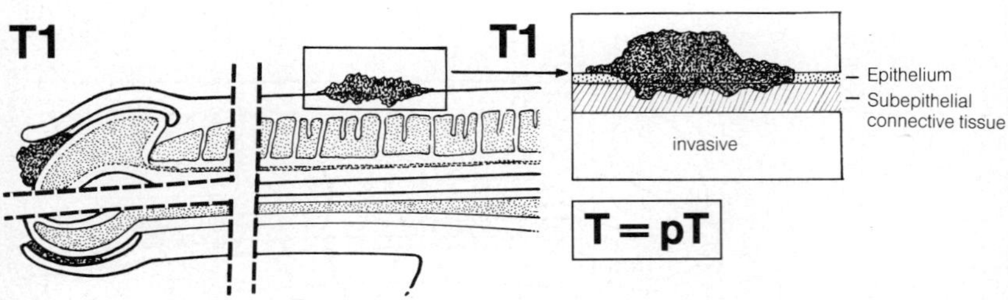

Fig. 321

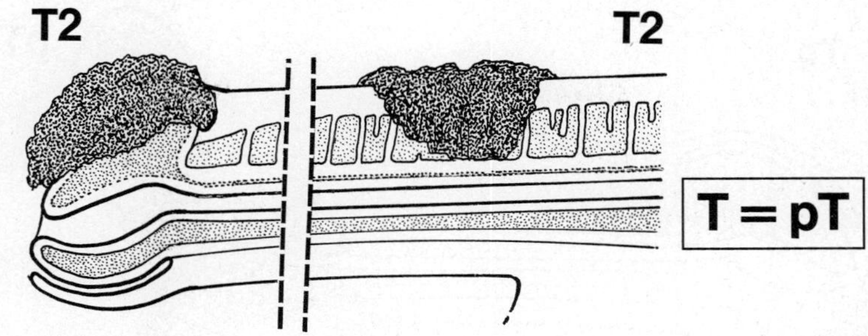

Fig. 322

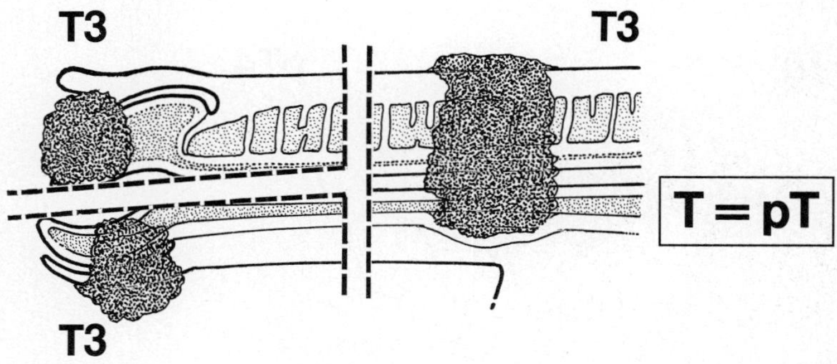

Fig. 323

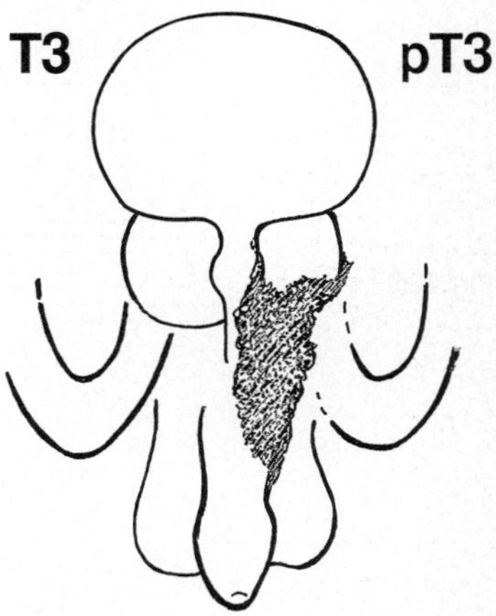

Fig. 324

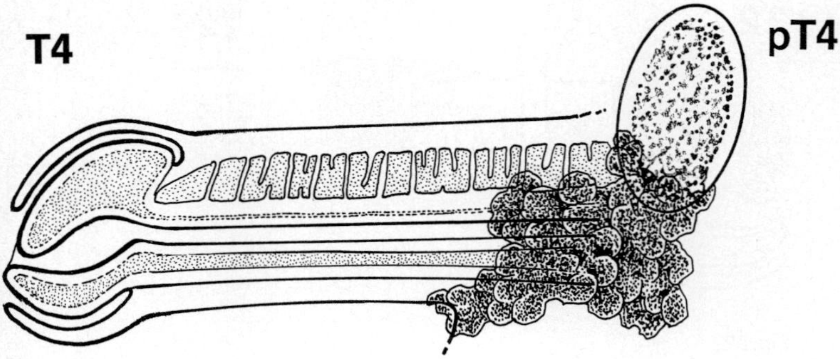

Fig. 325

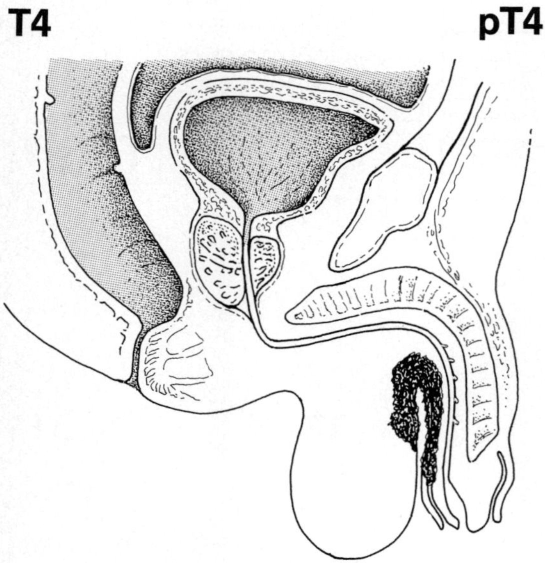

Fig. 326

N - Regional Lymph Nodes

NX Regional lymph nodes cannot be assessed
N0 No regional lymph node metastasis
N1 Metastasis in a single superficial inguinal lymph node (Fig. 327)

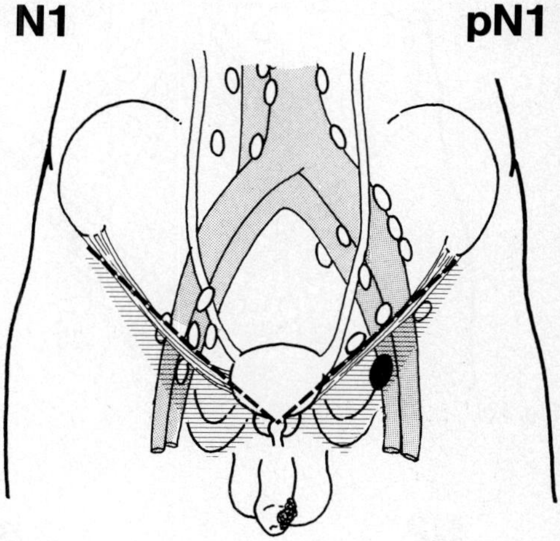

Fig. 327

N2 Metastasis in multiple (Fig. 328) or bilateral superficial inguinal lymph nodes (Fig. 329)

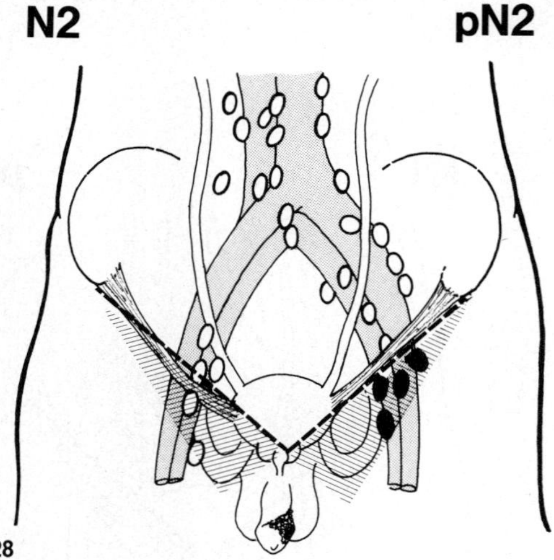

Fig. 328

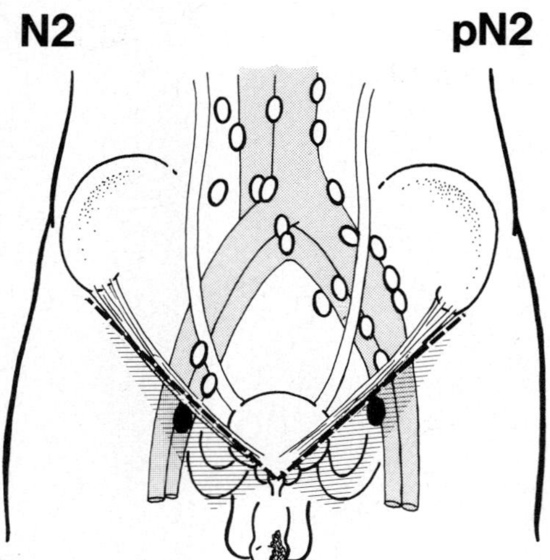

Fig. 329

N3 Metastasis in deep inguinal (Fig. 330) or pelvic lymph node(s), unilateral (Fig. 331) or bilateral (Fig. 332)

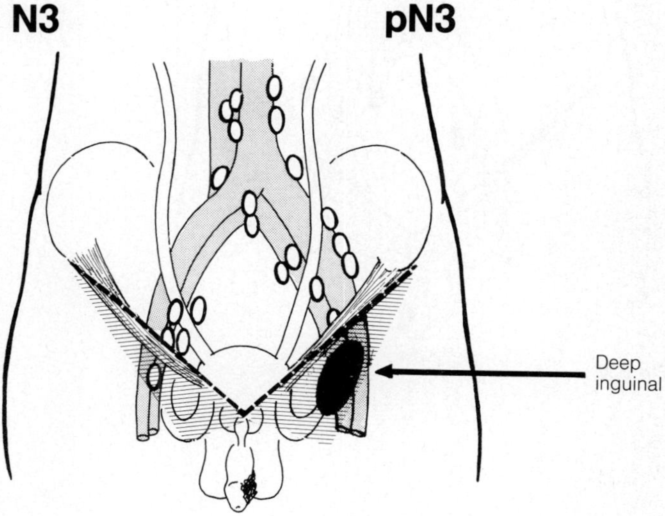

Fig. 330

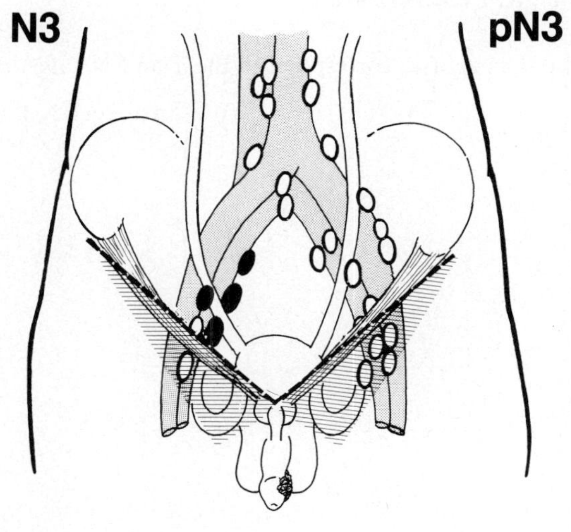

Fig. 331

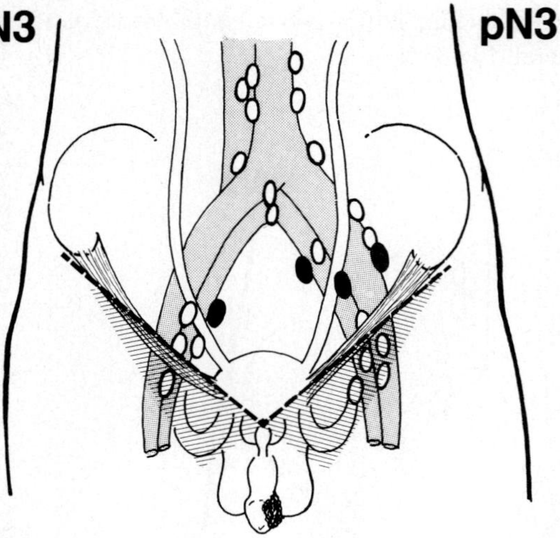

Fig. 332

pTN Pathological Classification

The pT and pN categories correspond to the T and N categories.

Urinary Bladder (ICD-O 188)

Rules for Classification

The classification applies only to carcinoma. Papilloma is excluded. There should be histological or cytological confirmation of the disease.

Anatomical Subsites (Fig. 333)

1. Trigone (188.0)
2. Dome (188.1)
3. Lateral wall (188.2)
4. Anterior wall (188.3)
5. Posterior wall (188.4)
6. Bladder neck (188.5)
7. Ureteral orifice (188.6)
8. Urachus (188.7)

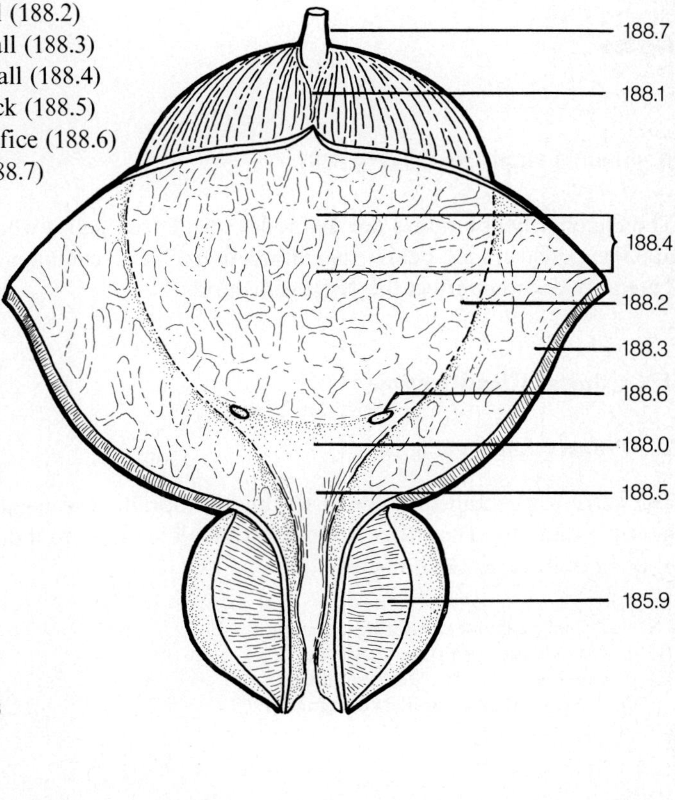

Fig. 333

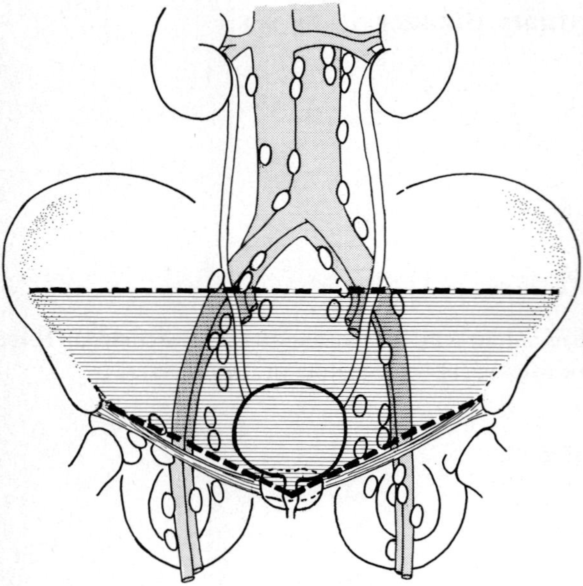

Fig. 334

Regional Lymph Nodes (Fig. 334)

The regional lymph nodes are the nodes of the true pelvis which essentially are the pelvic nodes below the bifurcation of the common iliac arteries. Laterality does not affect the N classification.

TN Clinical Classification

T – Primary Tumour (Fig. 335)

The suffix (m) should be added to the appropriate T category to indicate multiple tumours. The suffix (is) may be added to any T to indicate presence of associated carcinoma in situ.

TX Primary tumour cannot be assessed
T0 No evidence of primary tumour
Tis Carcinoma in situ: "flat tumour"
  Ta Non-invasive papillary carcinoma

T1 Tumour invades subepithelial connective tissue
T2 Tumour invades superficial muscle (inner half)
T3 Tumour invades deep muscle or perivesical fat
  T3a Tumour invades deep muscle (outer half)
  T3b Tumour invades perivesical fat
T4 Tumour invades any of the following: prostate, uterus, vagina, pelvic wall, abdominal wall

Note: If pathology report does not specify that tumour invades muscle, consider as invasion of subepithelial connective tissue. If depth of muscle invasion is not specified by the surgeon, code as T2.

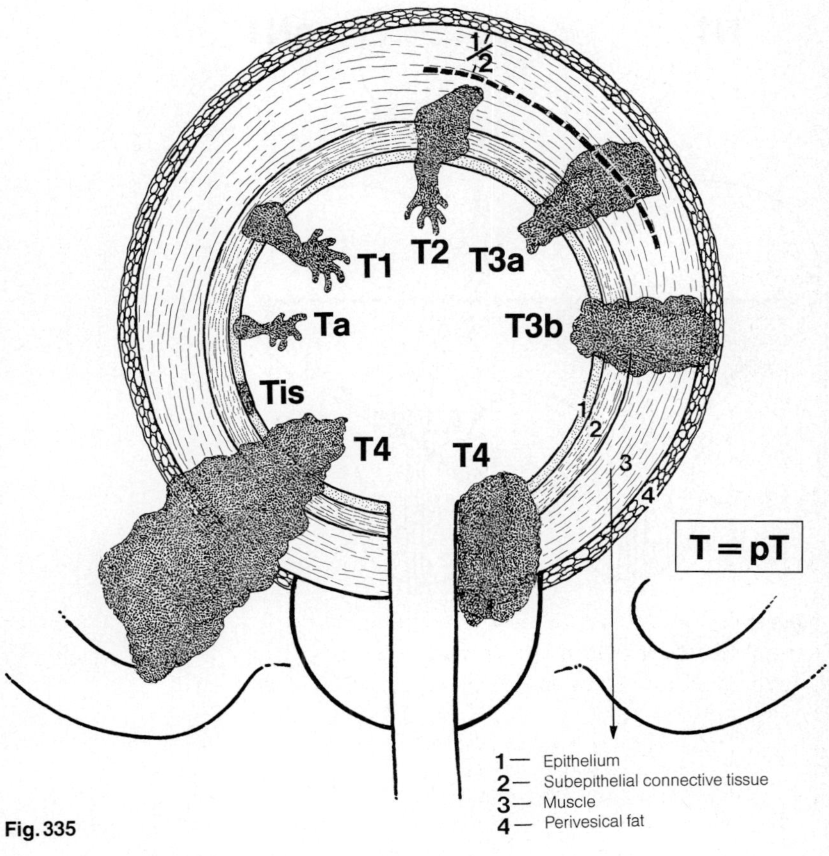

Fig. 335

N - Regional Lymph Nodes

NX Regional lymph nodes cannot be assessed
N0 No regional lymph node metastasis
N1 Metastasis in a single lymph node, 2 cm or less in greatest dimension (Fig. 336)
N2 Metastasis in a single lymph node, more than 2 cm but not more than 5 cm in greatest dimension (Fig. 337); *or* multiple lymph nodes, none more than 5 cm in greatest dimension (Fig. 338)
N3 Metastasis in a lymph node, more than 5 cm in greatest dimension (Figs. 339, 340)

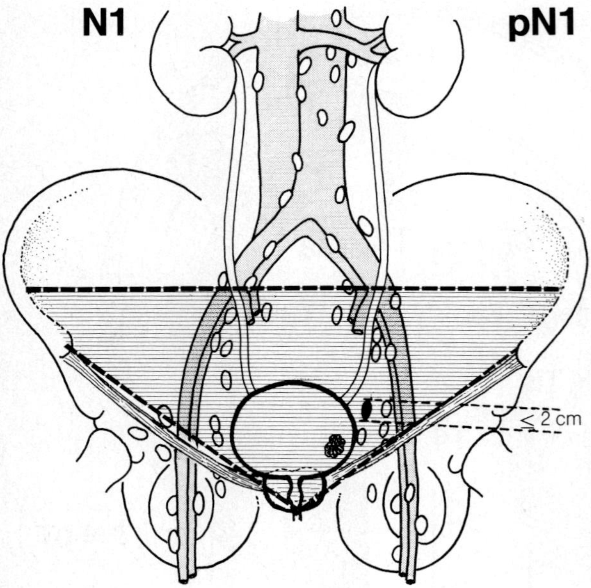

Fig. 336

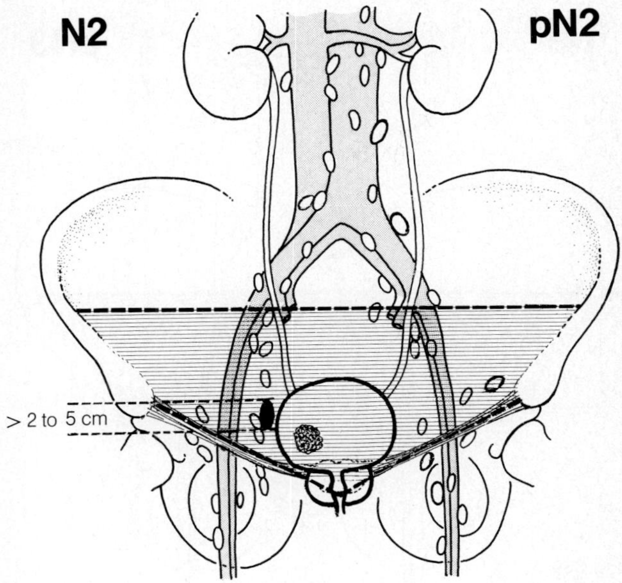

Fig. 337

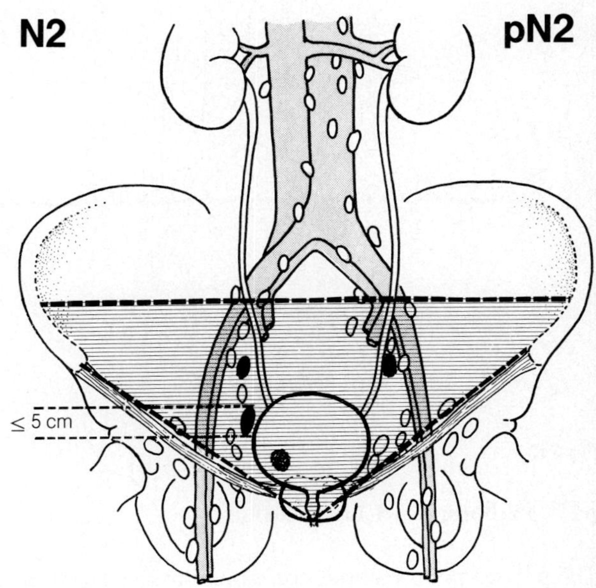

Fig. 338

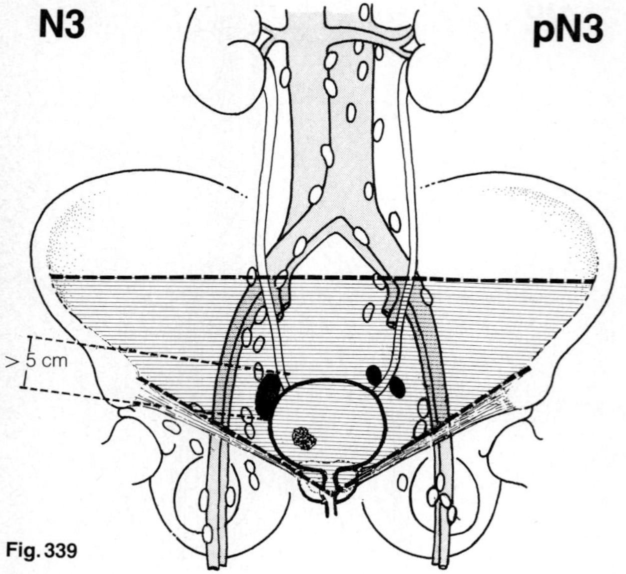

Fig. 339

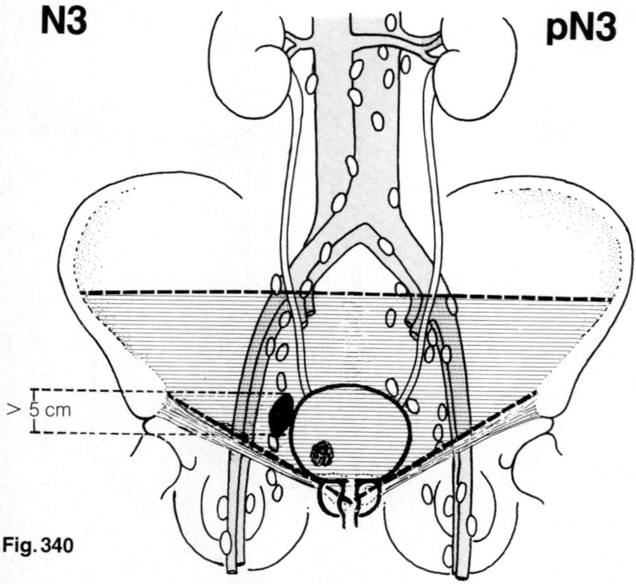

Fig. 340

pTN Pathological Classification

The pT and pN categories correspond to the T and N categories.

Kidney (ICD-O 189.0) (Fig. 341)

Rules for Classification

The classification applies only to renal cell carcinoma. Adenoma is excluded. There should be histological confirmation of the disease.

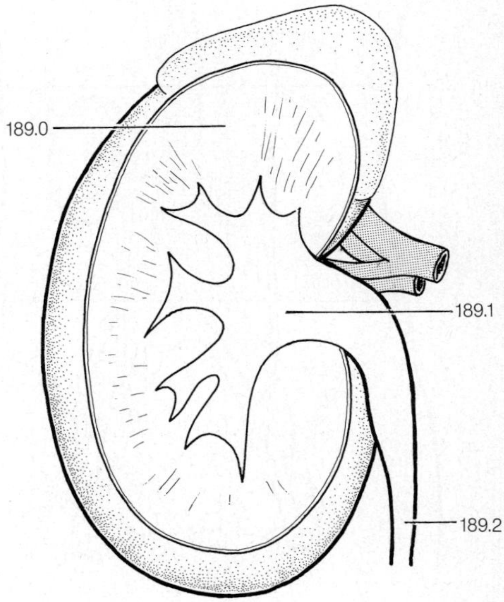

Fig. 341

Regional Lymph Nodes (Fig. 342)

The regional lymph nodes are the hilar, abdominal paraaortic and paracaval nodes. Laterality does not affect the N categories.

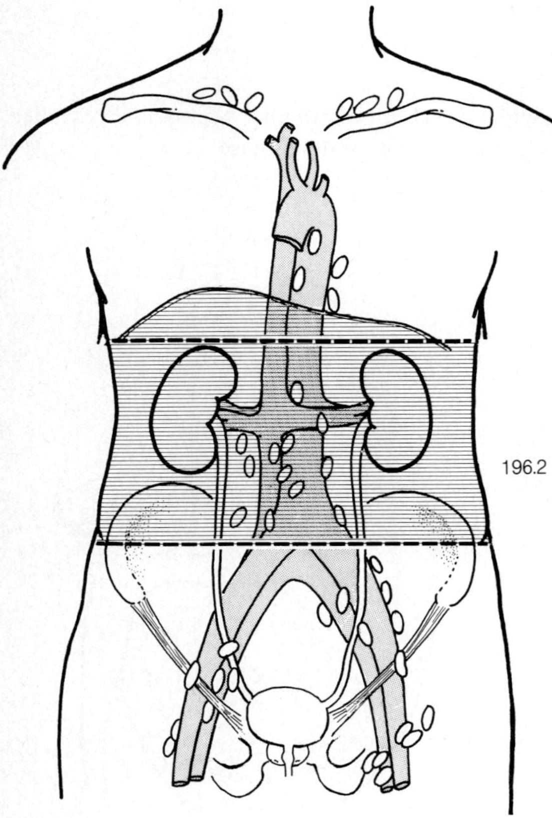

Fig. 342

TN Clinical Classification

T – Primary Tumour

TX Primary tumour cannot be assessed
T0 No evidence of primary tumour

T1 Tumour 2.5 cm or less in greatest dimension, limited to the kidney (Fig. 343)

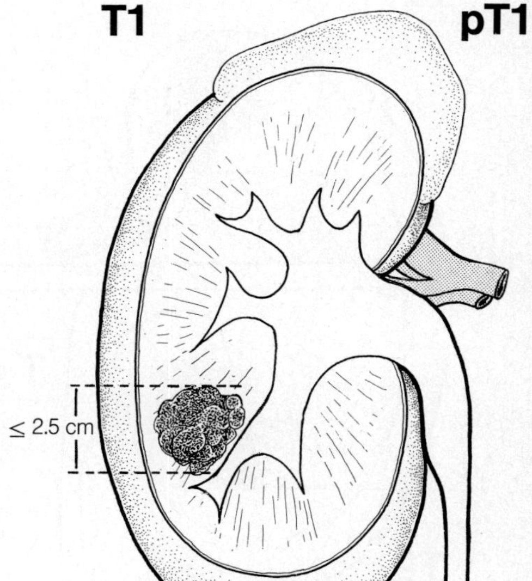

Fig. 343

T2 Tumour more than 2.5 cm in greatest dimension, limited to the kidney (Fig. 344)

T3 Tumour extends into major veins or invades adrenal gland or perinephric tissues but not beyond Gerota's fascia

- T3a Tumour invades adrenal gland or perinephric tissues but not beyond Gerota's fascia (Fig. 345)
- T3b Tumour grossly extends into renal vein(s) or vena cava (Fig. 346)

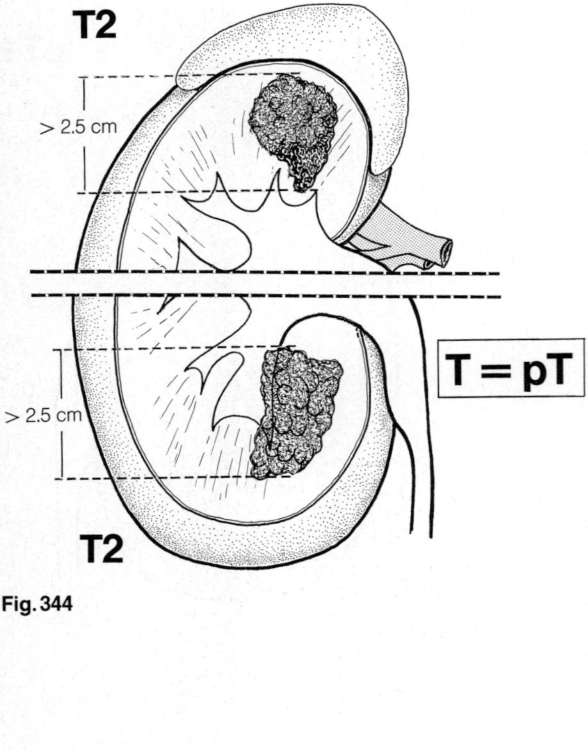

Fig. 344

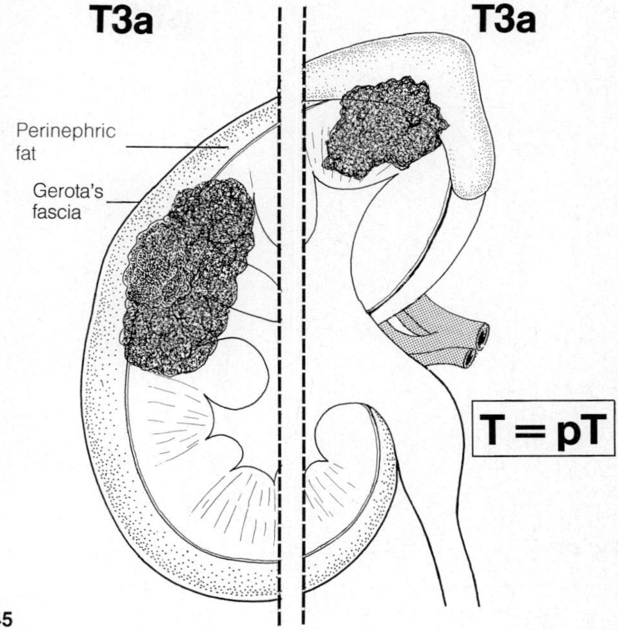

Fig. 345

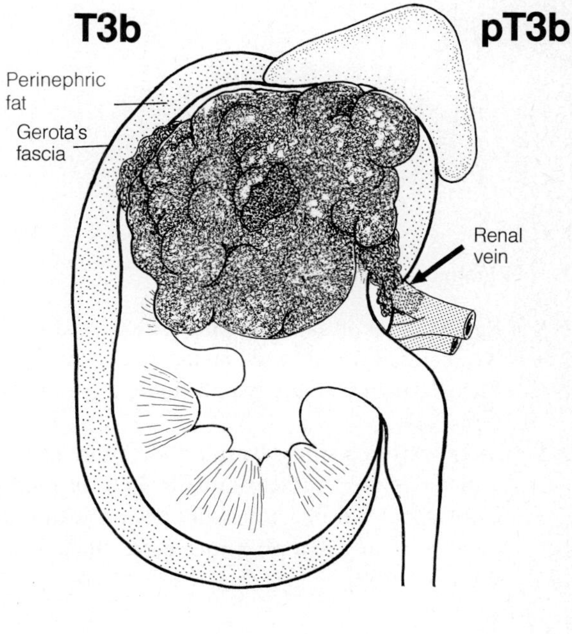

Fig. 346

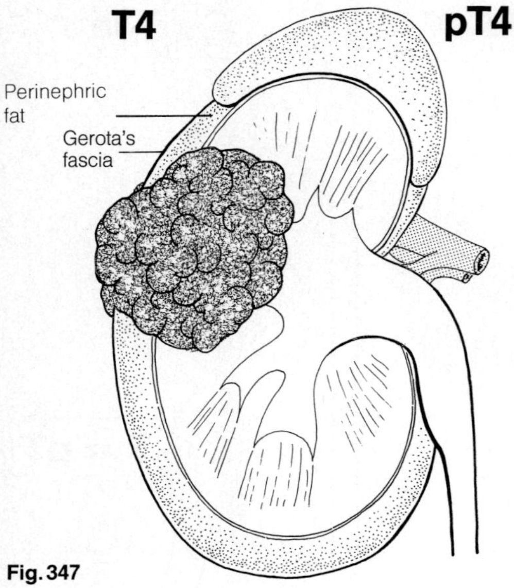

Fig. 347

T4 Tumour invades beyond Gerota's fascia (Fig. 347)

N – Regional Lymph Nodes

NX Regional lymph nodes cannot be assessed

N0 No regional lymph node metastasis

N1 Metastasis in a single lymph node, 2 cm or less in greatest dimension (Fig. 348)

N2 Metastasis in a single lymph node, more than 2 cm but not more than 5 cm in greatest dimension (Fig. 349), *or* multiple lymph nodes, none more than 5 cm in greatest dimension (Fig. 350)

N3 Metastasis in a lymph node, more than 5 cm in greatest dimension (Figs. 351, 352)

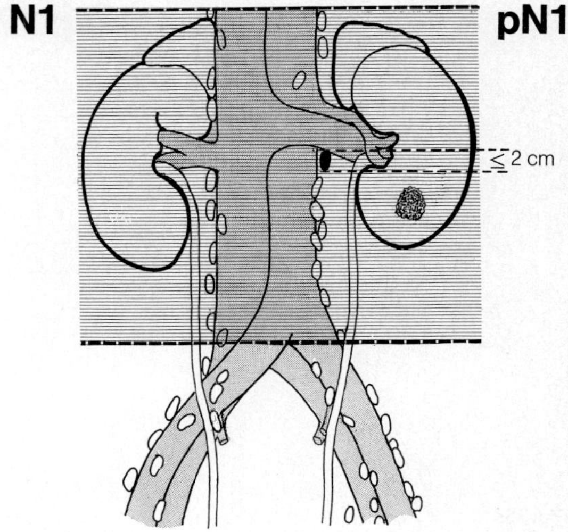

Fig. 348

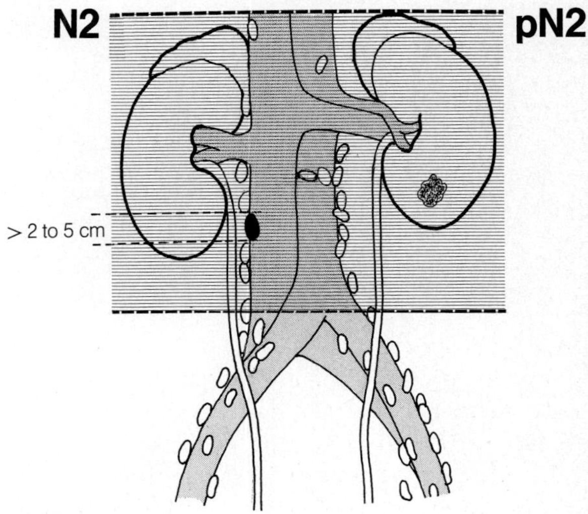

Fig. 349

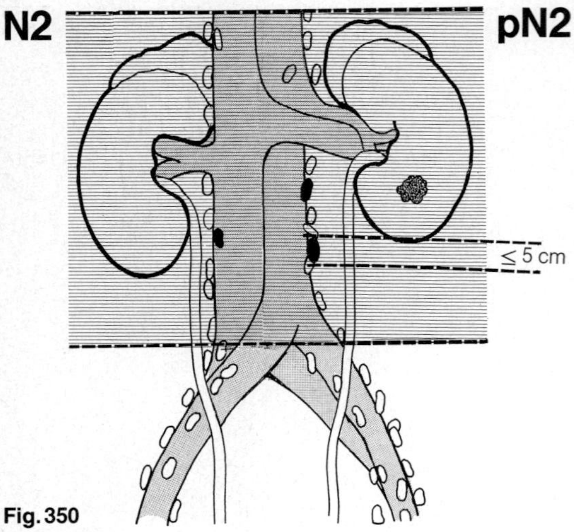

Fig. 350

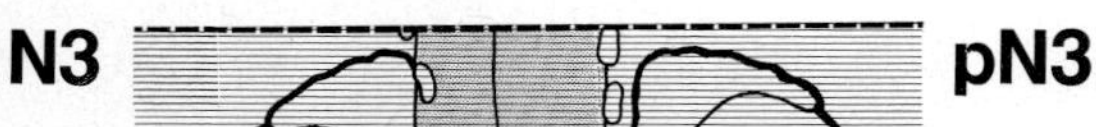

Fig. 351

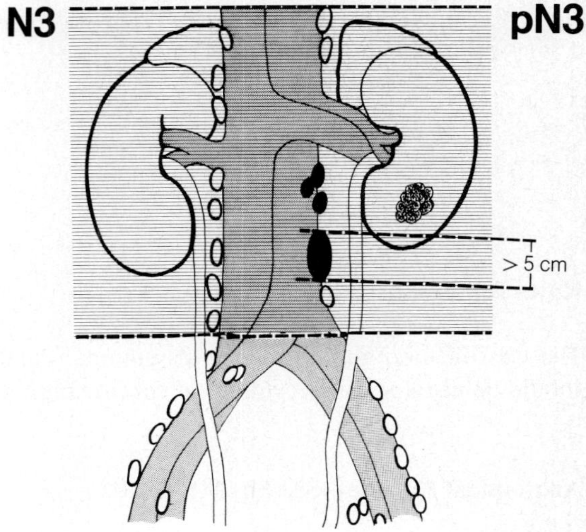

Fig. 352

pTN Pathological Classification

The pT and pN categories correspond to the T and N categories.

Renal Pelvis and Ureter (ICD-O 189.1,2)

Rules for Classification

The classification applies only to carcinoma. Papilloma is excluded. There should be histological or cytological confirmation of the disease.

Anatomical Subsites (See Fig. 341, p. 251)

1. Renal pelvis (189.1)
2. Ureter (189.2)

Regional Lymph Nodes (See Fig. 452, p. 343)

The regional lymph nodes are the hilar, abdominal paraaortic, paracaval and intrapelvic nodes. Laterality does not effect the N classification.

TN Clinical Classification

T – Primary Tumour

TX Primary tumour cannot be assessed
T0 No evidence of primary tumour
Tis Carcinoma in situ
  Ta Papillary non-invasive carcinoma (Fig. 353)
T1 Tumour invades subepithelial connective tissue (Fig. 353)
T2 Tumour invades muscularis (Fig. 353)
T3 Tumour invades beyond muscularis into peri-ureteric or peripelvic fat or renal parenchyma (Fig. 354)

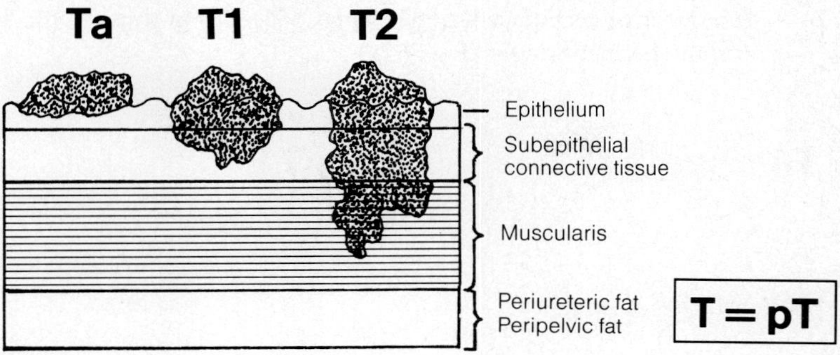

Fig. 353

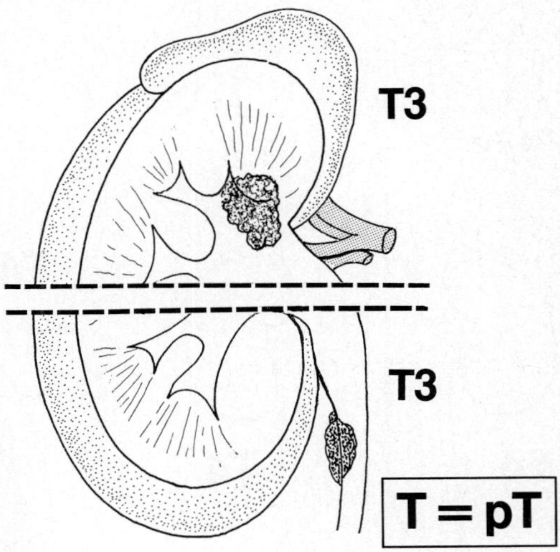

Fig. 354

T4 Tumour invades adjacent organs (Figs. 355, 356) or through the kidney into the perinephric fat (Fig. 357)

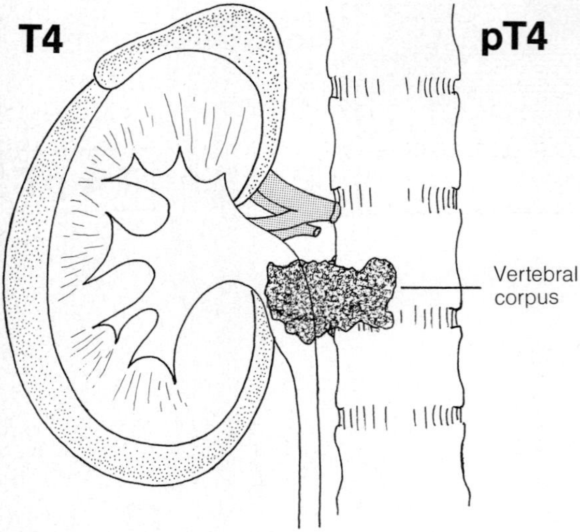

Fig. 355

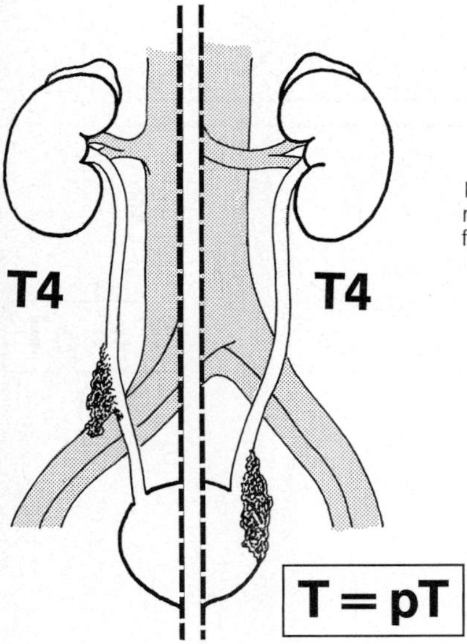

Fig. 356

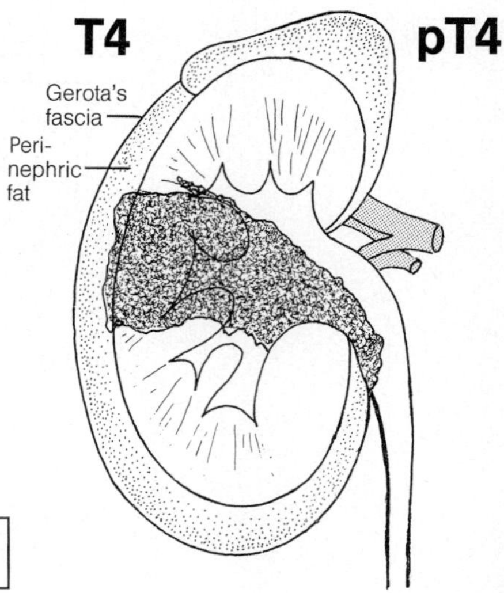

Fig. 357

N – Regional Lymph Nodes

NX Regional lymph nodes cannot be assessed
N0 No regional lymph node metastasis
N1 Metastasis in a single lymph node, 2 cm or less in greatest dimension (see Fig. 348, p. 257)
N2 Metastasis in a single lymph node, more than 2 cm but not more than 5 cm in greatest dimension (see Fig. 349, p. 257), *or* multiple lymph nodes, none more than 5 cm in greatest dimension (see Fig. 350, p. 258)
N3 Metastasis in a lymph node, more than 5 cm in greatest dimension (see Figs. 351, 352, pp. 258–259)

pTN Pathological Classification

The pT and pN categories correspond to the T and N categories.

Urethra (ICD-O 189.3)

Rules for Classification

The classification applies only to carcinoma. There should be histological or cytological confirmation of the disease.

Regional Lymph Nodes (See Fig. 452, p. 343)

The regional lymph nodes are the inguinal and the pelvic lymph nodes. Laterality does not affect the N classification.

TN Clinical Classification

T – Primary Tumour

TX Primary tumour cannot be assessed
T0 No evidence of primary tumour
Tis Carcinoma in situ
  Ta Non-invasive papillary, polypoid or verrucous carcinoma (Figs. 358, 359)

T1 Tumour invades subepithelial connective tissue (Figs. 358, 360)
T2 Tumour invades corpus spongiosum or prostate or periurethral muscle (Figs. 358, 361, 362)
T3 Tumour invades corpus cavernosum or beyond prostatic capsule (Fig. 363) or anterior vagina (Fig. 364) or bladder neck (Fig. 365)
T4 Tumour invades other adjacent organs (Fig. 366)

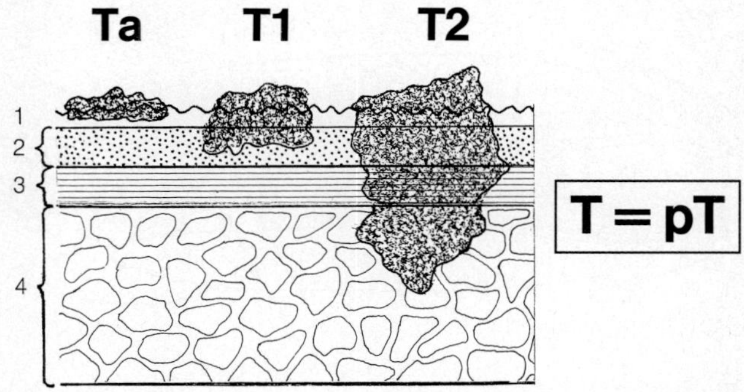

Fig. 358. *1* Epithelium; *2* subepithelial connective tissue; *3* urethral muscle; *4* urogenital diaphragm

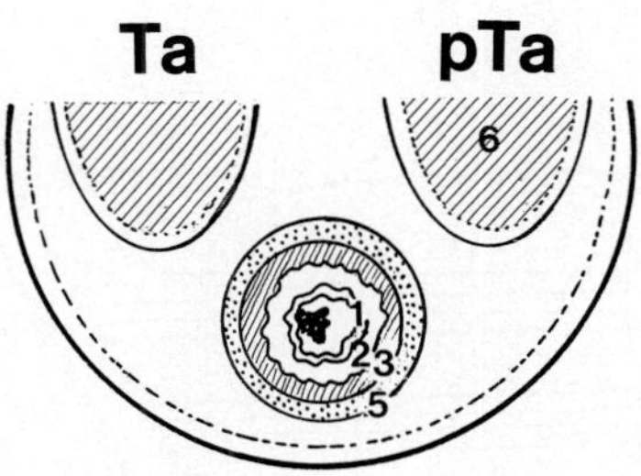

Fig. 359. *1* Epithelium; *2* subepithelial connective tissue; *3* urethral muscle; *5* corpus spongiosum; *6* corpus cavernosum

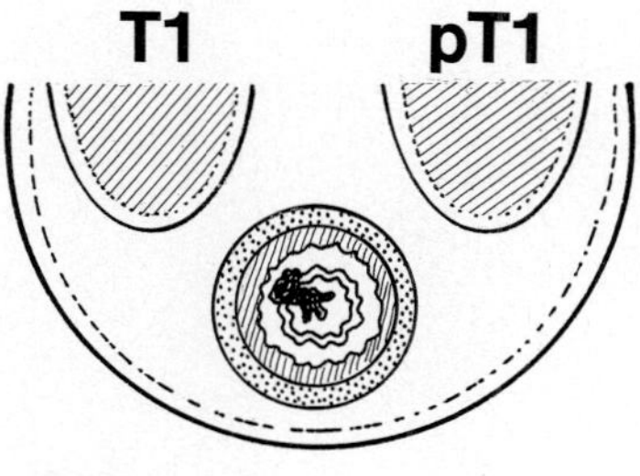

Fig. 360

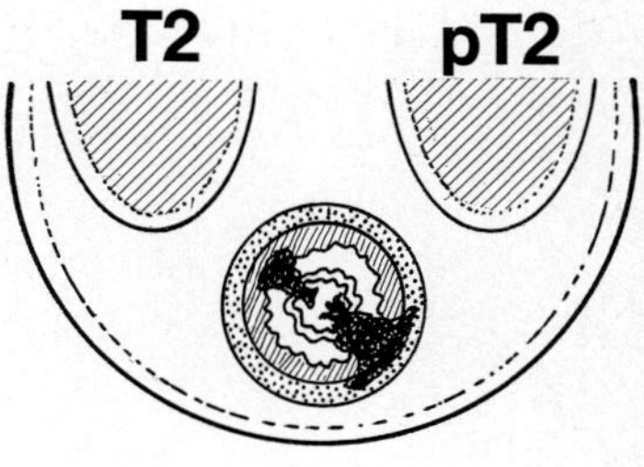

Fig. 361

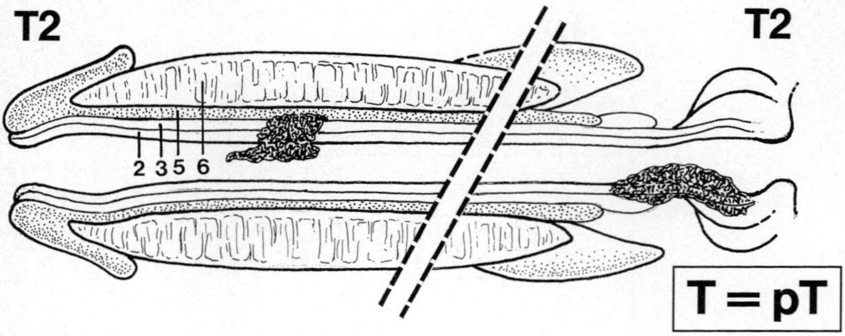

Fig. 362. *2, 3, 5, 6:* See Fig. 359

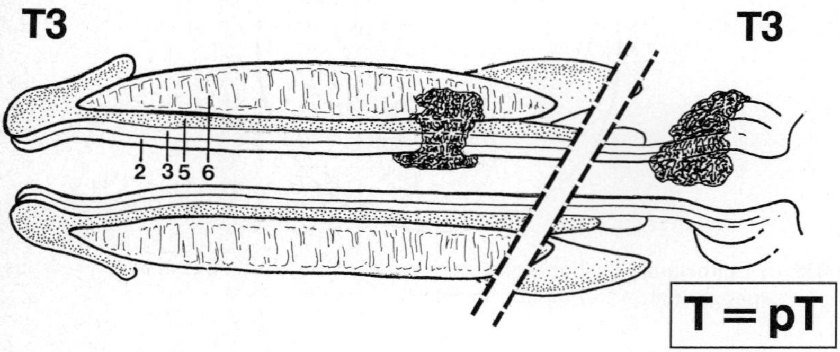

Fig. 363. *2, 3, 5, 6:* See Fig. 359

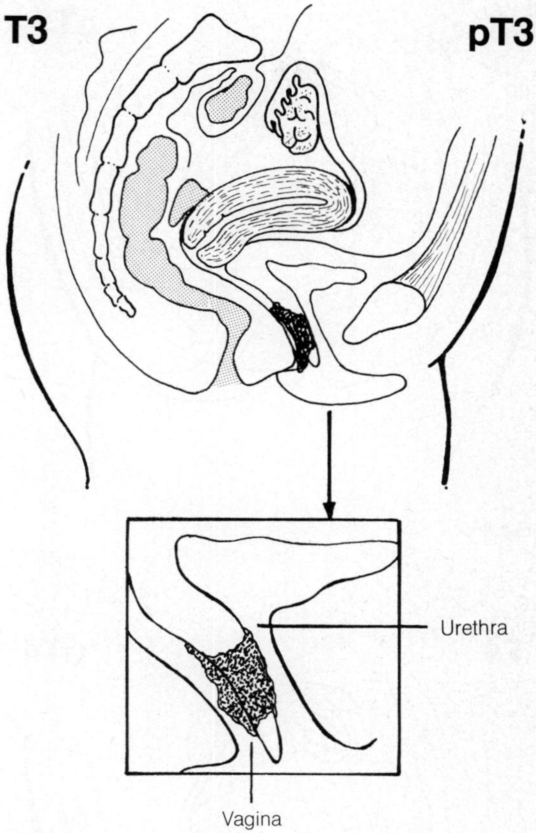

Fig. 364

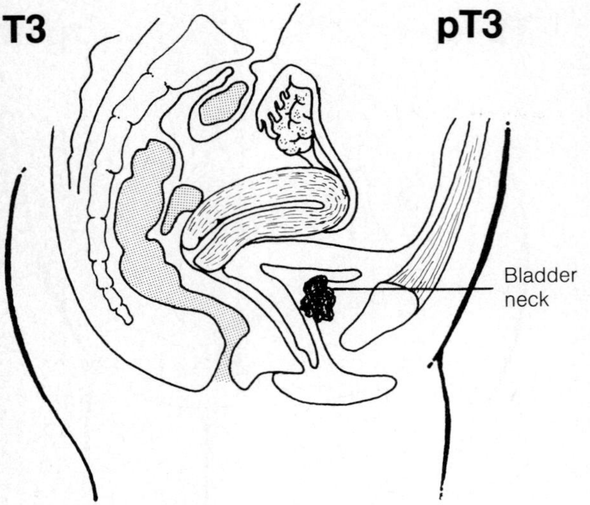

Fig. 365

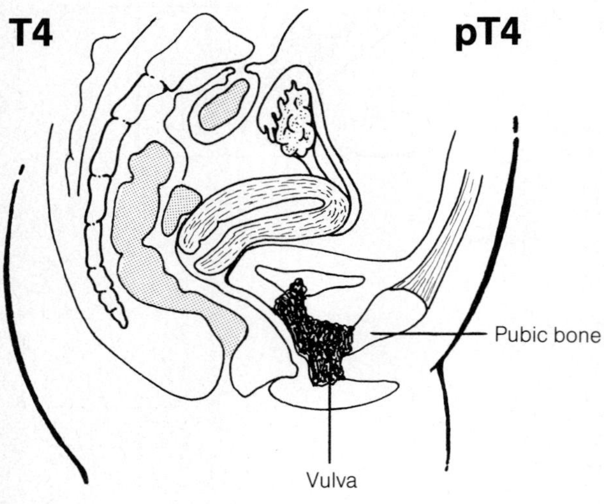

Fig. 366

N – Regional Lymph Nodes

NX Regional lymph nodes cannot be assessed
N0 No regional lymph node metastasis
N1 Metastasis in a single lymph node, 2 cm or less in greatest dimension (Fig. 367)

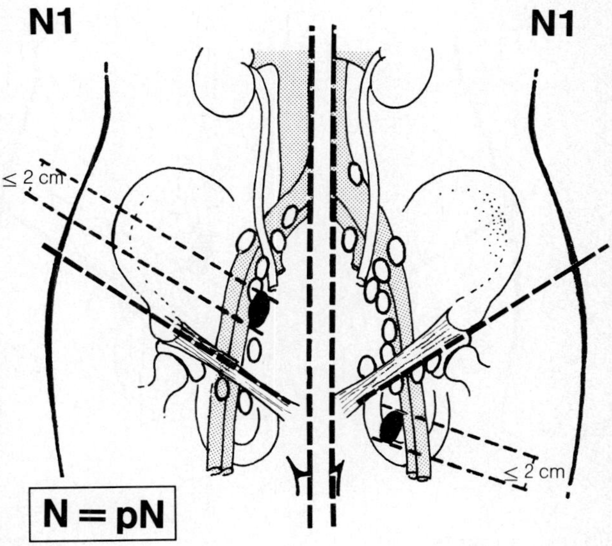

Fig. 367

N2 Metastasis in a single lymph node, more than 2 cm but not more than 5 cm in greatest dimension (Fig. 368), *or* multiple lymph nodes, none more than 5 cm in greatest dimension (Fig. 369)

N3 Metastasis in a lymph node, more than 5 cm in greatest dimension (Figs. 370, 371)

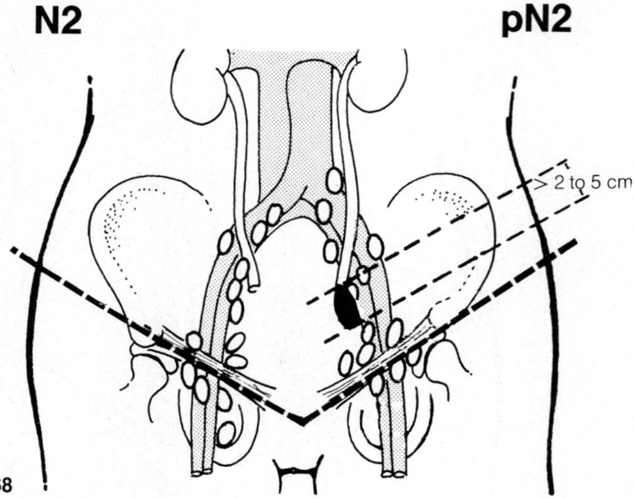

Fig. 368

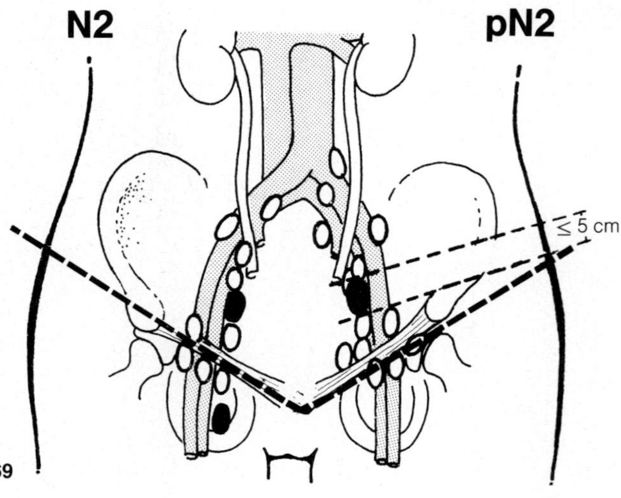

Fig. 369

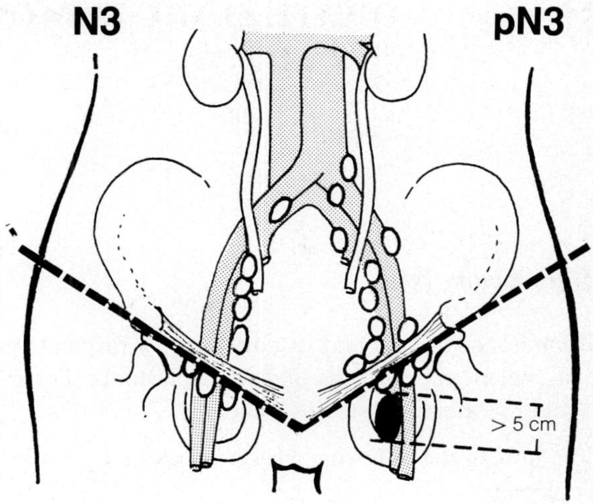

Fig. 370

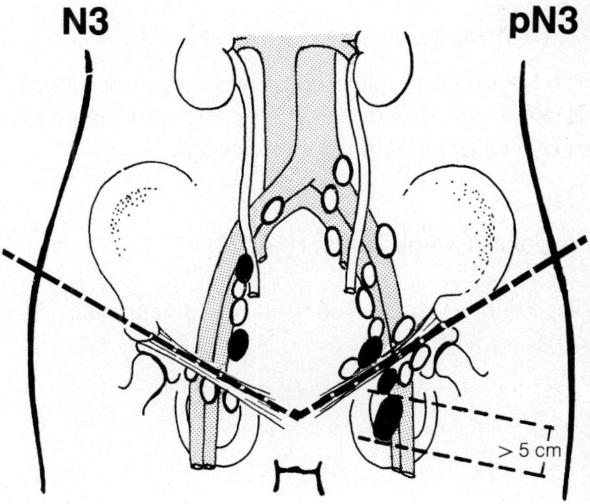

Fig. 371

pTN Pathological Classification

The pT and pN categories correspond to the T and N categories.

OPHTHALMIC TUMOURS

Introductory Notes

Tumours of the eye and its adnexa are a disparate group including carcinoma, melanoma, sarcoma and retinoblastoma. For clinical convenience they should be classified in one section.

Tumours in the following sites are classified:

- Eyelid
- Conjunctiva
- Uvea
- Retina
- Orbit
- Lacrimal gland

For histological nomenclature and diagnostic criteria, reference to the WHO classification (International Histological Classification of Tumours, No. 24, WHO, Geneva 1980) is recommended.

Regional Lymph Nodes (Fig. 372)

The regional lymph nodes are the preauricular *(1),* submandibular *(2)* and cervical *(3)* lymph nodes.

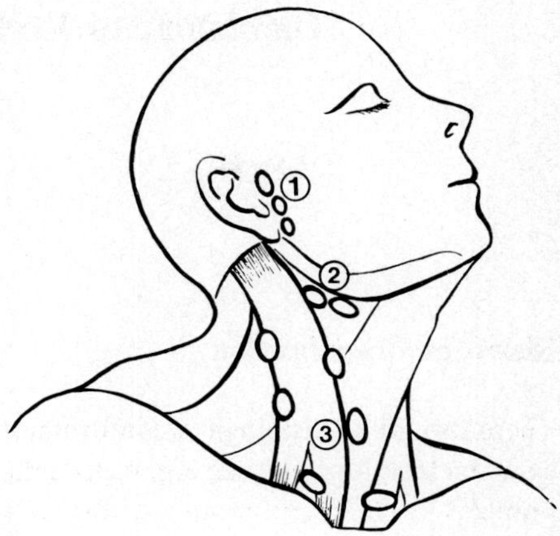

Fig. 372

The definitions of the N categories for ophthalmic tumours *excluding melanoma of eyelid* are:

N – Regional Lymph Nodes

NX Regional lymph nodes cannot be assessed
N0 No regional lymph node metastasis
N1 Regional lymph node metastasis

Carcinoma of Eyelid (ICD-O 173.1)

Rules for Classification

There should be histological confirmation of the disease to permit division of cases by histological type, e.g. basal cell, squamous cell and sebaceous carcinoma.

T Clinical Classification

T – Primary Tumour

TX	Primary tumour cannot be assessed
T0	No evidence of primary tumour
Tis	Carcinoma in situ
T1	Tumour of any size, not invading the tarsal plate; *or* at eyelid margin, 5 mm or less in greatest dimension (Fig. 373)

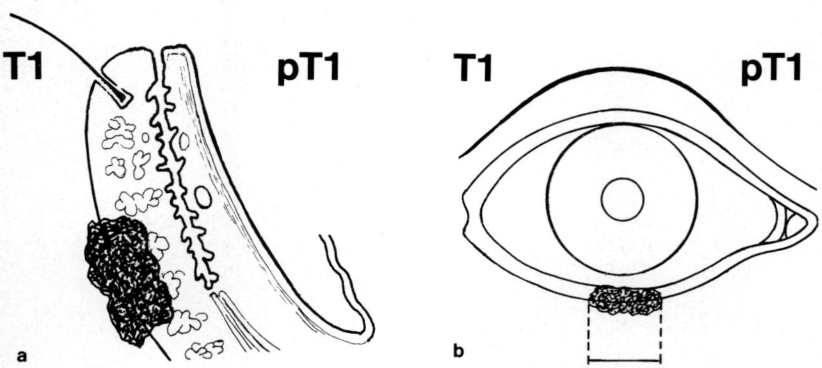

Fig. 373 a, b

T2 Tumour invades tarsal plate; *or* at eyelid margin, more than 5 mm but not more than 10 mm in greatest dimension (Fig. 374)

T3 Tumour involves full eyelid thickness; *or* at eyelid margin, more than 10 mm in greatest dimension (Fig. 375)

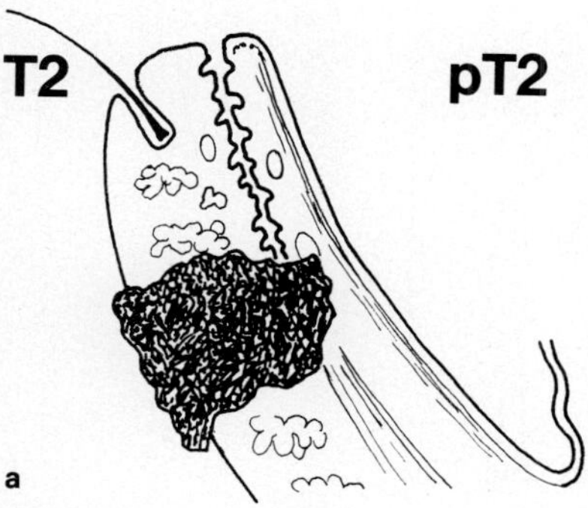

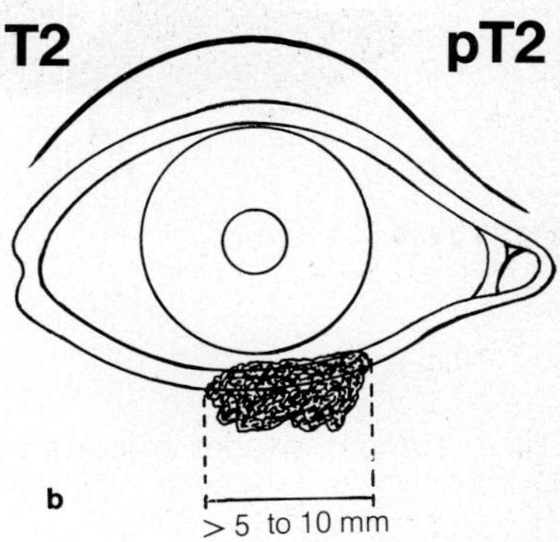

Fig. 374 a, b

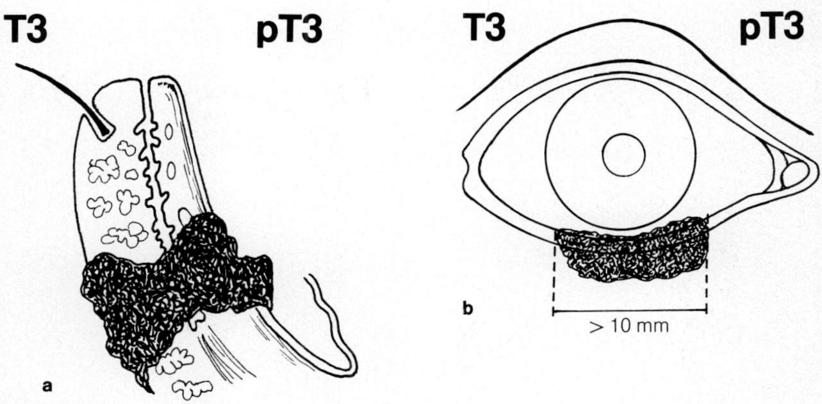

Fig. 375 a, b

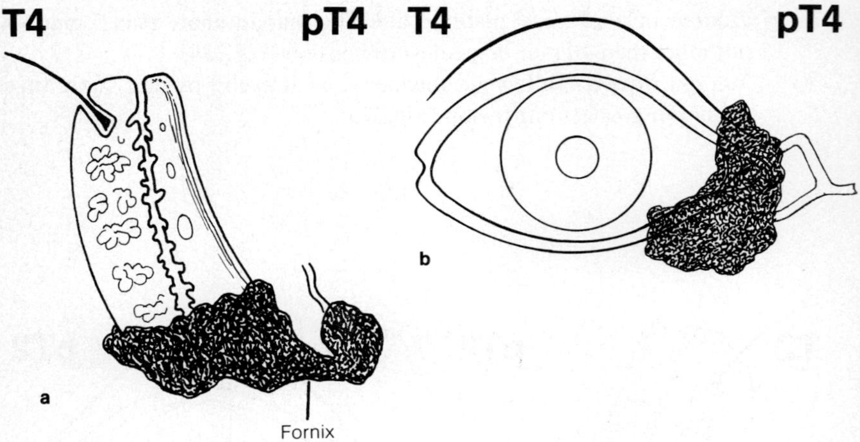

Fig. 376 a, b

T4 Tumour invades adjacent structures (Fig. 376)

pT Pathological Classification

The pT categories correspond to the T categories.

Malignant Melanoma of Eyelid (ICD-O 173.1)

Rules for Classification

The classification is identical to that of malignant melanoma of the skin (see p. 163 and Figs. 220–235, pp. 164–172). There should be histological confirmation of the disease.

Carcinoma of Conjunctiva (ICD-O 190.3)

Rules for Classification

There should be histological confirmation of the disease to permit division of cases by histological type, e.g. mucoepidermoid and squamous cell carcinoma.

T Clinical Classification

T – Primary Tumour

TX Primary tumour cannot be assessed
T0 No evidence of primary tumour
Tis Carcinoma in situ

T1 Tumour 5 mm or less in greatest dimension (Fig. 377)
T2 Tumour more than 5 mm in greatest dimension, without invasion of adjacent structures (Fig. 378)
T3 Tumour invades adjacent structures, excluding the orbit (Fig. 379)
T4 Tumour invades the orbit (Fig. 380)

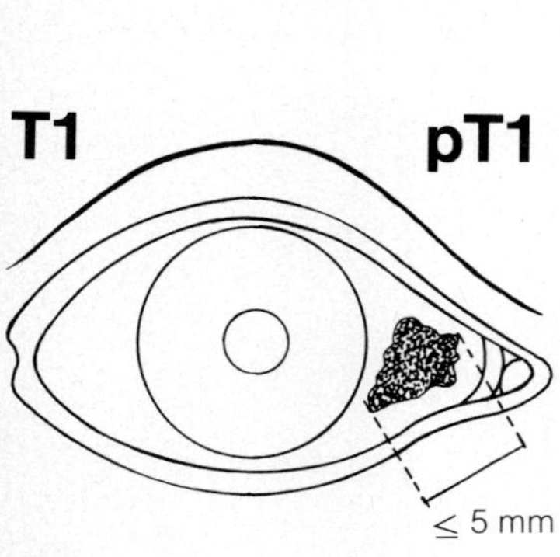

Fig. 377

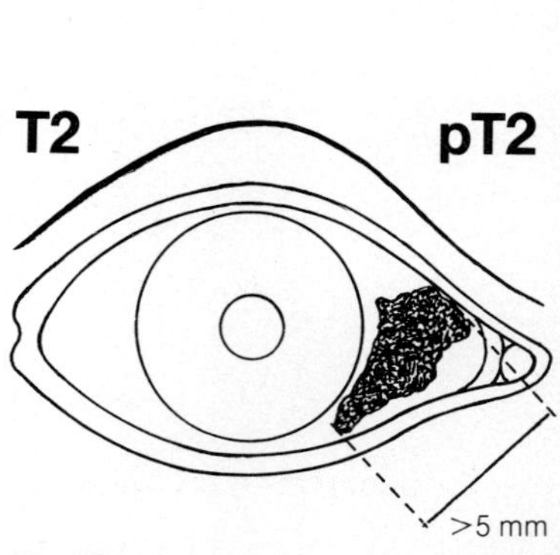

Fig. 378

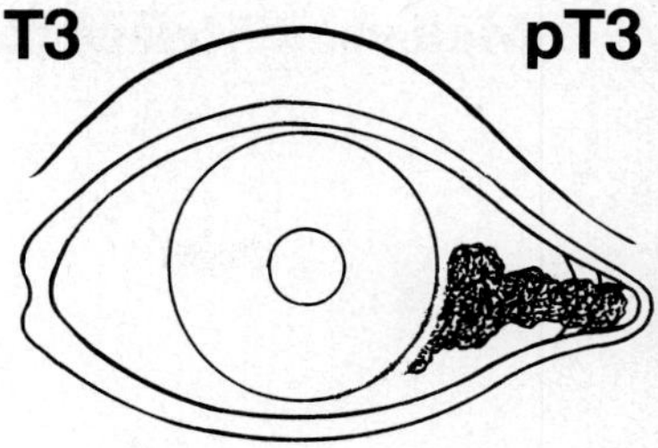

Fig. 379

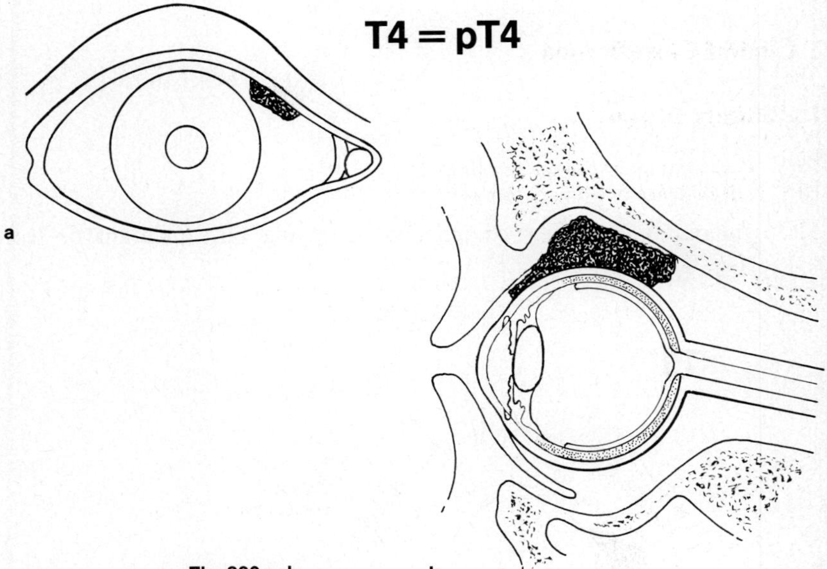

Fig. 380 a, b

pT Pathological Classification

The pT categories correspond to the T categories.

Malignant Melanoma of Conjunctiva (ICD-O 190.3)

Rules for Classification

There should be histological confirmation of the disease. The tumour should be distinguished from non-tumorous pigmentation. Primary acquired melanosis should be classified under the category T0; however, in case of histological and/or cytological confirmation such cases should be listed under G0.

T Clinical Classification

T – Primary Tumour

TX Primary tumour cannot be assessed
T0 No evidence of primary tumour
T1 Tumour(s) of bulbar conjunctiva occupying one quadrant or less (Fig. 381)

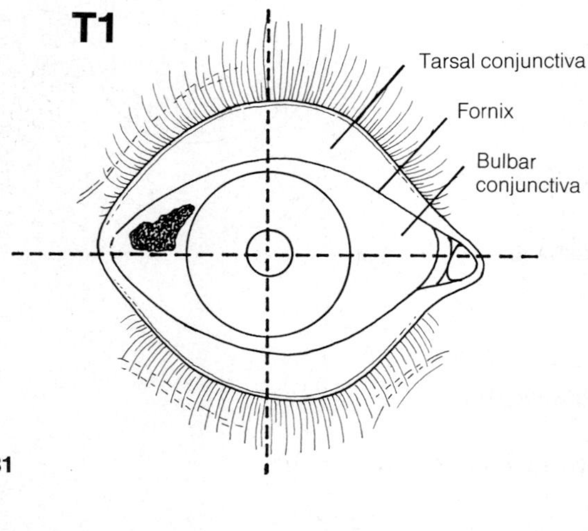

Fig. 381

T2 Tumour(s) of bulbar conjunctiva occupying more than one quadrant (Fig. 382)

T3 Tumour(s) of conjunctival fornix and/or palpebral conjunctiva and/or caruncle (Fig. 383)

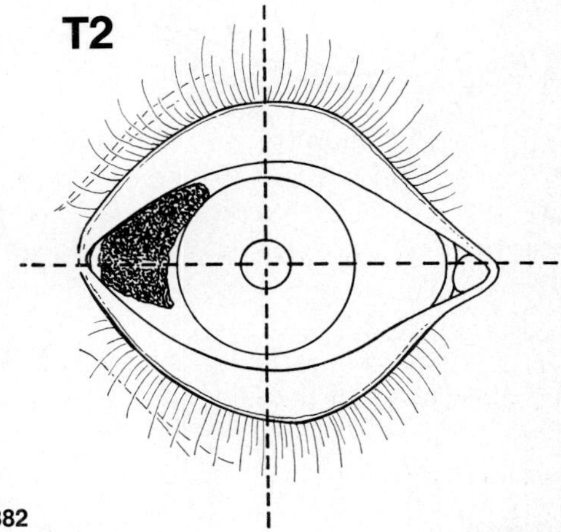

Fig. 382

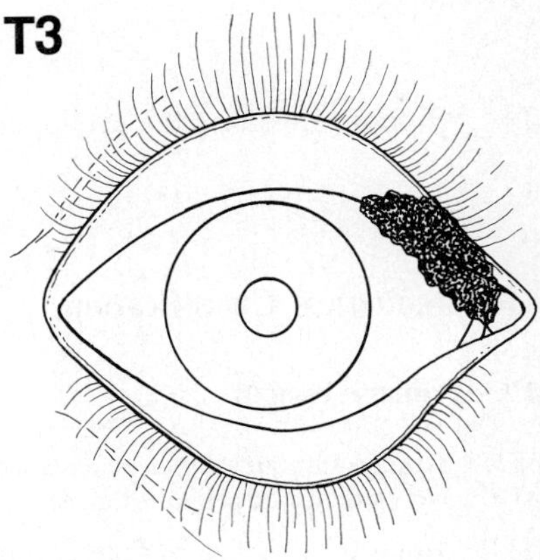

Fig. 383

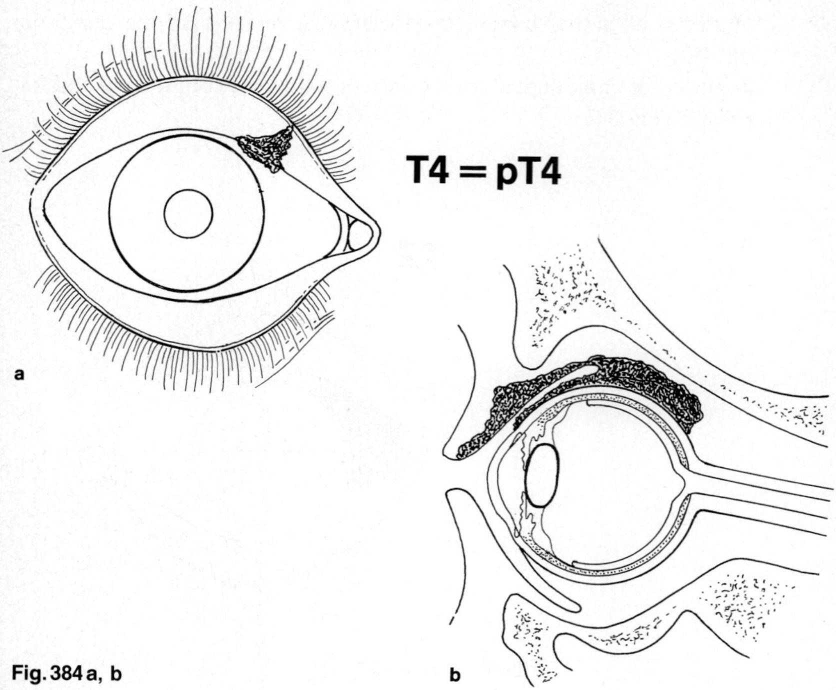

Fig. 384 a, b

T4 Tumour invading the eyelid, cornea and/or orbit (Fig. 384)

pT Pathological Classification

pT – Primary Tumour

pTX Primary tumour cannot be assessed
pT0 No evidence of primary tumour

pT1 Tumour(s) of the bulbar conjunctiva occupying one quadrant or less *and* 2 mm or less in thickness (Fig. 385)

pT2 Tumour(s) of the bulbar conjunctiva occupying more than one quadrant *and* 2 mm or less in thickness (Fig. 385)

pT3 Tumour(s) of the conjunctival fornix and/or palpebral conjunctiva and/or caruncle or tumour of the bulbar conjunctiva more than 2 mm in thickness (Fig. 386)

pT4 Tumour invading the eyelid, cornea and/or orbit (Fig. 384)

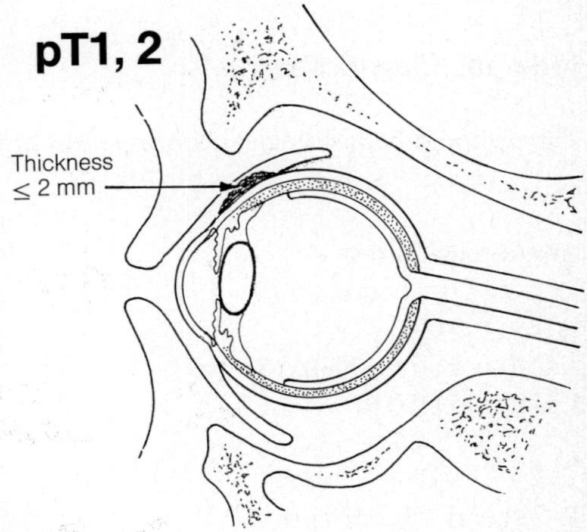

Fig. 385

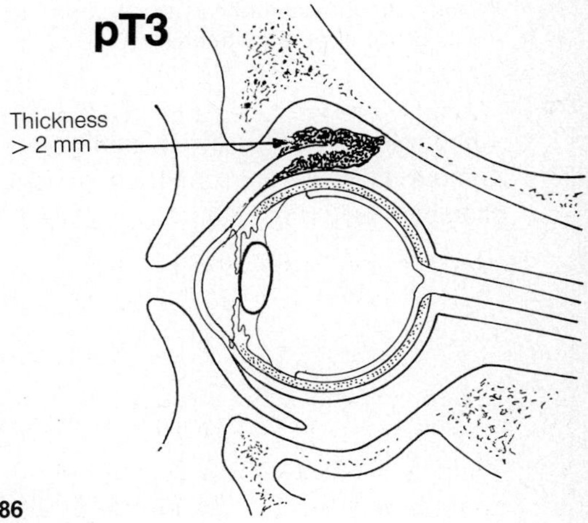

Fig. 386

Malignant Melanoma of Uvea (ICD-O 190.0,6)

Rules for Classification

There should be histological confirmation of the disease.

Anatomical Sites

1. Iris (190.0)
2. Ciliary body (190.0)
3. Choroid (190.6)

T Clinical Classification

T - Primary Tumour

TX Primary tumour cannot be assessed
T0 No evidence of primary tumour

Iris

T1 Tumour limited to the iris (Fig. 387)
T2 Tumour involves one quadrant or less, with invasion into anterior chamber angle (Fig. 388)

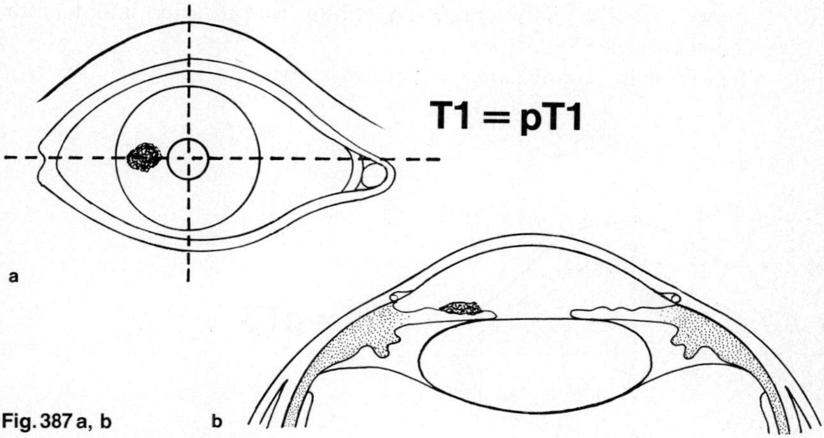

Fig. 387 a, b

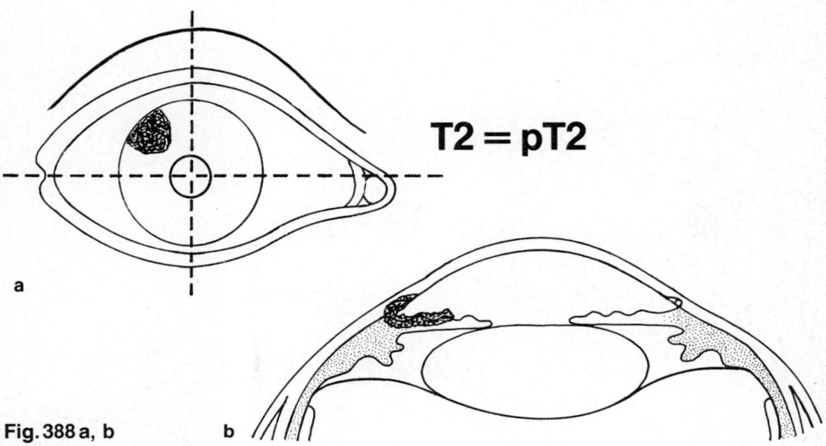

Fig. 388 a, b

T3 Tumour involves more than one quadrant, with invasion into anterior chamber angle (Fig. 389)

T4 Tumour with extraocular extension (Fig. 390)

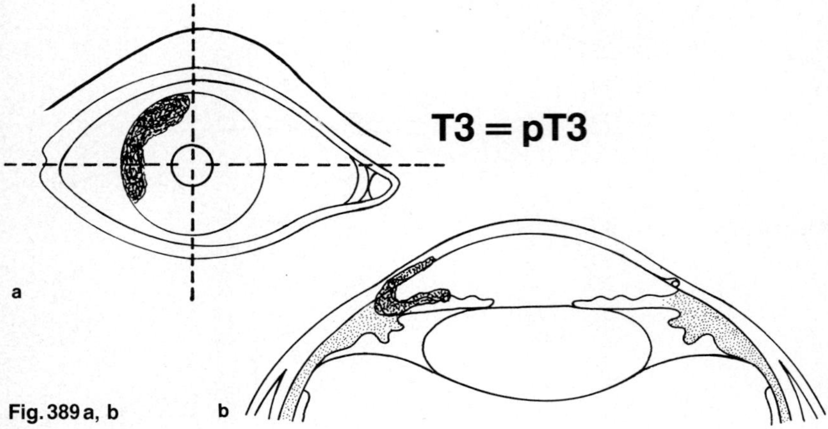

Fig. 389 a, b

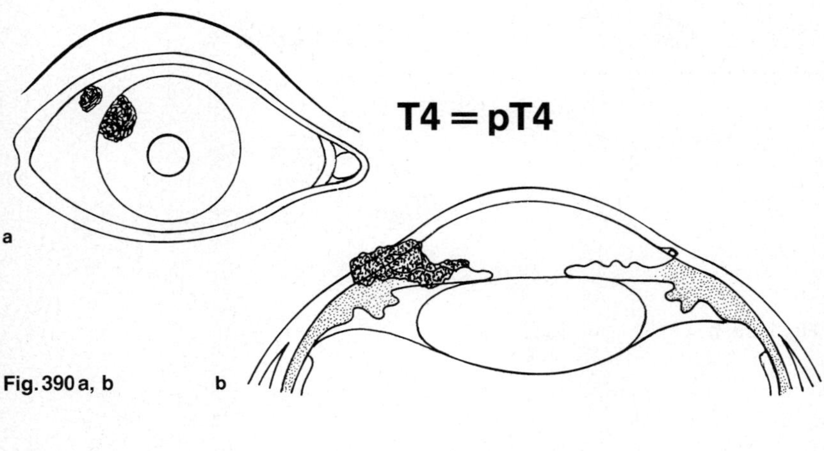

Fig. 390 a, b

Ciliary Body

T1 Tumour limited to the ciliary body (Fig. 391)
T2 Tumour invades into anterior chamber and/or iris (Fig. 392)
T3 Tumour invades choroid (Fig. 393)
T4 Tumour with extraocular extension (Fig. 394)

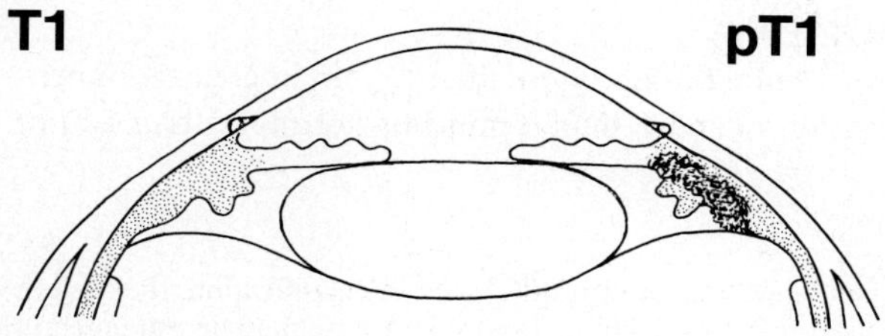

Fig. 391

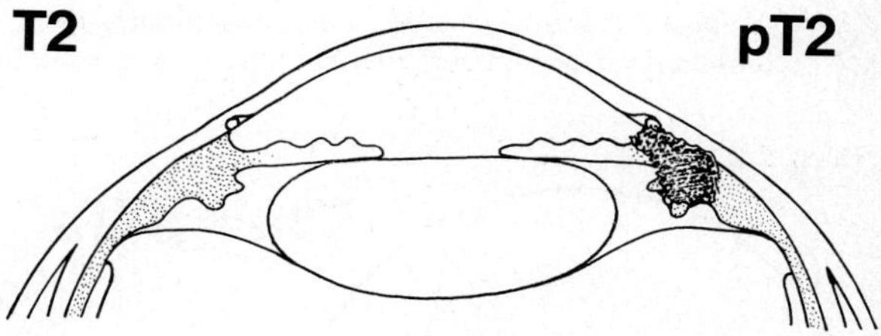

Fig. 392

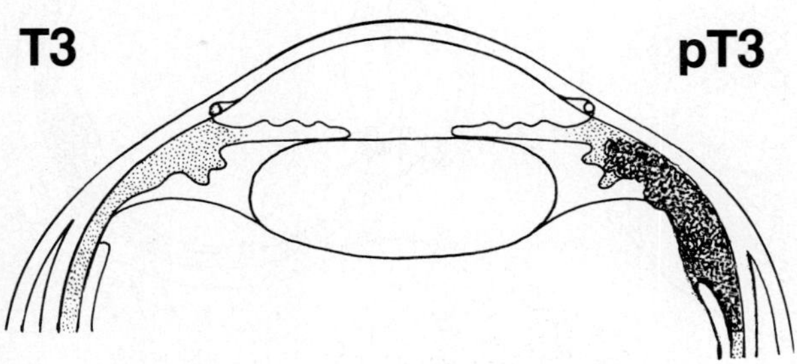

Fig. 393

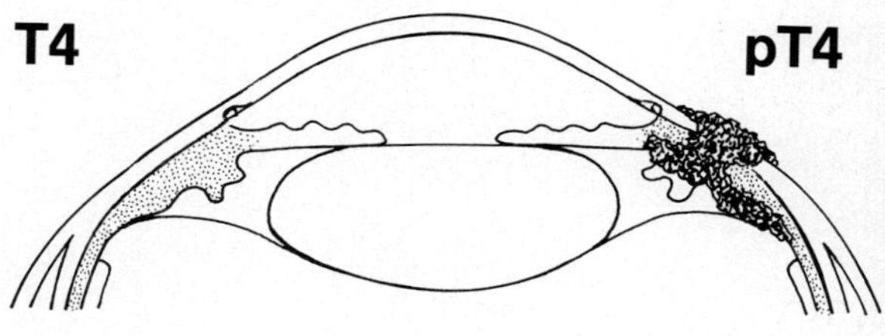

Fig. 394

Choroid

T1 Tumour 10 mm or less in greatest dimension with an elevation of 3 mm or less[1]

- T1a Tumour 7 mm or less in greatest dimension with an elevation of 2 mm or less (Fig. 395)
- T1b Tumour more than 7 mm but not more than 10 mm in greatest dimension with an elevation of more than 2 mm but not more than 3 mm (Fig. 396)

T2 Tumour more than 10 mm but not more than 15 mm in greatest dimension with an elevation of more than 3 mm but not more than 5 mm[1] (Fig. 397)

Note: [1] When dimension and elevation show a difference in classification, the highest category should be used for classification. The tumour base may be estimated in optic disc diameters (dd, average 1 dd = 1.5 mm) and the elevation in dioptres (average 3 dioptres = 1 mm); other techniques, such as ultrasonography and computerized stereometry, may provide a more accurate measurement.

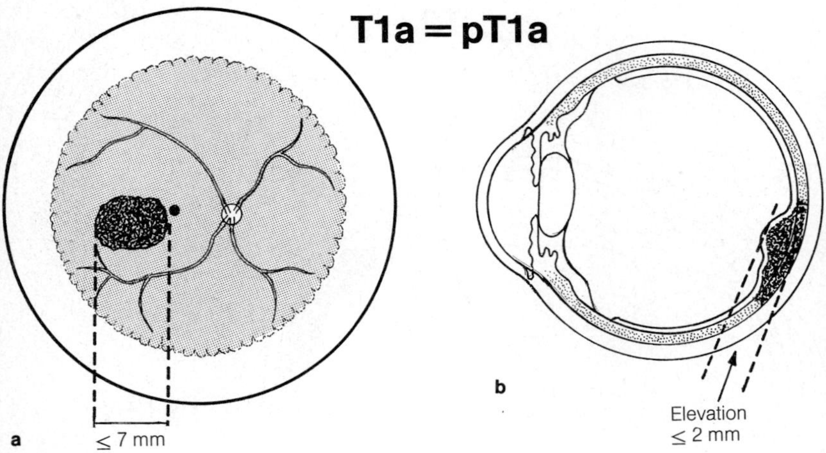

Fig. 395 a, b

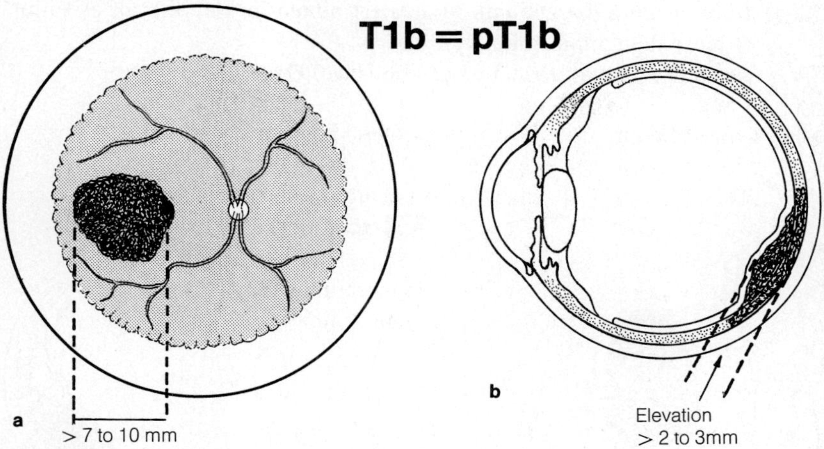

Fig. 396 a, b

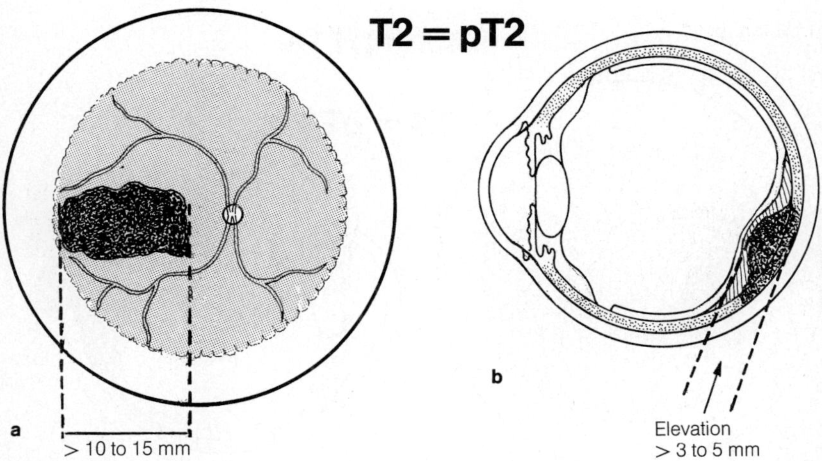

Fig. 397 a, b

T3 Tumour more than 15 mm in greatest dimension or with an elevation of more than 5 mm (Fig. 398)

T4 Tumour with extraocular extension (Fig. 399)

Note: See page 288

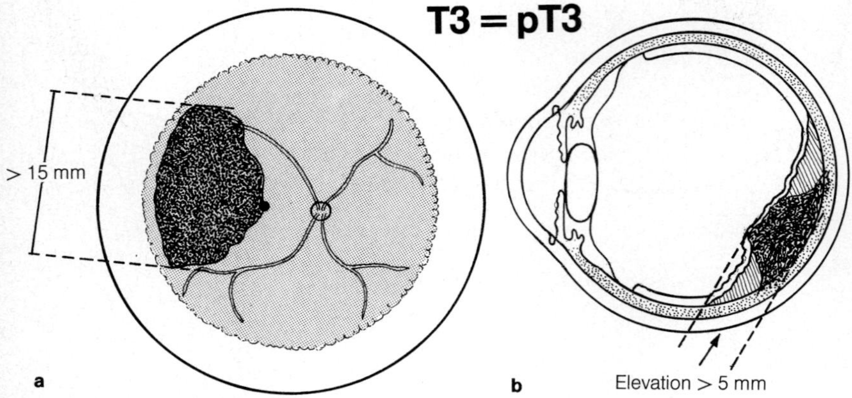

Fig. 398 a, b

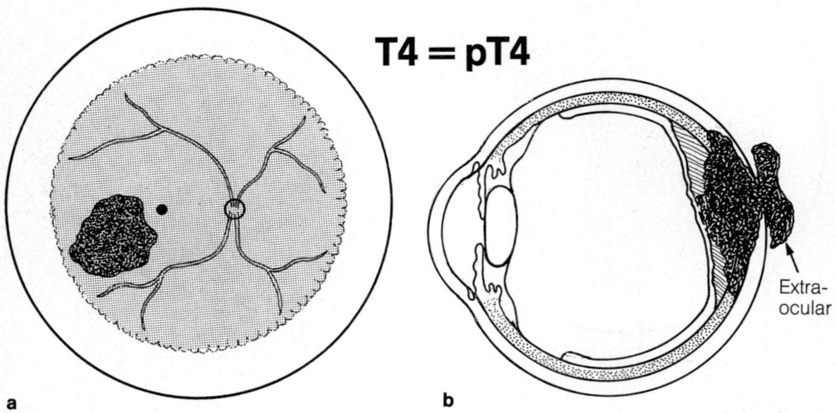

Fig. 399 a, b

pT Pathological Classification

The pT categories correspond to the T categories.

Retinoblastoma (ICD-O 190.5)

Rules for Classification

In bilateral cases, each eye should be classified separately. The classification does not apply to complete spontaneous regression of the tumour. There should be histological confirmation of the disease in an enucleated eye.

T Clinical Classification

T – Primary Tumour

The extent of retinal involvement is indicated as a percentage.

TX Primary tumour cannot be assessed
T0 No evidence of primary tumour

T1 Tumour(s) limited to 25% or less of the retina (Fig. 400)

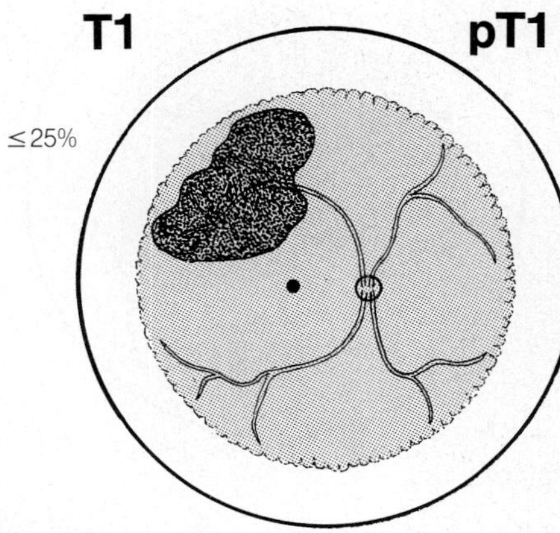

Fig. 400

T2 Tumour(s) involve(s) more than 25% but not more than 50% of the retina (Fig. 401)

T3 Tumour(s) involve(s) more than 50% of the retina and/or invade(s) beyond the retina but remain(s) intraocular

T3a Tumour(s) involve(s) more than 50% of the retina and/or tumour cells in the vitreous body (Fig. 402)

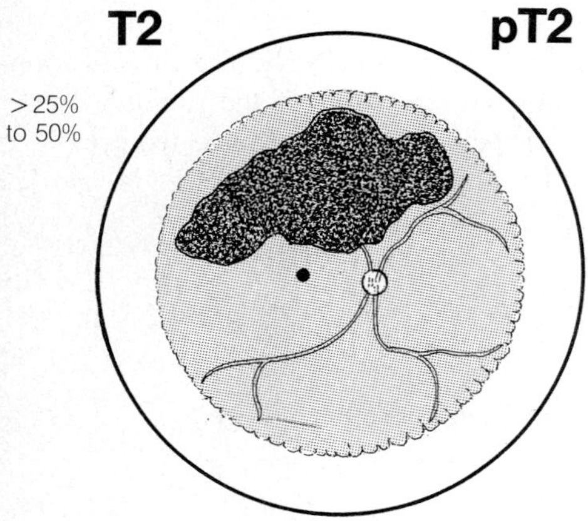

Fig. 401

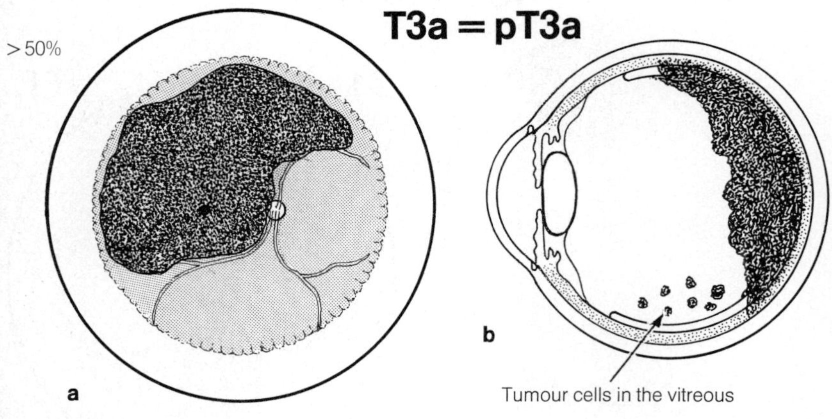

Fig. 402 a, b

T3b Tumour(s) involve(s) optic disc (Fig. 403)
T3c Tumour(s) involve(s) anterior chamber and/or uvea (Fig. 404)

T3b = pT3b

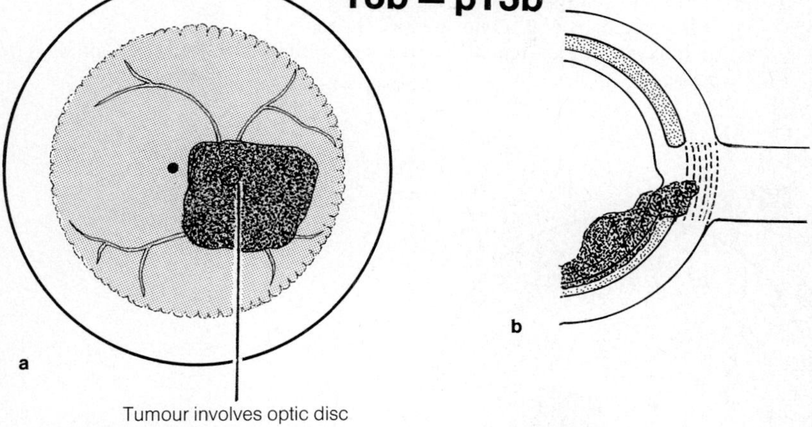

Fig. 403 a, b

T3c = pT3c

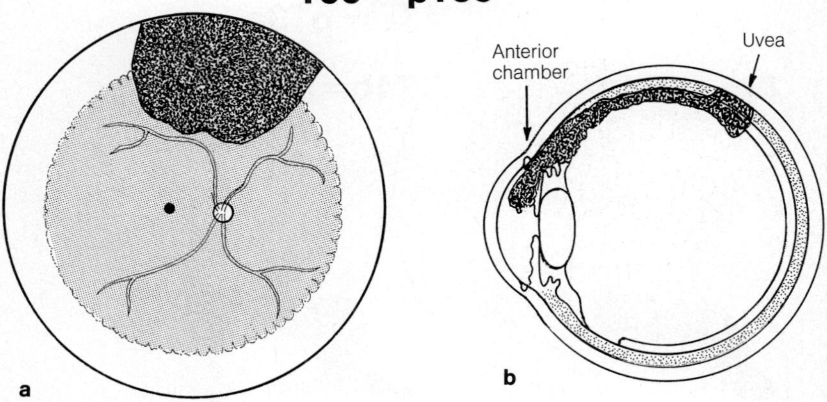

Fig. 404 a, b

T4 Tumour with extraocular invasion (Figs. 405, 406)

- T4a Tumour invades retrobulbar optic nerve (Fig. 405)
- T4b Extraocular extension other than invasion of optic nerve (Fig. 406)

Note: The following suffixes may be added to the appropriate T categories:

(m) to indicate multiple tumours, e.g. T2(m)
(f) to indicate cases with a known family history
(d) to indicate diffuse retinal involvement without the formation of discrete masses

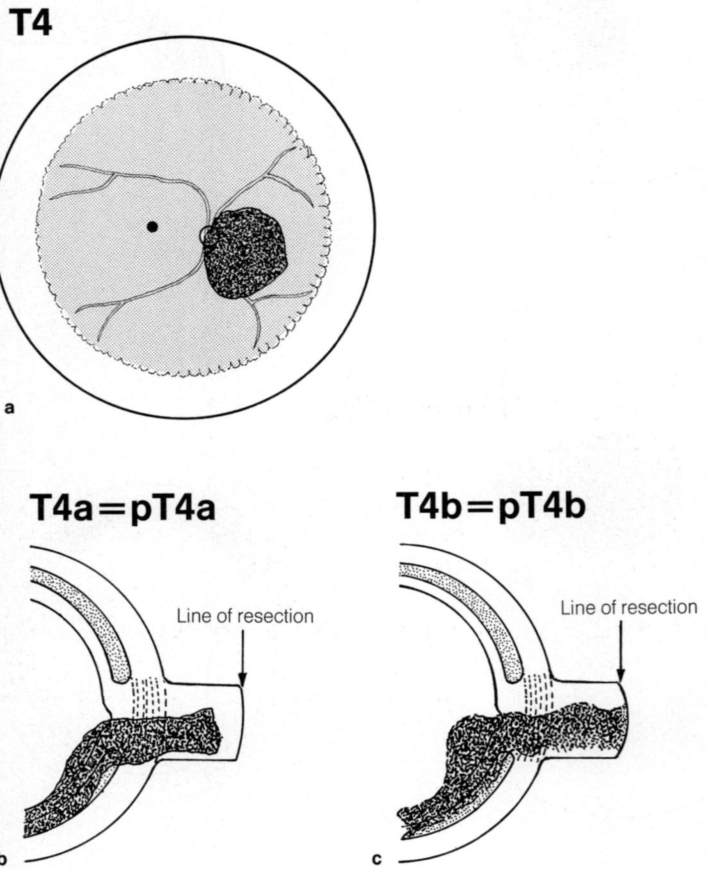

Fig. 405a–c

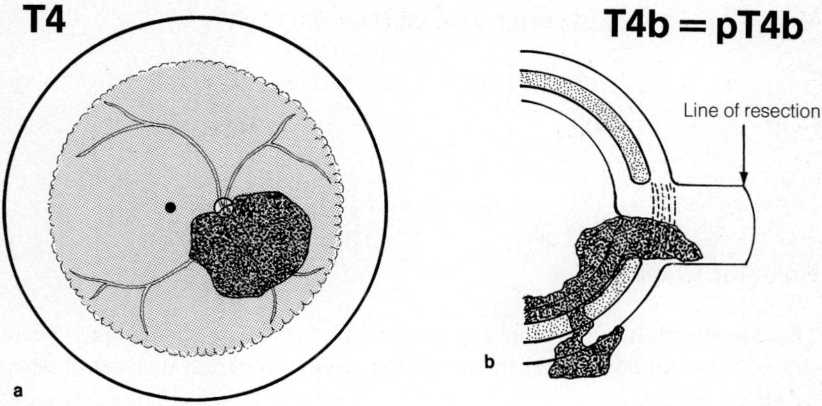

Fig. 406 a, b

pT Pathological Classification

pT – Primary Tumour

pTX Primary tumour cannot be assessed
pT0 No evidence of primary tumour
pT1 Corresponds to T1 (Fig. 400, see p. 291)
pT2 Corresponds to T2 (Fig. 401, see p. 292)
pT3 Corresponds to T3
  pT3a Corresponds to T3a (Fig. 402)
  pT3b Tumour invades optic nerve as far as lamina cribrosa (Fig. 403)
  pT3c Tumour in anterior chamber and/or invasion with thickening of uvea and/or intrascleral invasion (Fig. 404)
pT4 Corresponds to T4
  pT4a Intraneural tumour beyond lamina cribrosa, but not at line of resection (Fig. 405 b)
  pT4b Tumour at line of resection or other extraocular extension (Figs. 405 c, 406 b)

Sarcoma of Orbit (ICD-O 190.1)

Rules for Classification

The classification applies only to sarcomas of soft tissue and bone. There should be histological confirmation of the disease to permit division of cases by histological type.

T Clinical Classification

T – Primary Tumour

TX Primary tumour cannot be assessed
T0 No evidence of primary tumour

T1 Tumour 15 mm or less in greatest dimension (Fig. 407)
T2 Tumour more than 15 mm in greatest dimension (Fig. 408)
T3 Tumour of any size with diffuse invasion of orbital tissues and/or bony walls (Fig. 409)
T4 Tumour invades beyond the orbit to adjacent sinuses and/or to cranium (Fig. 410)

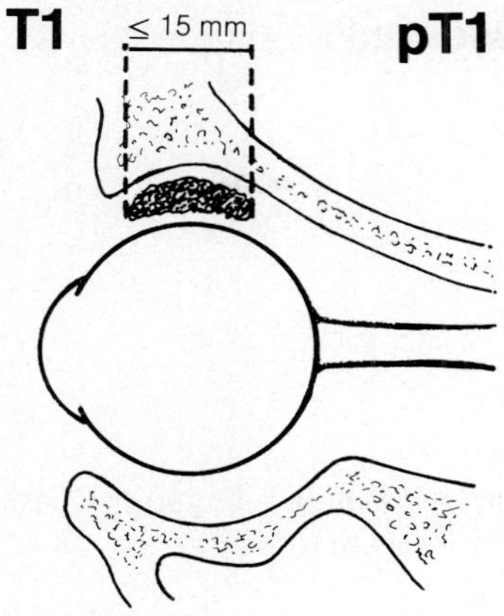

Fig. 407

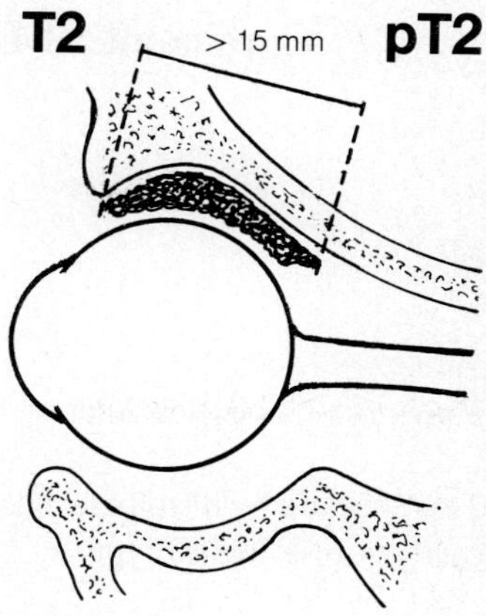

Fig. 408

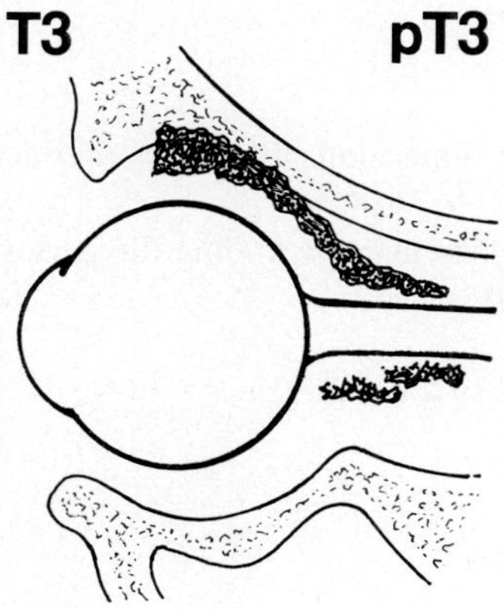

Fig. 409

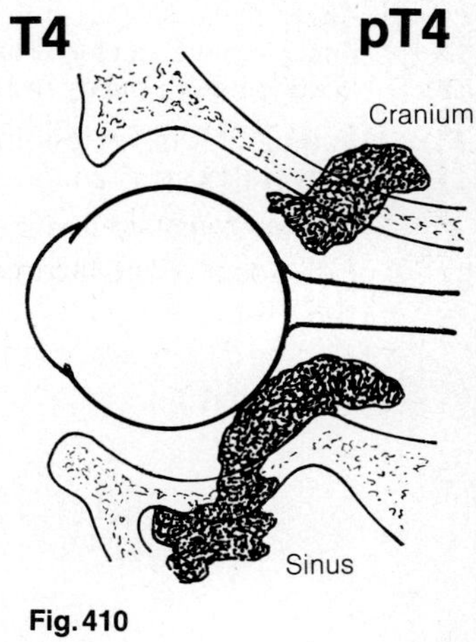

Fig. 410

pT Pathological Classification

The pT categories correspond to the T categories.

Carcinoma of Lacrimal Gland (ICD-O 190.2)

Rules for Classification

There should be histological confirmation of the disease to permit division of cases by histological type.

T Clinical Classification

T – Primary Tumour

TX Primary tumour cannot be assessed
T0 No evidence of primary tumour
T1 Tumour 2.5 cm or less in greatest dimension, limited to the lacrimal gland (Fig. 411)
T2 Tumour 2.5 cm or less in greatest dimension, invading the periosteum of the fossa of the lacrimal gland (Fig. 412)

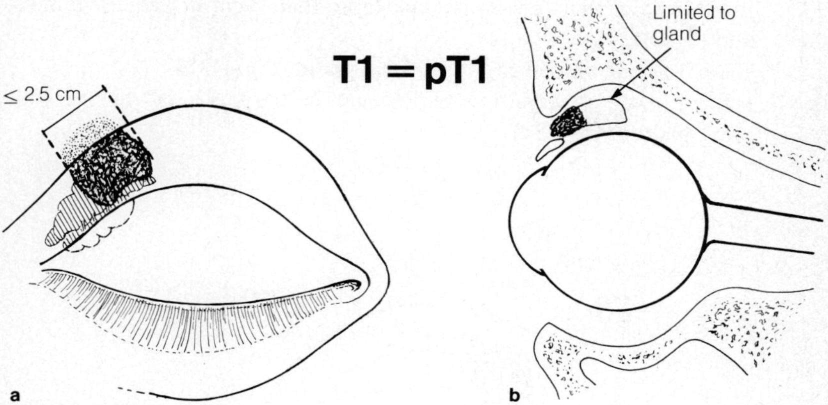

Fig. 411 a, b

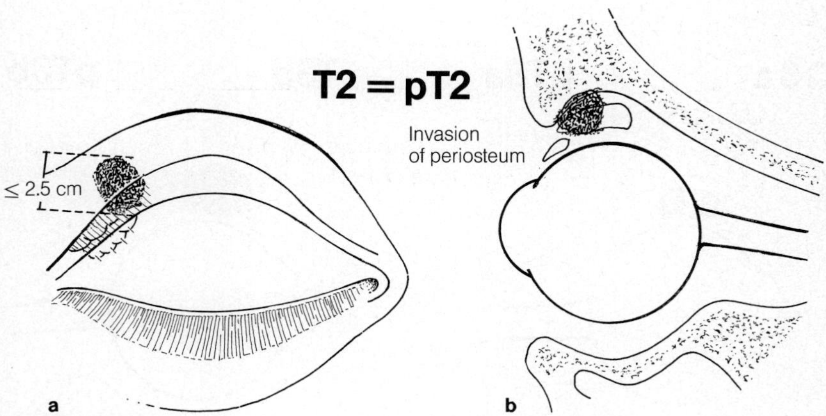

Fig. 412 a, b

T3 Tumour more than 2.5 cm but not more than 5 cm in greatest dimension (Fig. 413 a)

T3a Tumour limited to the lacrimal gland (Fig. 413 b)

T3b Tumour invades the periosteum of the fossa of the lacrimal gland (Fig. 413 c)

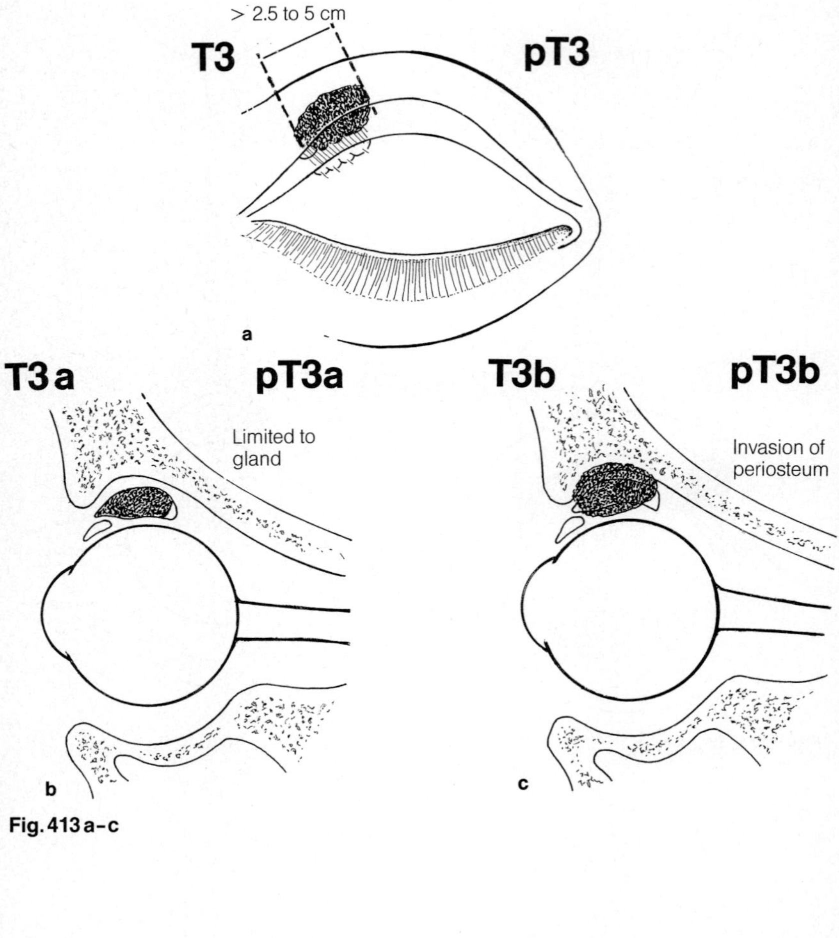

Fig. 413 a–c

T4 Tumour more than 5 cm in greatest dimension (Fig. 414 a)
- T4a Tumour invades orbital soft tissues, optic nerve, or globe *without* bone invasion (Fig. 414 b)
- T4b Tumour invades orbital soft tissues, optic nerve, or globe *with* bone invasion (Fig. 414 c)

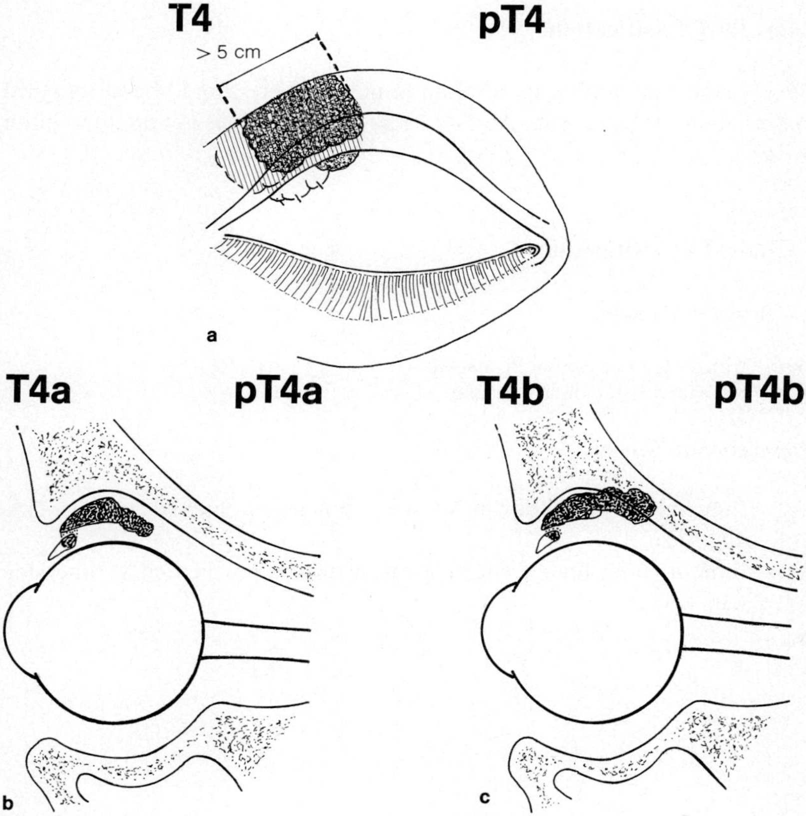

Fig. 414 a–c

pT Pathological Classification

The pT categories correspond to the T categories.

BRAIN TUMOURS (ICD-O 191)

Rules for Classification

The classification applies to all brain tumours. There should be histological confirmation of the disease. An N/pN classification does not apply to brain tumours.

T Clinical Classification

T – Primary Tumour

TX Primary tumour cannot be assessed
T0 No evidence of primary tumour

Supratentorial Tumours

T1 Tumour 5 cm or less in greatest dimension, limited to one side (Fig. 415)
T2 Tumour more than 5 cm in greatest dimension, limited to one side (Fig. 416)

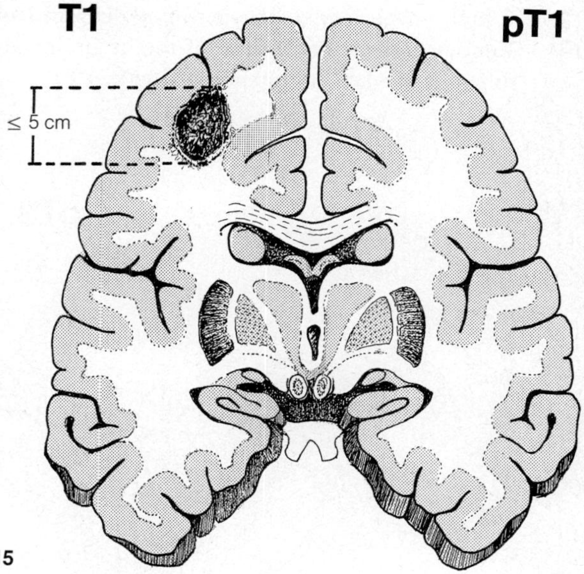

Fig. 415

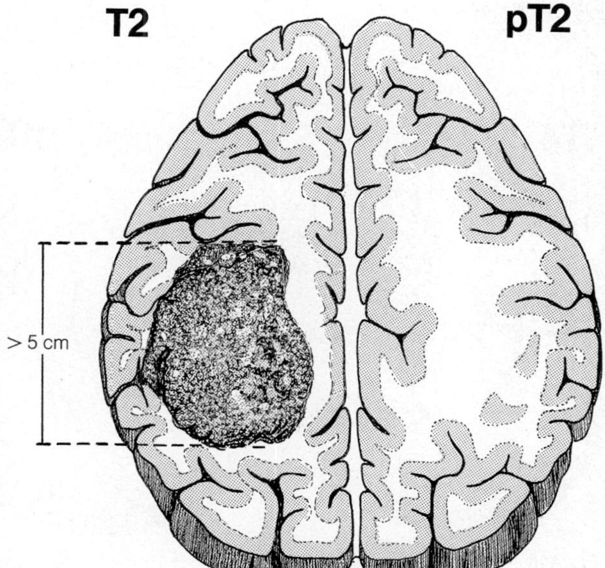

Fig. 416

T3 Tumour invades or encroaches upon the ventricular system (Fig. 417)

T4 Tumour crosses the midline of the brain, invades the opposite hemisphere, or invades infratentorially (Fig. 418)

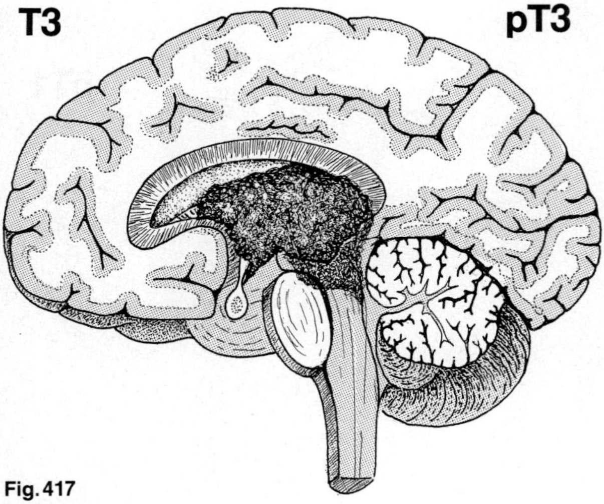

Fig. 417

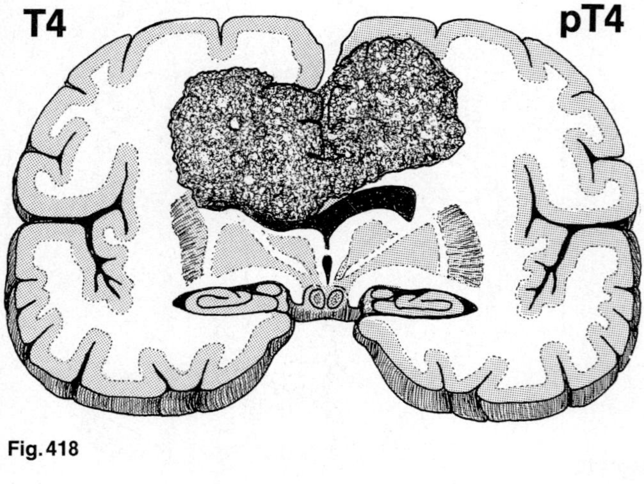

Fig. 418

Infratentorial Tumours

T1 Tumour 3 cm or less in greatest dimension, limited to one side (Fig. 419)

T2 Tumour more than 3 cm in greatest dimension, limited to one side (Fig. 420)

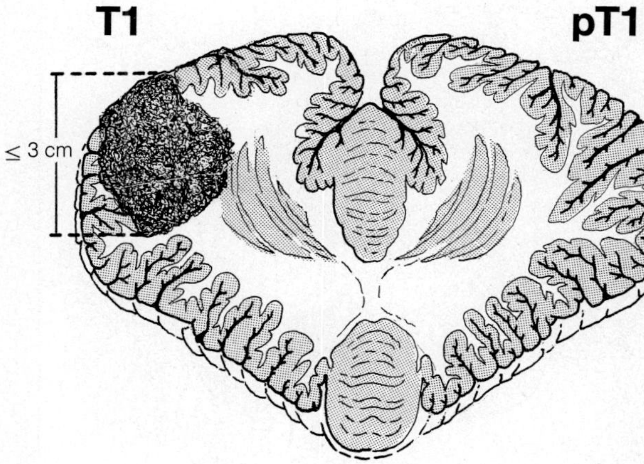

Fig. 419

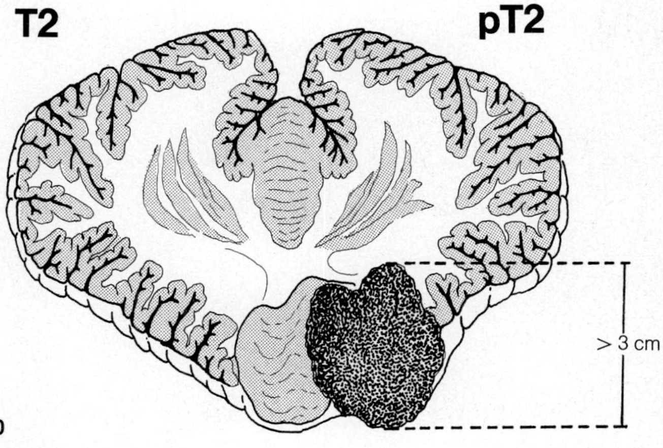

Fig. 420

T3 Tumour invades or encroaches upon the ventricular system (Fig. 421)
T4 Tumour crosses the midline of the brain, invades the opposite hemisphere (Fig. 422), or invades supratentorially (Fig. 423)

T3 **pT3**

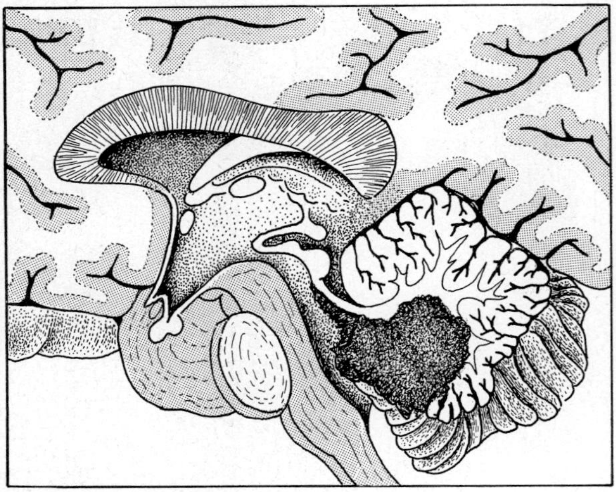

Fig. 421

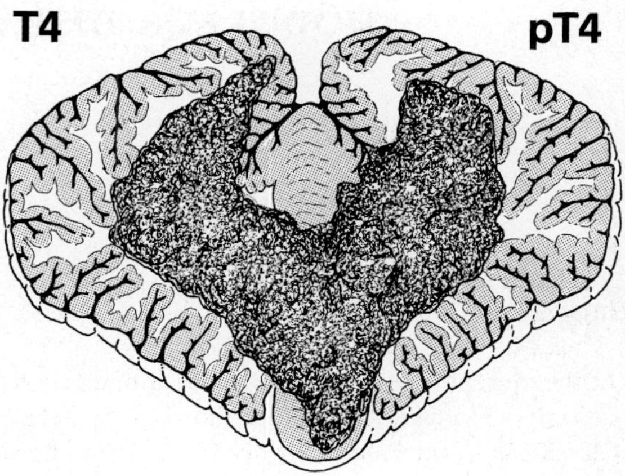

Fig. 422

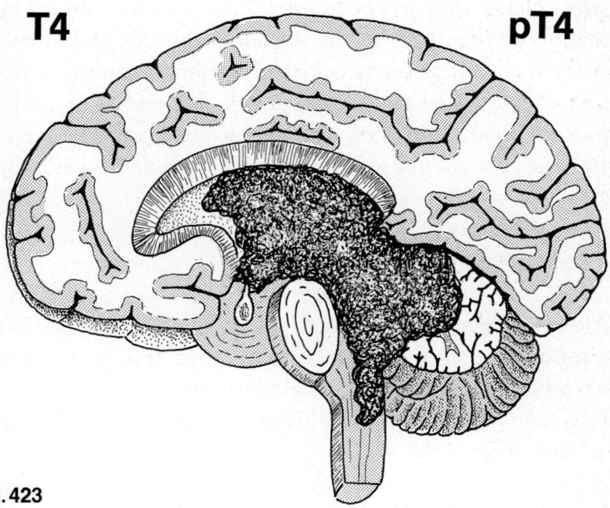

Fig. 423

pT Pathological Classification

The pT categories correspond to the T categories.

HODGKIN'S DISEASE

Introductory Notes

At the present time it is not considered practical to propose a TNM classification for Hodgkin's disease. Following the development of the Ann Arbor Classification for Hodgkin's disease in 1971, the significance of two important observations with major impact on staging has been appreciated. First, extralymphatic disease, if localized and related to adjacent lymph node disease, does not adversely affect the survival of patients. Secondly, laparotomy with splenectomy has been introduced as a method for obtaining more information on the extent of the disease within the abdomen.
A stage classification based on information from histopathological examination of the spleen and lymph nodes obtained at laparotomy cannot be compared with another done without such exploration. Therefore, two systems of classification are presented, a clinical (cS) and a pathological (pS).

Clinical Staging (cS)

Although recognized as incomplete, this is easily performed and should be reproducible from one centre to another. It is determined by history, clinical examination, imaging, blood analysis and the initial biopsy report. Bone marrow biopsy must be taken from a clinically or radiologically non-involved area of bone.

Liver Involvement. Clinical evidence of liver involvement must include either enlargement of the liver and at least an abnormal serum alkaline phosphatase level and two different liver function test abnormalities, or an abnormal liver demonstrated by imaging and one abnormal liver function test.

Spleen Involvement. Clinical evidence of spleen involvement is accepted if there is palpable enlargement of the spleen confirmed by imaging.

Lymphatic and Extralymphatic Disease. The lymphatic structures are as follows:

Lymph nodes	Waldeyer's ring
Spleen	Appendix
Thymus	Peyer's patches

The lymph nodes are grouped into regions, and one or more (2, 3 etc.) may be involved. The spleen is designated S and extralymphatic organs or sites E.

Lung involvement limited to one lobe, or perihilar extension associated with ipsilateral lymphadenopathy, or unilateral pleural effusion with or without lung involvement but with hilar lymphadenopathy are considered *localized* extralymphatic diseases.

Liver involvement is always considered as *diffuse* extralymphatic disease.

Pathological Staging (pS)

This takes into account additional data and has a higher degree of precision. It should be applied whenever possible. The various categories should be subscripted − (minus) or + (plus) according to the results of histopathological examination.

Histopathological Information

This is classified by notations indicating the tissue sampled. The following notation is common to the distant metastases (or M1 categories) of all regions classified by the TNM system. However, in order to conform with the Ann Arbor classification, the initial letters used in that system are also given.

Pulmonary	PUL or L	Bone marrow	MAR or M
Osseous	OSS or O	Pleura	PLE or P
Hepatic	HEP or H	Peritoneum	PER
Brain	BRA	Skin	SKI or D
Lymph nodes	LYM or N	Other	OTH

Clinical Stages (cS)

Stage I Involvement of a single lymph node region (I) (Figs. 424–427), or localized involvement of a single extralymphatic organ or site (I_E) (Fig. 428)

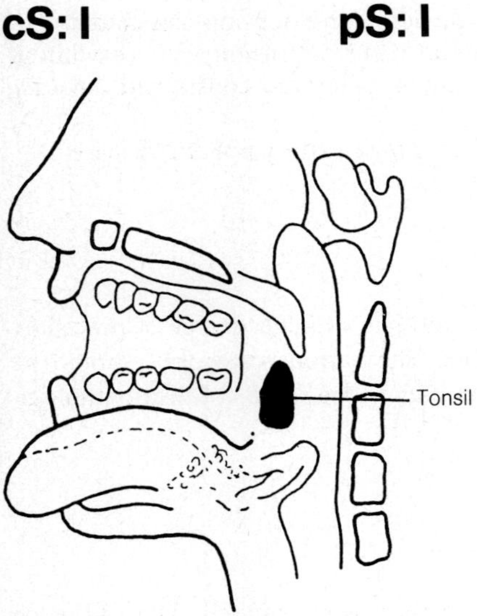

Fig. 424

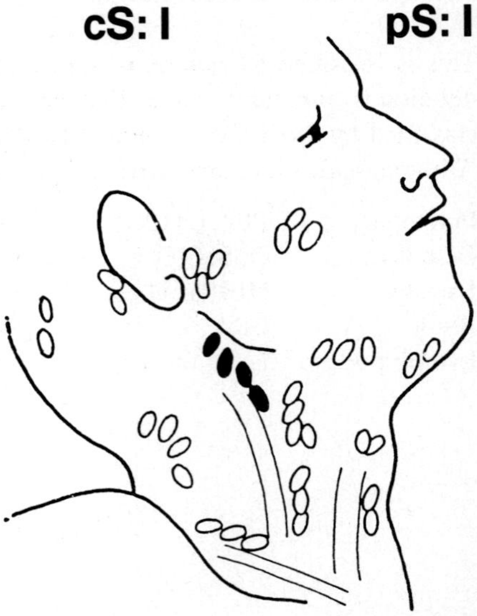

Fig. 425

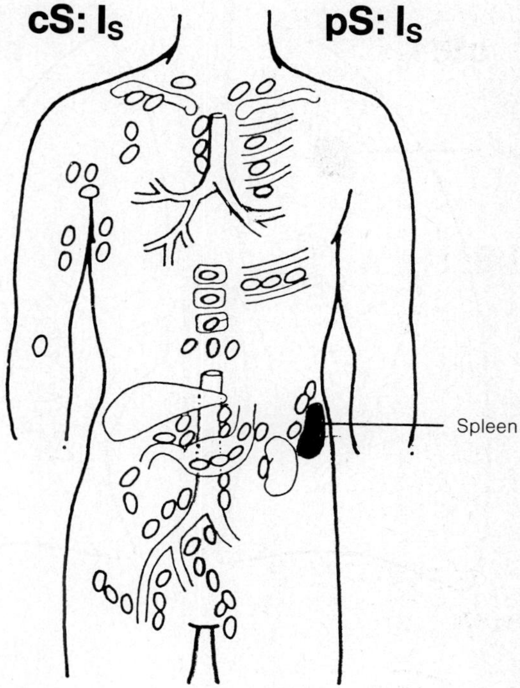

Fig. 426

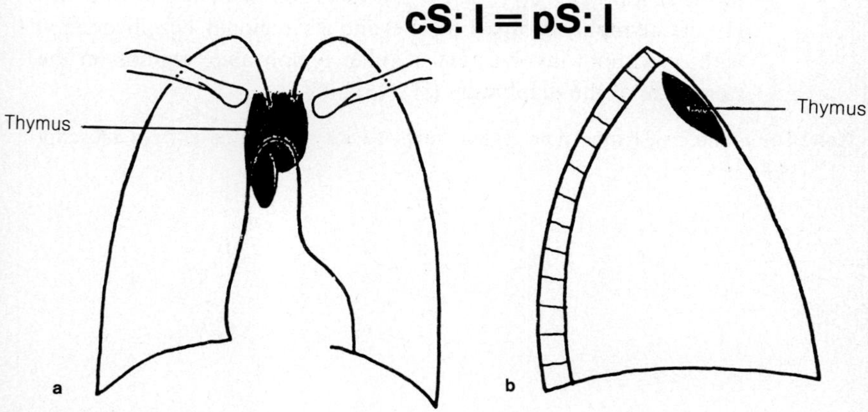

Fig. 427 a, b

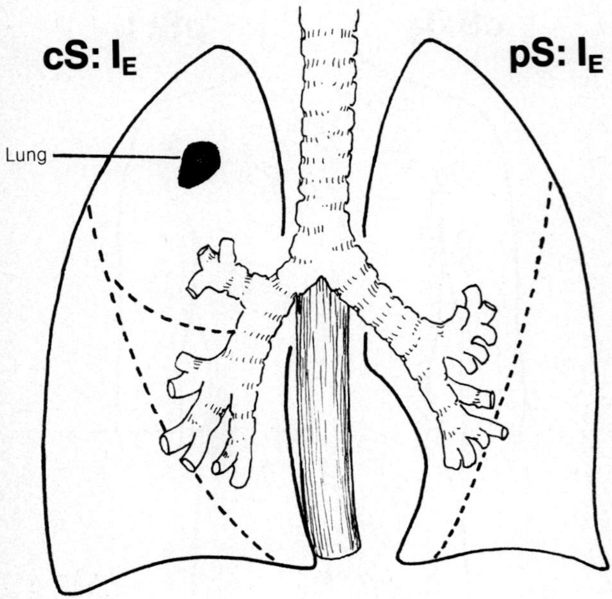

Fig. 428

Stage II Involvement of two or more lymph node regions on the same side of the diaphragm (II) (Fig. 429), or localized involvement of a single extralymphatic organ or site and its regional lymph node(s) with or without involvement of other lymph node regions on the same side of the diaphragm (II_E) (Fig. 430)

Note: The number of lymph note regions involved may be indicated by a subscript (e.g., II_5).

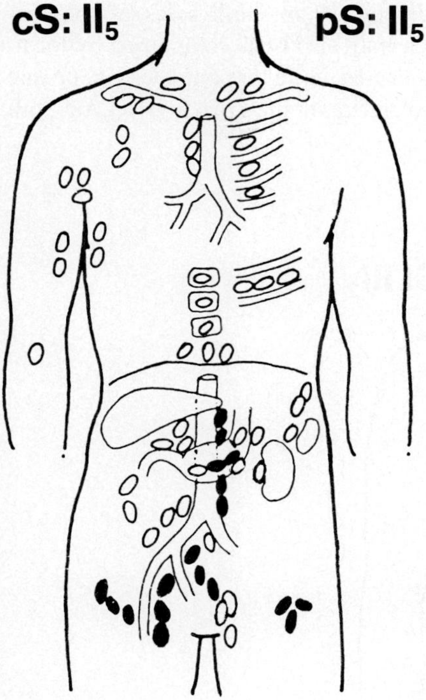

Fig. 429

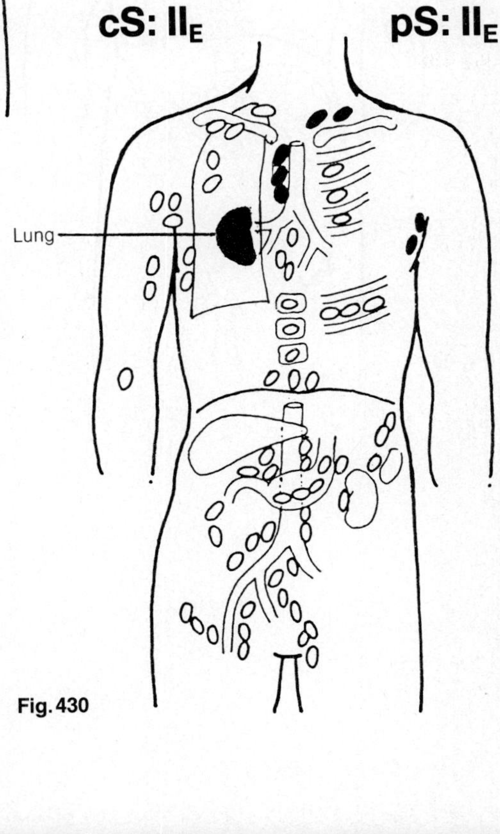

Fig. 430

Stage III Involvement of lymph node regions on both sides of the diaphragm (III) (Fig. 431), which may also be accompanied by localized involvement of an associated extralymphatic organ or site (III_E) (Fig. 432), or by involvement of the spleen (III_S), or both (III_{E+S}) (Fig. 433)

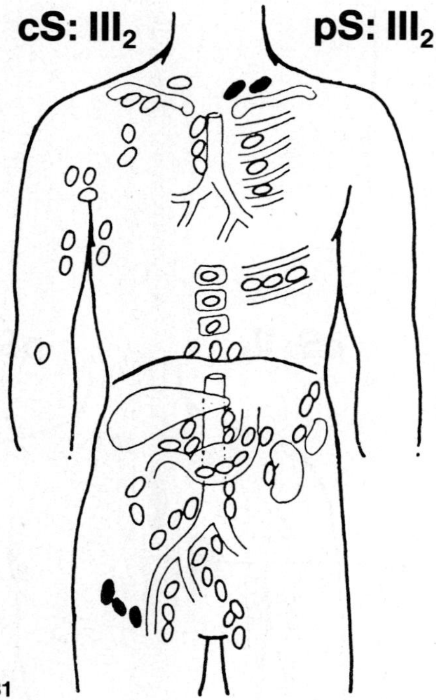

Fig. 431

cS: III_E **pS: III_E**

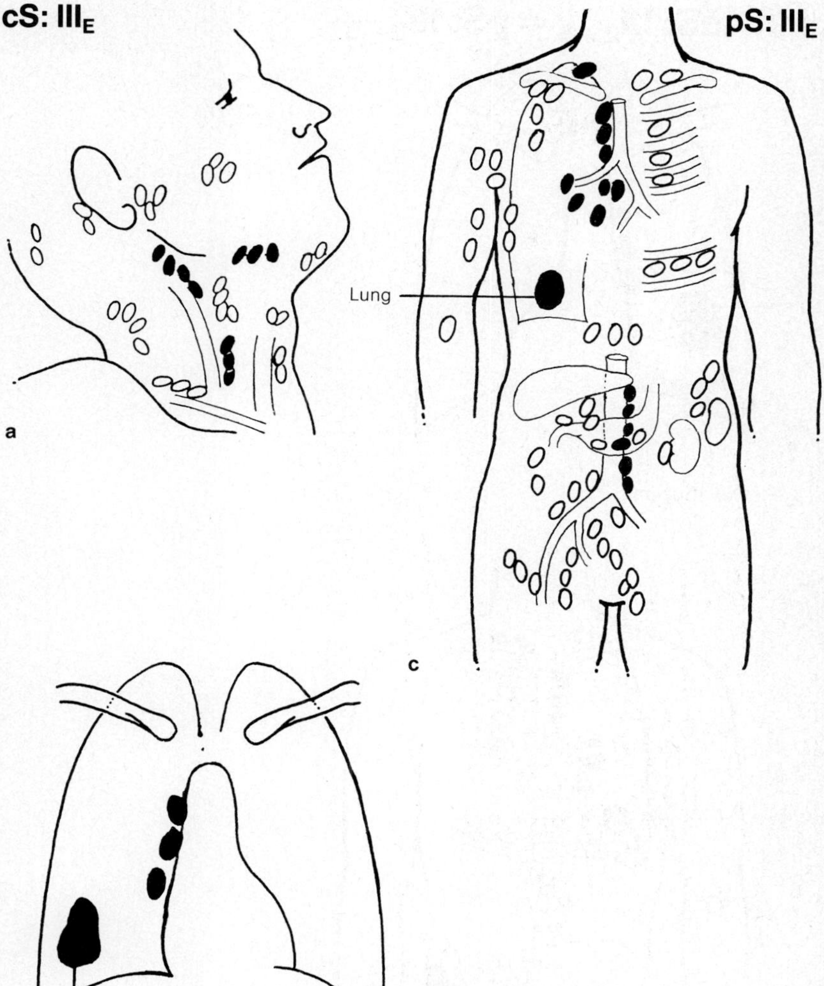

Fig. 432 a–c

$cS: III_{E+S} = pS: III_{E+S}$

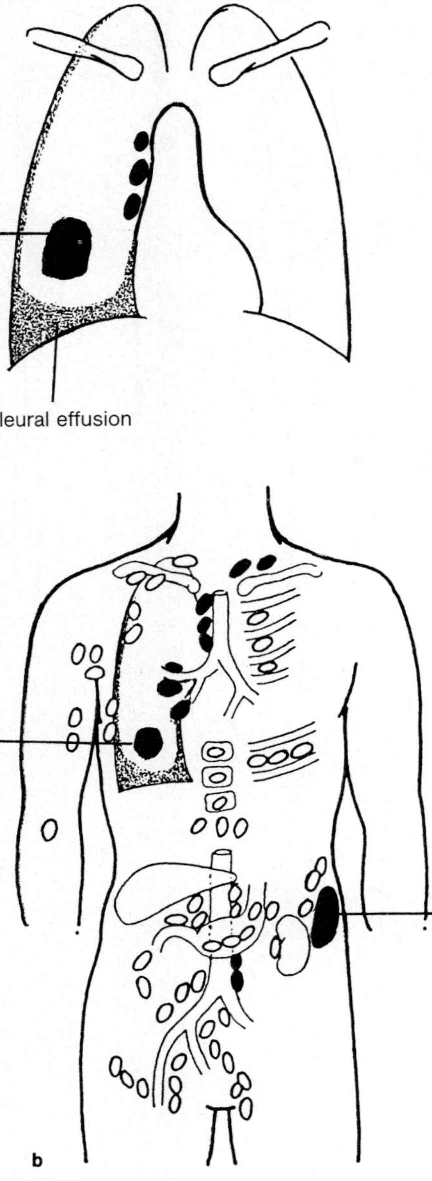

Fig. 433 a, b

Stage IV Disseminated (multifocal) involvement of one or more extralymphatic organs, with or without associated lymph node involvement (Figs. 434, 435), or isolated extralymphatic organ involvement with distant (non-regional) nodal involvement (Fig. 436)

Note: The site of Stage IV disease is identified further by specifying sites according to the notations listed on p. 309.

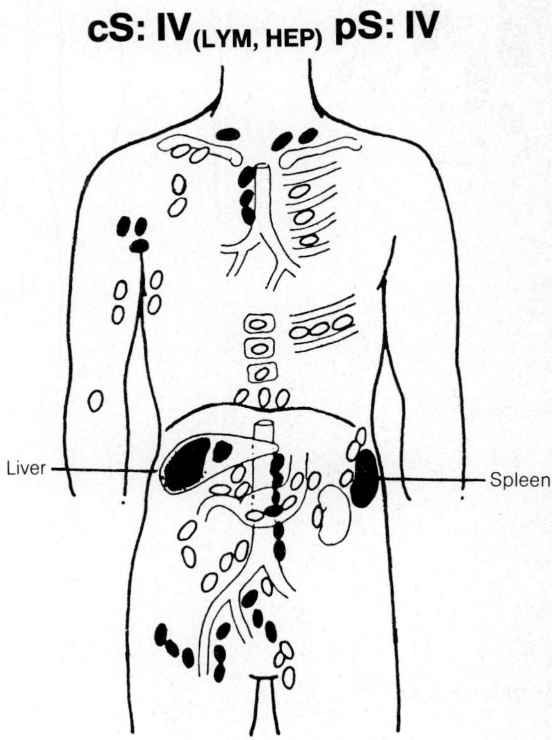

Fig. 434

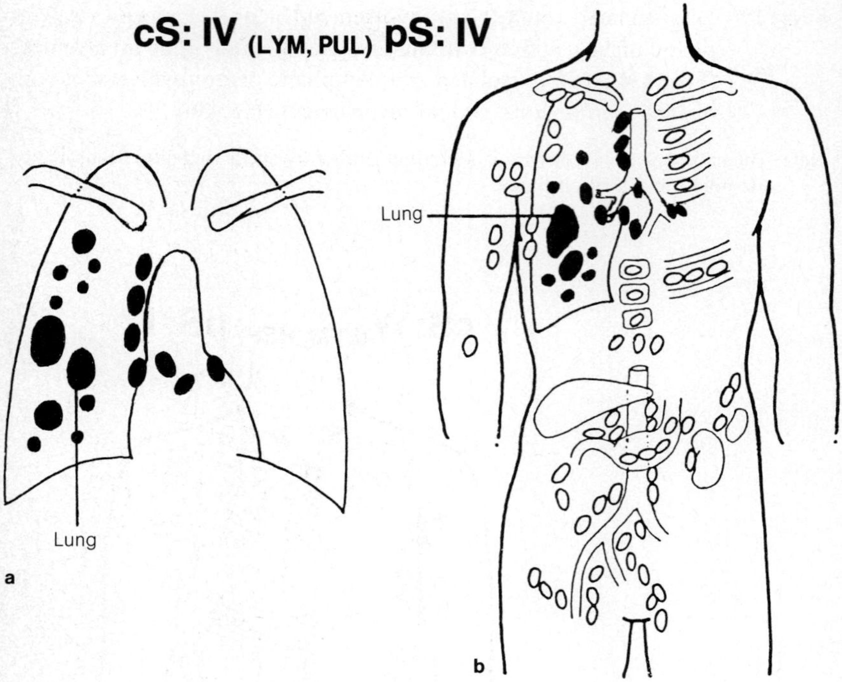

Fig. 435 a, b

Symptoms A and B

Each stage should be divided into A and B according to the absence or presence of defined general symptoms. These are:

1. Unexplained weight loss of more than 10% of the usual body weight in the 6 months prior to first attendance
2. Unexplained fever with temperature above 38 °C
3. Night sweats

Note: Pruritus alone does not qualify for B classification nor does a short, febrile illness associated with a known infection.

$cS: IV_{(LYM, HEP)}$ $pS: IV$

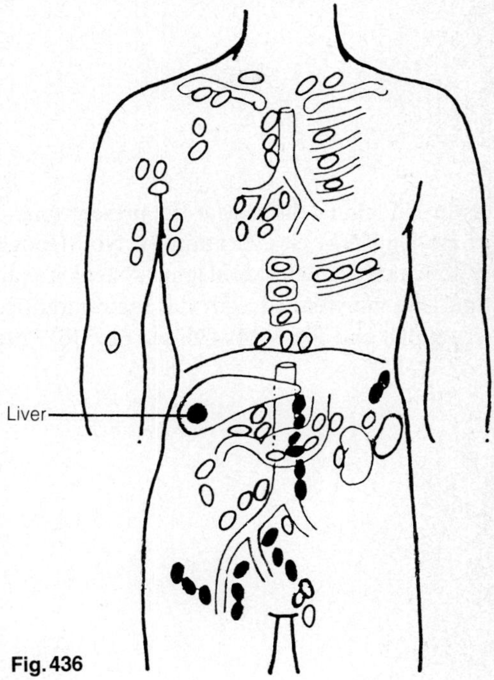

Fig. 436

Pathological Stages (pS)

The definitions of the four stages follow the same criteria as the clinical stages but with the additional information obtained following laparotomy. Splenectomy, liver biopsy, lymph node biopsy and marrow biopsy are mandatory for the establishment of pathological stages. The results of these biopsies are recorded as indicated above (see p. 309 and Figs. 424–436, see p. 310).

NON-HODGKIN'S LYMPHOMAS

As in Hodgkin's disease, at the present time it is not considered practical to propose a TNM classification for Non-Hodgkin's lymphomas. Since no other convincing and tested staging system is available, the Ann Arbor classification is recommended with the same modification as for Hodgkin's disease (see p. 308 and Figs. 424–436, see pp. 310–319).

PAEDIATRIC TUMOURS

Introductory Notes

The tumours classified are nephroblastoma, neuroblastoma and soft tissue sarcomas of childhood. These tumours are classified according to the recommendations of the Société Internationale d'Oncologie Pédiatrique (SIOP). They have the approval of UICC and the national TNM committees including AJCC.

The rules for the classification of paediatric tumours differ in one respect from those applicable to other sites. It is necessary to include a category for those cases in which a surgical exploration is done and in which a non-resectable tumour is found. Such cases are designated pT3c or, if following previous non-surgical treatment, ypT3c.

Nephroblastoma (Wilms' Tumour) (ICD-O 189.0)

Rules for Classification

There should be histological confirmation of the disease.

Regional Lymph Nodes (Fig. 437)

The regional lymph nodes are the hilar *(1)*, para-aortic *(2)* and paracaval *(3)* nodes between the diaphragm and the bifurcation of the aorta. Other lymph nodes involved are considered distant metastases.

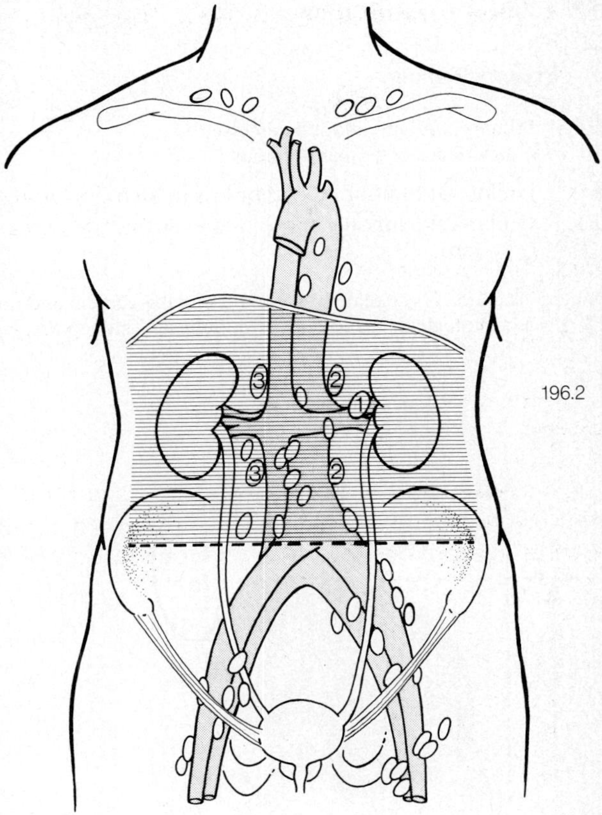

196.2

Fig. 437

TN Clinical Classification

T – Primary Tumour

TX Primary tumour cannot be assessed

T0 No evidence of primary tumour

T1 Unilateral tumour 80 cm^2 or less in area (including kidney)[1] (Fig. 438)

T2 Unilateral tumour more than 80 cm^2 in area (including kidney) (Fig. 439)

Note: [1] The area is calculated by multiplying the vertical and horizontal dimensions of the radiological shadow of the tumour and kidney *(a × b)*.

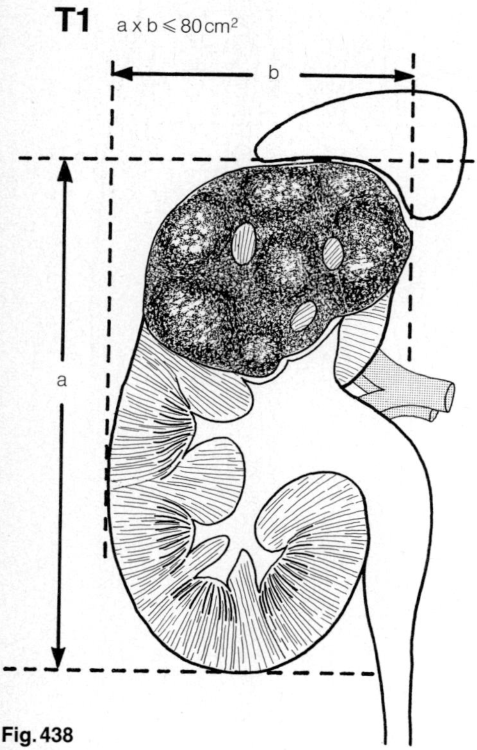

Fig. 438

T2 a x b > 80 cm²

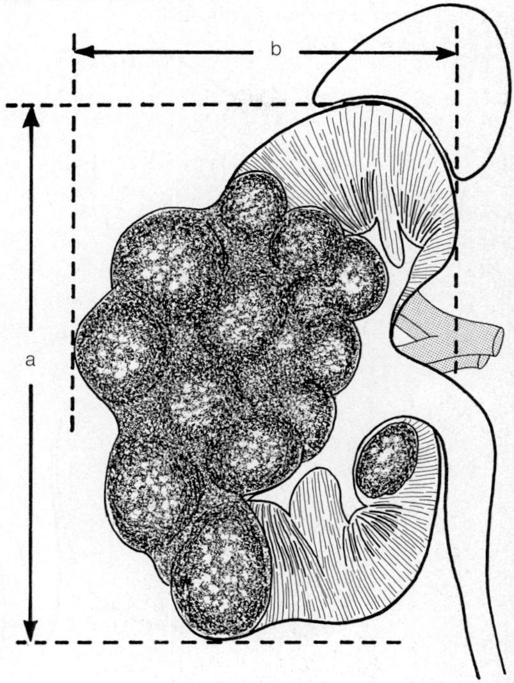

Fig. 439

T3 Unilateral tumour rupture before treatment (Fig. 440)

T4 Bilateral tumours (Fig. 441)

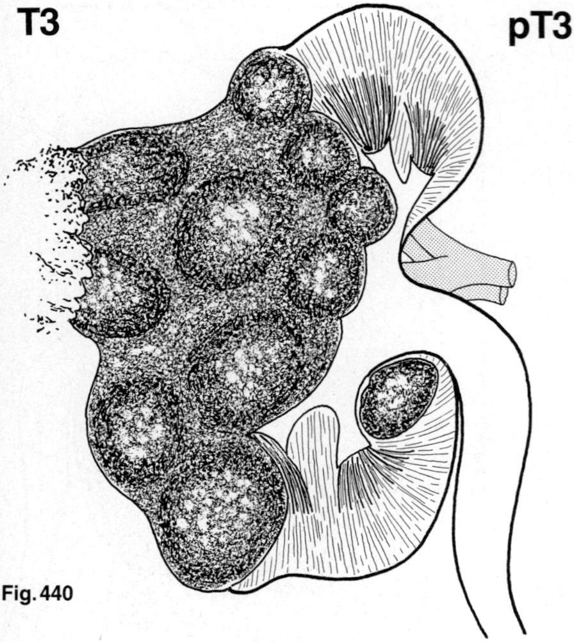

Fig. 440

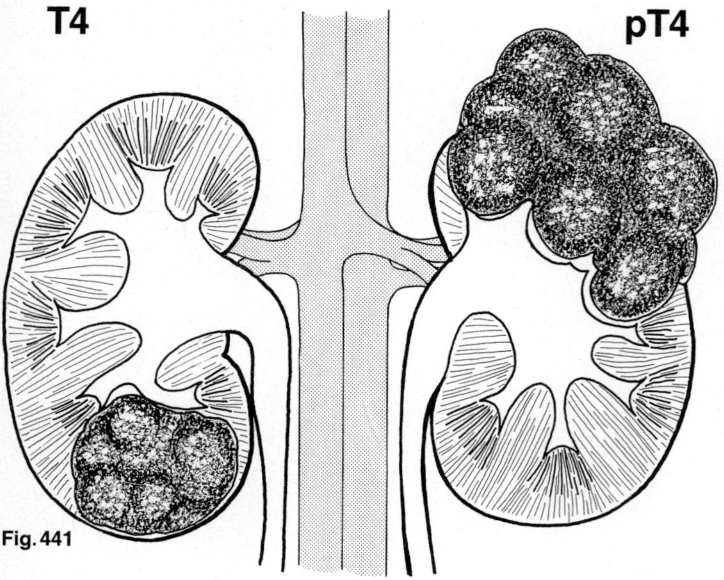

Fig. 441

N – Regional Lymph Nodes

NX Regional lymph nodes cannot be assessed
N0 No regional lymph node metastasis
N1 Regional lymph node metastasis (Fig. 442)

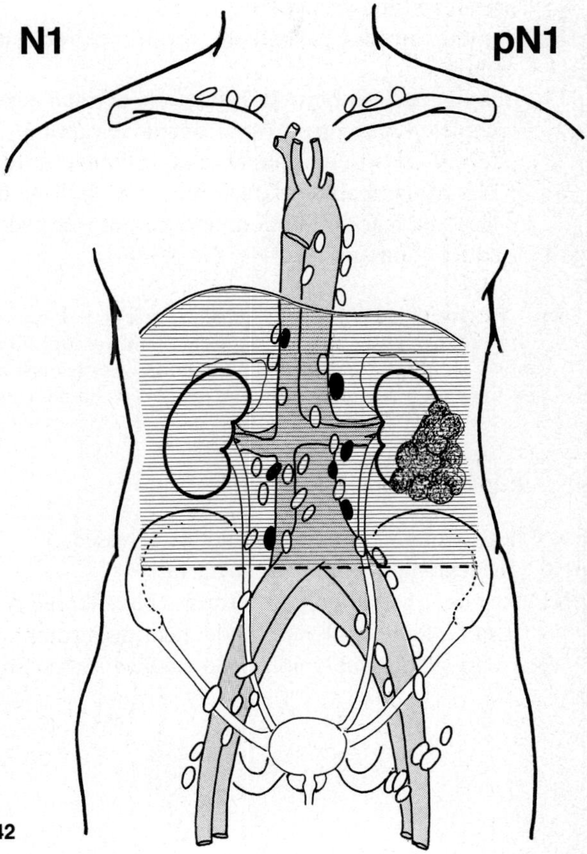

Fig. 442

pTN Pathological Classification

pT – Primary Tumour

pTX Primary tumour cannot be assessed
pT0 No evidence of primary tumour

pT1 Intrarenal tumour completely encapsulated, excision complete and margins histologically free
pT2 Tumour invades beyond the capsule or renal parenchyma[2], excision complete
pT3 Tumour invades beyond the capsule or renal parenchyma[2], excision incomplete *or* pre-operative or operative rupture
  pT3a Microscopic residual tumour limited to tumour bed
  pT3b Macroscopic residual tumour or spillage or malignant ascites
  pT3c Surgical exploration, tumour not resected
pT4 Bilateral tumours (Fig. 441, see p. 326)

Note: [2] This includes breach of the renal capsule and/or tumours seen microscopically outside the capsule; tumour adhesions microscopically confirmed, infiltrations of, or tumour thrombus within, the renal vessels outside the kidney; infiltration of the renal pelvis and/or ureter, peripelvic and pericalyceal fat.

pN – Regional Lymph Nodes

pNX Regional lymph nodes cannot be assessed
pN0 No regional lymph node metastasis
pN1 Regional lymph node metastasis (Fig. 442, see p. 327)
  pN1a Regional lymph node metastasis completely resected
  pN1b Regional lymph node metastasis incompletely resected

Neuroblastoma

The same principles apply to ganglioneuroblastoma.

Rules for Classification

There should be histological confirmation of the disease and/or confirmation by biochemical tests.

Anatomical Regions

The primary tumour site should be indicated according to the following notation:

Cervical	CER	Pelvic	PEL
Thoracic	THO	Other	OTH
Abdominal	ABD		

Note: Dumbbell tumours should be identified by the prefix D.

Regional Lymph Nodes

The regional lymph nodes are as follows:

Cervical region	Cervical and supraclavicular nodes
Thoracic region	Intrathoracic and infraclavicular nodes
Abdominal and pelvic regions	Subdiaphragmatic, intra-abdominal and pelvic nodes, including the external iliac nodes
Other regions	The appropriate regional lymph nodes

TN Clinical Classification

T – Primary Tumour

Because it is often impossible to differentiate between the primary tumour and the adjacent lymph nodes, the T assessment relates to the total mass. When there is doubt between multicentricity and metastasis, the latter is presumed.

Note: Size is estimated clinically and/or radiologically. For classification the larger measurement should be used.

TX Primary tumour cannot be assessed
T0 No evidence of primary tumour

T1 Single tumour 5 cm or less in greatest dimension (Fig. 443)
T2 Single tumour more than 5 cm but not more than 10 cm in greatest dimension (Fig. 444)
T3 Single tumour more than 10 cm in greatest dimension (Fig. 445)
T4 Multicentric tumours occurring simultaneously (Fig. 446)

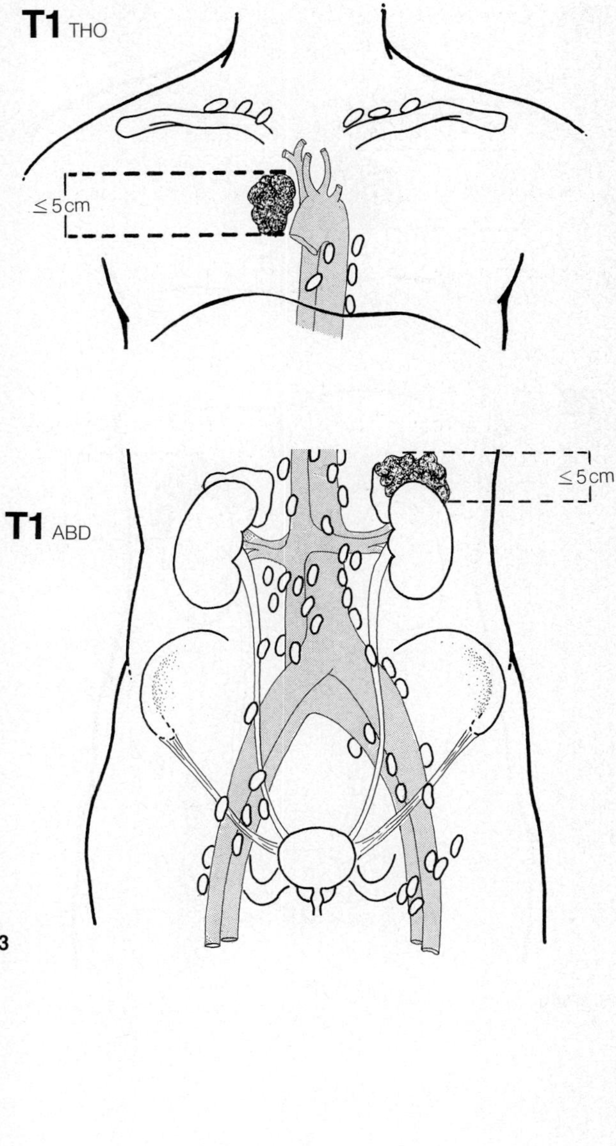

Fig. 443

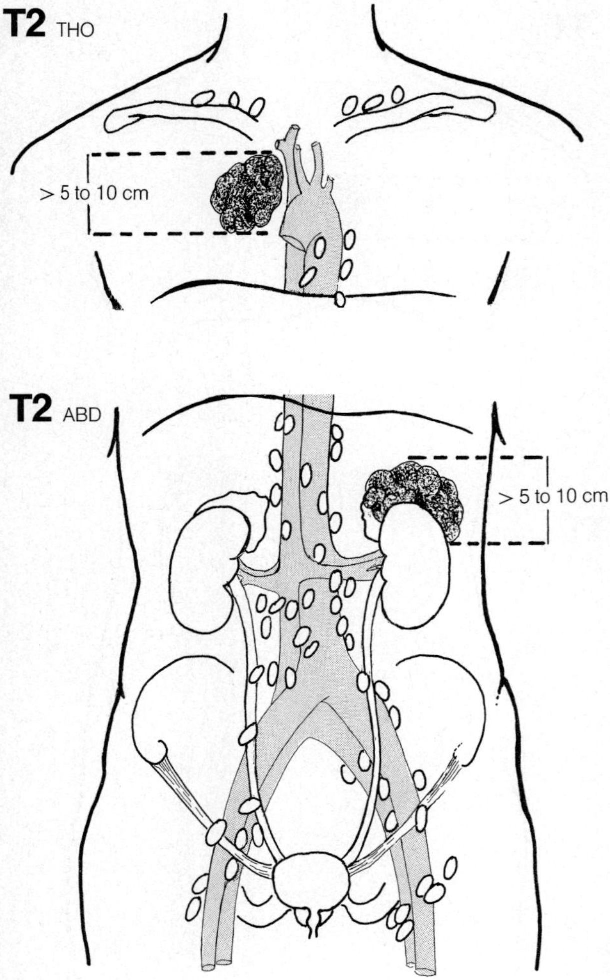

Fig. 444

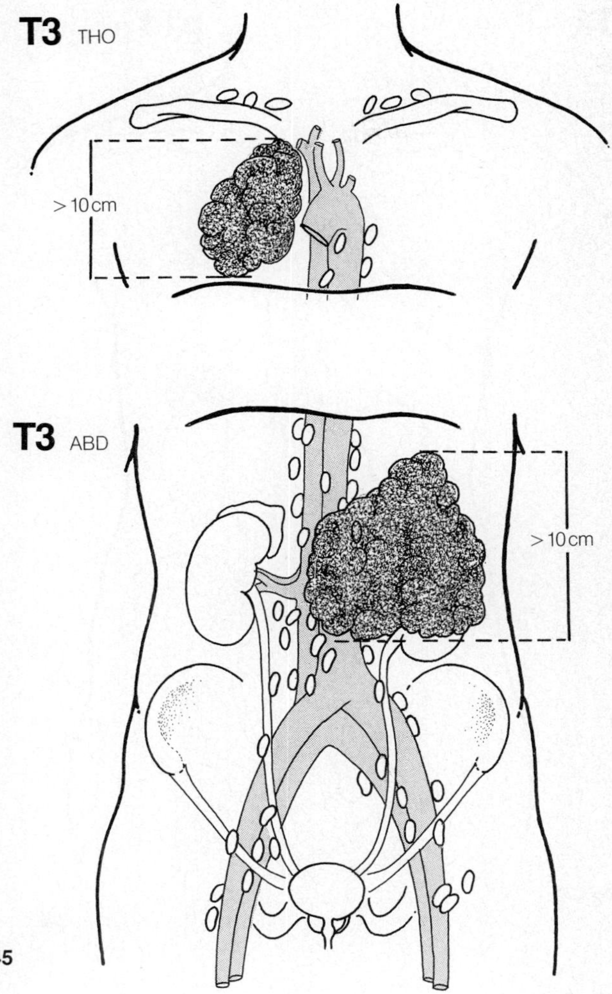

Fig. 445

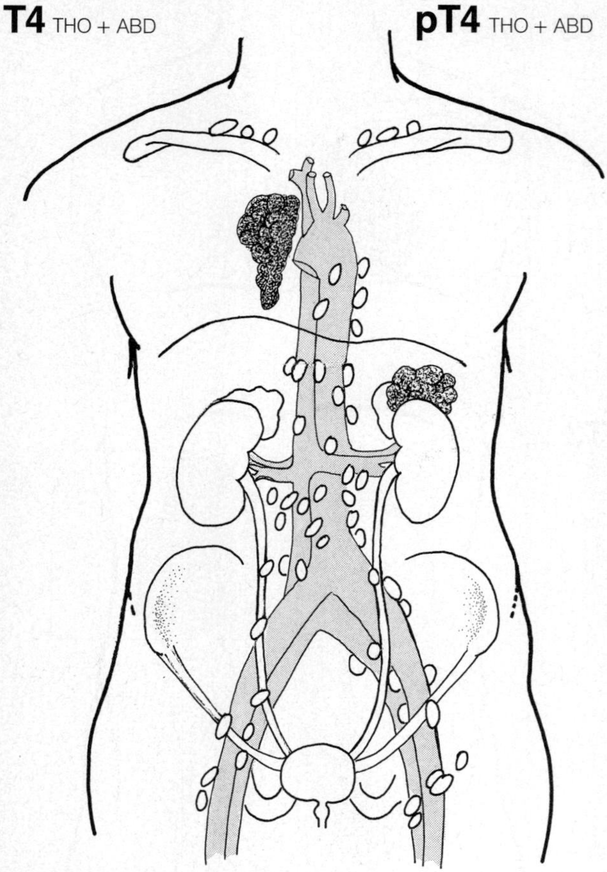

Fig. 446

N – Regional Lymph Nodes

NX Regional lymph nodes cannot be assessed
N0 No regional lymph node metastasis
N1 Regional lymph node metastasis (Fig. 447)

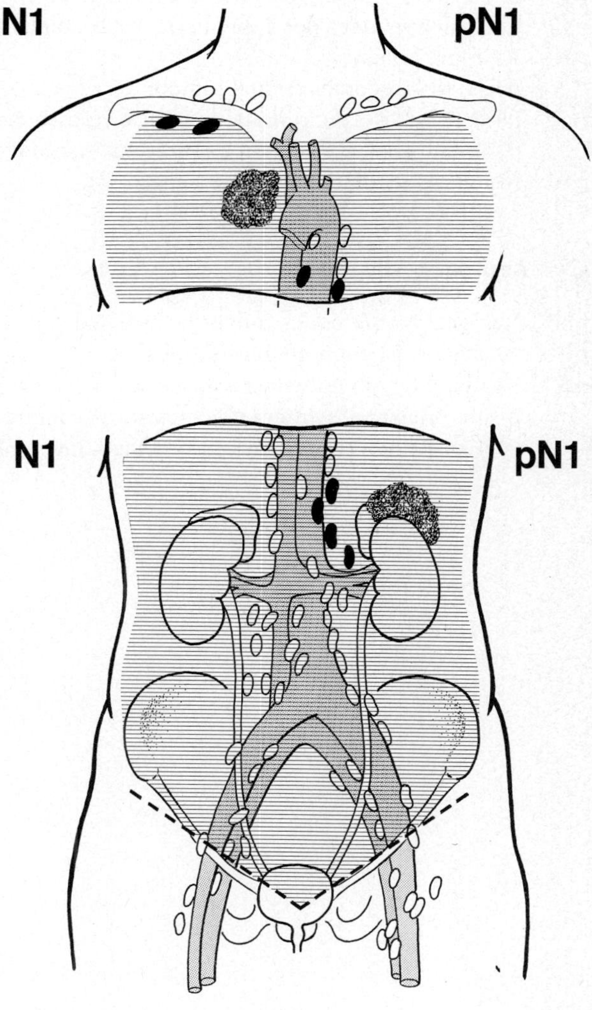

Fig. 447

pTN Pathological Classification

pT – Primary Tumour

pTX Primary tumour cannot be assessed
pT0 No evidence of primary tumour

pT1 Excision of tumour complete and margins histologically free
pT2 The category does not apply to neuroblastoma
pT3 Residual tumour
- pT3a Microscopic residual tumour
- pT3b Macroscopic residual tumour or grossly incomplete excision
- pT3c Surgical exploration, tumour not resected

pT4 Multicentric tumour (Fig. 446, see p. 334)

pN – Regional Lymph Nodes

pNX Regional lymph nodes cannot be assessed
pN0 No regional lymph node metastasis
pN1 Regional lymph node metastasis (Fig. 447, see p. 335)
- pN1a Regional lymph node metastasis completely resected
- pN1b Regional lymph node metastasis incompletely resected

Soft Tissue Sarcomas - Paediatric

Rules for Classification

The classification is designed to apply particularly to rhabdomyosarcoma in childhood (ICD-O M 8900/3) but may be used for other soft tissue sarcomas in childhood (listed on p. 148).
There should be histological confirmation of the disease.

Anatomical Regions

The primary tumour site should be indicated according to the following notation:

Orbit	ORB
Head and neck	HEA
Limbs	LIM
Pelvis (including walls, genital tract and viscera)	PEL
Abdomen (including walls and viscera)	ABD
Thorax (including walls, diaphragm and viscera)	THO
Other	OTH

Regional Lymph Nodes (See Fig. 452, p. 343)

The regional lymph nodes are those appropriate to the situation of the primary tumour, for example:

Head and neck	Cervical and supraclavicular lymph nodes
Abdominal and pelvic	Subdiaphragmatic, intra-abdominal and ilio-inguinal lymph nodes
Upper limbs	Ipsilateral epitrochlear and axillary lymph nodes
Lower Limbs	Ipsilateral popliteal and inguinal lymph nodes

In the case of unilateral tumours, all contralateral involved lymph nodes are considered to be distant metastasis.

TN Clinical Classification

T - Primary Tumour

TX Primary tumour cannot be assessed
T0 No evidence of primary tumour

T1 Tumour limited to organ or tissue of origin
- T1a Tumour 5 cm or less in greatest dimension (Fig. 448)
- T1b Tumour more than 5 cm in greatest dimension (Fig. 449)

T2 Tumour invades contiguous organ(s) or tissue(s) and/or with adjacent malignant effusion
- T2a Tumour 5 cm or less in greatest dimension (Fig. 450)
- T2b Tumour more than 5 cm in greatest dimension (Fig. 451)

Note: The categories T3 and T4 do not apply. The existence of more than one tumour is generally considered a primary tumour with distant metastasis.

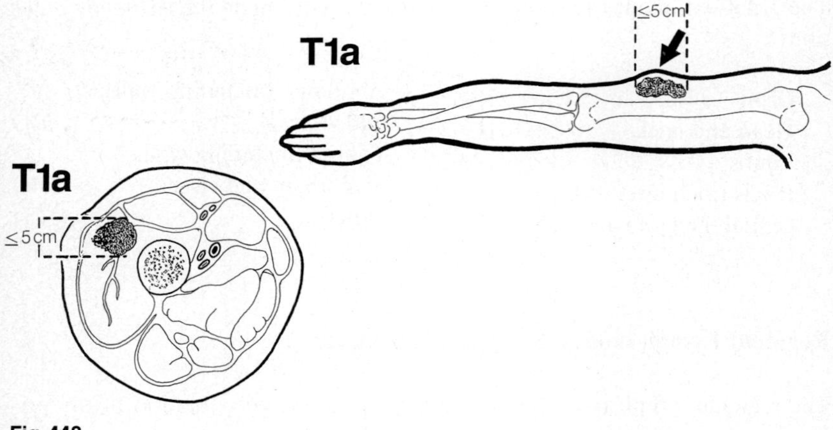

Fig. 448

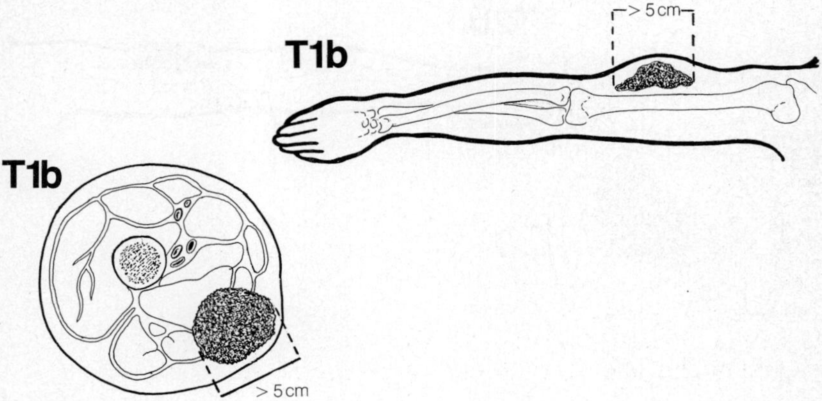

Fig. 449

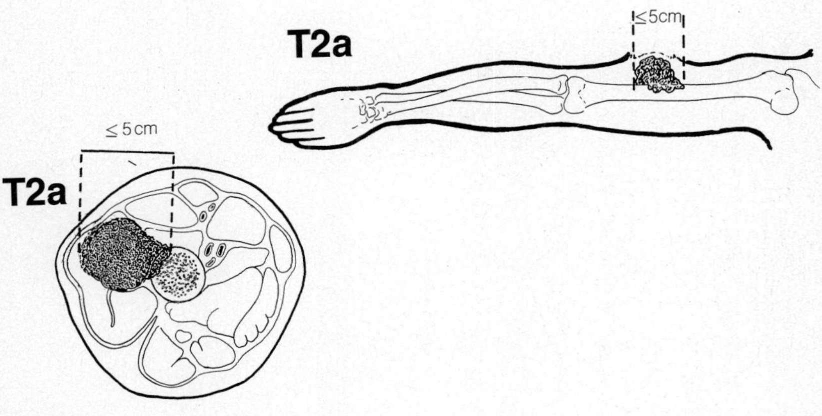

Fig. 450

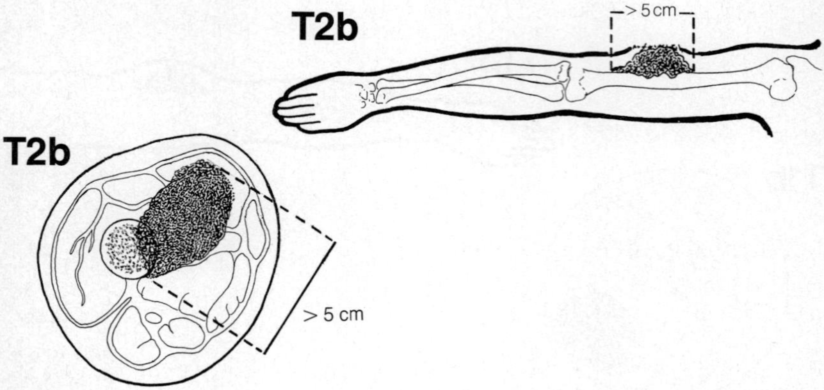

Fig. 451

N - Regional Lymph Nodes

NX Regional lymph nodes cannot be assessed
N0 No regional lymph node metastasis
N1 Regional lymph node metastasis

pTN Pathological Classification

pT - Primary Tumour

pTX Primary tumour cannot be assessed
pT0 No evidence of primary tumour
pT1 Tumour limited to organ or tissue of origin; excision complete and margins histologically free
pT2 Tumour invades beyond organ or tissue of origin; excision complete and margins histologically free
pT3 Tumour invades beyond the organ or tissue of origin; excision incomplete
 pT3a Microscopic residual tumour
 pT3b Macroscopic residual tumour or adjacent malignant effusion
 pT3c Surgical exploration, tumour not resected

pN - Regional Lymph Nodes

pNX Regional lymph nodes cannot be assessed
pN0 No regional lymph node metastasis
pN1 Regional lymph node metastasis
 pN1a Regional lymph node metastasis completely resected
 pN1b Regional lymph node metastasis incompletely resected

AREAS OF REGIONAL LYMPH NODES (Fig. 452)

A↑[1]	Head and neck, cervical oesophagus, ophthalmic tumours
A–B[2]	Lung
A–B	Intrathoracic oesophagus
B–C (partly)	Stomach
B–C (partly)	Liver, gall bladder, extrahepatic bile ducts, ampulla of Vater, pancreas
B–C	Kidney
B–C[3]	Colon
B–E	Renal pelvis and ureter
B–E[4]	Testis
B–E and E↓	Ovary
C–E (partly)[5]	Rectum
C–E	Corpus uteri, cervix uteri, upper two-thirds of vagina
D–E	Urinary bladder, prostate
D–E and E↓	Penis, urethra, vulva
D–E (partly) and E↓	Anal canal
F[6]	Breast
Skin	See Figs. 207–213, pp. 152–158.

---

[1] Plus the upper anterior mediastinal lymph nodes for thyroid tumours.

[2] Plus the scalene and supraclavicular lymph nodes.

[3] Plus lymph nodes located inferior to the level of the aorta bifurcation, along the branching of the ileocolic and sigmoid arteries.

[4] After previous scrotal or inguinal operations, the inguinal lymph nodes (E↓) are also considered regional lymph nodes.

[5] The lymph nodes along the trunk of the inferior mesenteric artery are also considered regional lymph nodes.

[6] Plus the ipsilateral internal mammary lymph nodes.

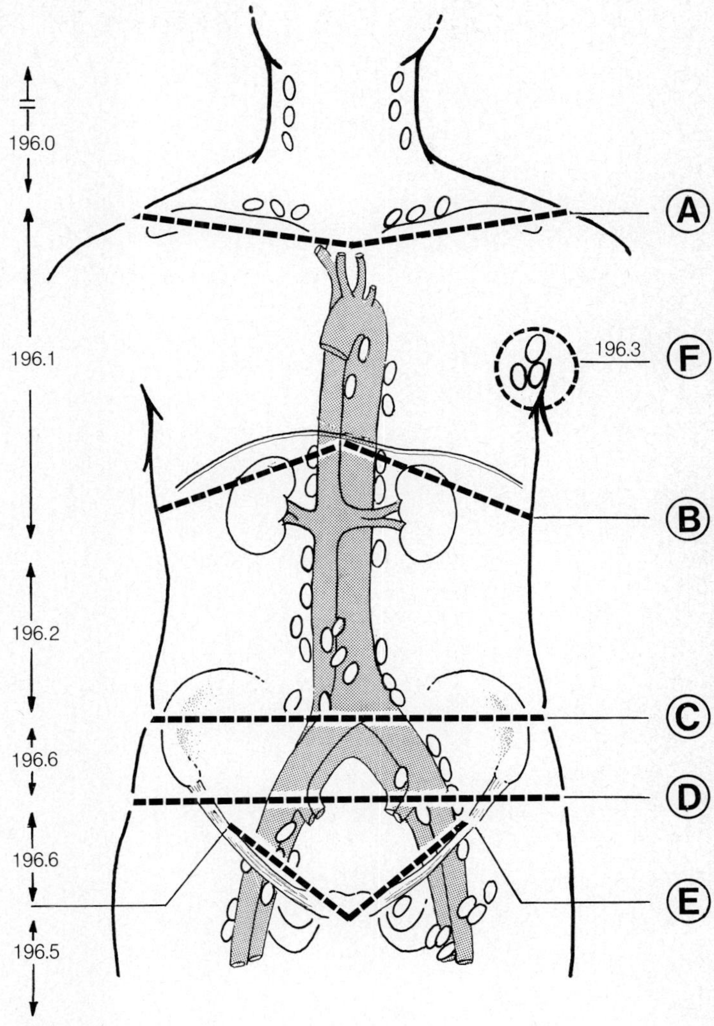

Fig. 452